BREAST CANCER INSIDE OUT

Medical Humanities: Criticism and Creativity
Vol 1

Series Editors: Maria Vaccarella, MA, PhD, Lecturer in
Medical Humanities, University of Bristol and
Kimberly R. Myers, MA, PhD, Professor of Humanities and
Medicine, Penn State College of Medicine

PETER LANG
Oxford • Bern • Berlin • Bruxelles • New York • Wien

BREAST CANCER INSIDE OUT

BODIES, BIOGRAPHIES & BELIEFS

Edited by Kimberly R. Myers

PETER LANG
Oxford • Bern • Berlin • Bruxelles • New York • Wien

Bibliographic information published by Die Deutsche Nationalbibliothek.
Die Deutsche Nationalbibliothek lists this publication in the Deutsche
National-bibliografie; detailed bibliographic data is available on the Internet at
http://dnb.d-nb.de.

A catalogue record for this book is available from the British Library.

Library of Congress Cataloging-in-Publication Data
Names: Myers, Kimberly R. (Kimberly Rena), 1962- editor.
Title: Breast cancer inside out : bodies, biographies & beliefs / [edited
  by] Kimberly R. Myers.
Description: Oxford ; New York : Peter Lang, [2021] | Series: Medical
  humanities ; vol. 1, 2504-5229 | Includes bibliographical references and
  index.
Identifiers: LCCN 2020017753 (print) | LCCN 2020017754 (ebook) | ISBN
  9781788747332 (hardback) | ISBN 9781788747349 (ebook) | ISBN
  9781788747356 (epub) | ISBN 9781788747363 (mobi)
Subjects: MESH: Breast Neoplasms | Breast Neoplasms--psychology | Self Care
  | Social Support | Personal Narrative
Classification: LCC RC280.B8 (print) | LCC RC280.B8 (ebook) | NLM WP 870
  | DDC 616.99/449--dc23
LC record available at https://lccn.loc.gov/2020017753
LC ebook record available at https://lccn.loc.gov/2020017754

Cover design: Deb Tomazin.

ISBN 978-1-78874-733-2 (print) • ISBN 978-1-78874-734-9 (ePDF)
ISBN 978-1-78874-735-6 (ePub) • ISBN 978-1-78874-736-3 (mobi)

© Peter Lang Group AG 2021

Published by Peter Lang Ltd, International Academic Publishers,
52 St Giles, Oxford, OX1 3LU, United Kingdom
oxford@peterlang.com, www.peterlang.com

Kimberly R. Myers has asserted her right under the Copyright, Designs and Patents Act, 1988,
to be identified as Editor of this Work.

All rights reserved.
All parts of this publication are protected by copyright.
Any utilisation outside the strict limits of the copyright law, without
the permission of the publisher, is forbidden and liable to prosecution.
This applies in particular to reproductions, translations, microfilming,
and storage and processing in electronic retrieval systems.

This publication has been peer reviewed.

For George R. Simms, MD, PhD, MTS, SP,
who made the journey with me.
Every step of the way.
ILDBIDE

Contents

Acknowledgements — xiii

Introduction — 1

PART I   A Trajectory of Breast Cancer: Diagnosis, Treatment and Beyond — 15

KIMBERLY R. MYERS AND JULIE A. MACK
When the Patient Knows What the Doctor Does Not (Yet) Know — 17

MARK STOUT AND LYNN FANTOM
A Step-by-Step Guide through Breast Cancer Diagnosis and Radiation — 29

GORDON L. KAUFFMAN, JR.
Communion — 43

LISA KATZ
Reconstruction — 50

JOHN D. POTOCHNY
Gauging Too Much Information: Discussing a Young Mother's Options for Reconstructive Surgery — 53

KATE JOLLIE
Flashpoints: Wisdom from the Trenches — 61

KEVIN B. KNOPF
Another Catcher in the Rye: Oncology Care at the County Hospital   67

DAVID CARNISH
Reflections on Solidarity   77

IAN R. ROSS
When Chaos Comes: The Role of a Hospitalist   85

ELIANA V. HEMPEL
Best-Laid Plans: When Follow-Up Fails   89

JEFFREY M. KOWALESKI
Always on Your Side: What All Patients Should Know about Palliative Care   97

GEORGE R. SIMMS
How Hospice Can Heal   103

MARK L. HUNNICUTT
A Steward of Suffering: One Man's Story of Breast Cancer   107

PART II Enhancing Your Health by Honoring Your Self   123

MICHAEL HAYES
Our Many Teachers: Wisdom for Psychological Health during Breast Cancer   125

Contents ix

DEBRA REX GEORGE AND DANIEL R. GEORGE
All You Need Is Love ... and Research: A Mother-Son Team
Navigate a Non-Aggressive Approach to Breast Cancer   135

KATHRYN H. SCHMITZ
I Promise You Will Feel Better: The Importance of Exercising
During and After Cancer Treatment   151

ELIZABETH REID
Food as Medicine: How to Eat During and After Treatment for
Breast Cancer   155

AMY HOLIDAY
A Future on Ice   171

ELVA J. WINTER
Intimacy and Sexuality in the Context of Breast Cancer   179

PART III   Shaping Cancer, (Re)Shaping Self   193

DEBORAH BOWMAN
On Being Constant and Changed: Breast Cancer in Six Acts   195

JOHANNA SHAPIRO
Women's Breast Cancer Poetry: Voice, Identity, Contingency
and Death   213

JENNIFER HAYDEN
Under the Birdcage   249

KIMBERLY R. MYERS

Breast Cancer Comics in the Classroom and the Clinic   255

RACHEL O'CONNOR

A Curator's Interpretation of *Edges of Light*   273

KIMBERLY R. MYERS AND WENDY PALMER

Edges of Light: Images of Breast Transformation   277

LISA KATZ

The Form   327

PART IV   Breast Cancer over Time: Evolutions in Understandings, Representations, Tools and Treatments   329

SIOBHAN CONATY

Milestones in the Depiction of Breasts and Breast Cancer in Art History   331

LISA KATZ

Breast Art   369

MICHAEL BAUM

An Historical Overview of Breast Cancer and Its Treatments   371

HENRY WAGNER

Radiation Therapy: Evolutions in Treatment, Consultations in Clinic   397

Contents

MICHAEL BAUM

Understanding How Cancer Behaves: Implications for
Paradigm Shifts in Treatment — 413

MARIA J. BAKER

Genetic Counseling and Testing for Hereditary Breast
Cancer: A Genetic Counselor's Perspective — 425

VICTORIA O'DONNELL

The Marketing of Metastatic Breast Cancer: A Cultural
Analysis of the Ibrance Commercial — 439

ARIANE B. ANDERSON

The New Normal: Metastatic Breast Cancer Experiences of
Survivor Identity — 461

LISA KATZ

Support Group — 465

Notes on Contributors — 467

Index — 477

Acknowledgements

I am grateful to the generous individuals who have shared their professional expertise and personal experiences in order to help others understand how breast cancer impacts individuals, families and communities. Thanks to Deb Tomazin for creating the cover we'd hoped for and to Dr. Carly Smith and friends whose insights while floating on Lake Bowen led to the subtitle of this book. For their photographic talent and kind support, I thank Wendy Palmer, who helped me discover edges of light in the darkness, and Dr. Dan Shapiro. Thanks to The Pennsylvania State University and Penn State College of Medicine for providing sabbatical time away to complete this work. I am grateful to Dr. Laurel Plapp, Senior Commissioning Editor for Peter Lang Oxford, who guided this project with skill, patience and encouragement, and to Dr. Maria Vaccarella, Lecturer in Medical Humanities at the University of Bristol, for incisive commentary and conversation that helped sculpt the manuscript. As always, heartfelt appreciation to my husband, Professor Jim Thomas, for constructive comments, generosity of time and talent in proofreading, nourishment and companionship the whole way through. Finally, I want to thank the many excellent physicians, nurses, therapists and staff members who make living with breast cancer easier – and the scientists and scholars, artists, advocates and activists whose visionary work gives us hope.

Permissions:

Illustrations from *Cancer Vixen: A True Story*, by Marisa Acocella Marchetto, copyright © 2006 by Marisa Acocella Marchetto. Used by permission of Alfred A. Knopf, an imprint of the Knopf Doubleday Publishing Group, a division of Penguin Random House LLC. All rights reserved.

The three photographs comprising "Choice" and "Excognito" in the *Edges of Light* sequence are used with the permission of Dr. Dan Shapiro.

The four poems by Lisa Katz – "Breast Art," "Reconstruction," "Support Group," and "The Form" – first appeared as a group entitled "Breast Art" in *Illness in the Academy: A Collection of Pathographies by Academics*, Ed. Kimberly R. Myers, copyright © 2007 by Purdue University Press. All rights reserved.

"When the Patient Knows What the Doctor Does Not (Yet) Know" first appeared in *Atrium: A Publication of the Medical Humanities and Bioethics Program, Northwestern University Feinberg School of Medicine* 11 (Winter 2013).

Six original drawings in "Breast Cancer in the Classroom and the Clinic" are used with the permission of artist Pamela Wagar Smith, MD.

Introduction

When patients become people and doctors become healers, story becomes the focus of attention. Shared stories give understanding, guidance, hope and wisdom to societies, cultures, families and individuals. It is the way healing has always taken place.
George R. Simms, M.D., Ph.D.

The Story of This Book

"Breast cancer." These words are among the most dreaded any woman – or man – can hear. I know. I heard the words from a kind physician on a winter afternoon in 2012.

Upon receiving this diagnosis, I felt an urgent need to know a lot that I didn't know – not only about various components of diagnosis and treatments, but also about people who shared my illness and about the kinds of people who would be caring for me. And I didn't just want to know how these people coped and what they did. I wanted to know who they are as individuals because, to me, that matters. I wanted to consider breast cancer in wider contexts, too – scientific, historical, cultural, academic, artistic – because I knew these contexts would have everything to do with my own personal contexts and how I lived into this "brave new world, that has such people in 't" in the short and long terms. I needed stories, both sweeping and intimate, because stories show us alternatives for how to live; they show us options we might otherwise never have considered. As physician-author Rachel Naomi Remen says, "Facts bring us to knowledge, but stories lead to wisdom" (xxx). Ultimately, stories provide us – or can, at least – with a sense of community and thereby potentially lessen the fear and isolation that a diagnosis of breast cancer often brings. I searched for the best book I could find, one that included the kind of information I needed all in one place. I found no such book. So six years after my diagnosis, I decided to create it. This is the book I wish I'd had.

Students, professionals whose work involves breast disease, and general readers who seek a wide-ranging understanding of how breast cancer impacts individuals and communities currently have a wide array of resources available to them. On the one hand, medical journals contain up-to-date reports on the state of diagnosis, treatment and outcomes; but most non-medical readers find these texts too technical to understand in a meaningful way. At the other end of the spectrum, a plethora of self-help books offer advice to patients on how best to navigate diagnosis and treatment, but offer little in the way of understanding how various healthcare providers go about their work – and how they think and feel as they care for patients. Somewhere in between lie theoretical books about breast cancer. These are written primarily for academic, non-medical researchers and scholars and, as such, are perhaps not well suited to most healthcare professionals, patients and general readers. Trying to decide among dozens of texts for a holistic understanding of breast cancer can be overwhelming.

Remarkably, even though I work in an academic medical center, teach medical students of all levels and socialize with many physician friends, when I received my diagnosis I knew of no one – *no* one – who had had direct experience with breast cancer. Or at least no one I knew had shared that information with me. But I needed to talk with someone who had been through what I now faced. I wanted to be prepared before meeting with various healthcare providers so that I could make the most well-informed decisions for my particular physiological, psychological and existential situation – in short, the best decisions for me as an individual.

I had full access to medical literature through our college of medicine's library and a relatively strong (lay person's) ability to interpret it accurately; and I had colleagues who generously offered to answer – or find answers to – any questions I might have. However, in part because they *are* my friends and they confide in me *as* a friend, I know that they can be bombarded with questions about health-related matters from people all the time. This knowledge made me especially reticent to impose on them not only because my questions would be "more work," but because being a friend to one who has a serious illness carries its own personal weight.

Introduction

Now, having gone through the various phases of diagnosis, treatment and surveillance as a patient, and through intensive work around breast cancer as a health humanities scholar, I have come to know much more about the various dimensions of this illness. I have listened to hundreds of stories from patients and healthcare providers, and I have researched breast cancer from a number of disciplinary perspectives. This personal and professional experience has led me to select particular artifacts for our book – the best information from the best individuals who do this work. I now know all these people personally, and I want you to meet them.

The Contexts of This Book

Here you will find patients, healthcare professionals and scholars from different walks of life and with varying perspectives. As I say when I speak about breast cancer publicly, "If you've known one person with breast cancer, you've known ... *one person* with breast cancer." Everyone's experience is unique, and that singularity is reflected in this volume. I am committed to inclusivity and have endeavored to incorporate as many different experiences – and people who have had those experiences – as possible. This means, therefore, that not all details will be relevant to all readers, nor will any given circumstance be true for everyone. Experiences of cancer – for both patients and healthcare providers – differ according to geographic location (nation or even region of a given country), race and ethnicity, social class, insurance status, to name a few. Readers from the UK might never have encountered a nurse navigator or fully understand the degree to which having no health insurance restricts a person's access to even basic, much less specialist, healthcare in the US – or, by contrast, how having private health insurance can sometimes afford a person seemingly limitless healthcare options. Readers from the US might not understand how breast surgery is triaged in the UK or know about the National Health Service's (NHS) provision for free prescriptions for medications via an exemption certificate – or that someone caring for a person with cancer in the UK may be entitled to a Carer's Allowance. As you read this book, it will be helpful to refer to the contributors' biographical sketches for a clearer sense of an individual's personal and professional contexts.

Scholars have a broad range of theoretical perspectives to choose from as they decide how to frame their work, so a few words about the philosophical and theoretical underpinnings of our book are in order. Terminology (and jargon) abound, but I'd like to streamline this section with some brief and straightforward comments on three key interdisciplinary movements or groupings of which this volume is a part: health humanities, medical humanities and critical humanities. "Applied humanities" and "expressive humanities" would also be appropriate descriptors.

In *Health Humanities* (2015), considered the manifesto for the field worldwide, Paul Crawford and colleagues argue that health humanities has arisen because many important stakeholders in healthcare "have been largely left out of the medical humanities," which is "more narrowly defined" (1,4). Craig M. Klugman and Erin Gentry Lamb clarify Crawford's meaning in their Introduction to *Research Methods in Health Humanities* (2019):

> The medical humanities focuses on how humanities and fine arts perspectives can aid physicians and medical students in becoming better healers: the humanities are a valuable tool used in medical education and practice. In contrast, health humanities puts the humanities, arts, and social sciences in the center, rather than as an add-on to clinical and basic science ... As a field the health humanities draws on the methodologies of the humanities, fine arts and social sciences to provide insight, understanding, and meaning to people facing illness including professional care providers, lay care providers, patients, policy-makers and others concerned with the suffering of humans." (3)

In short, as an inclusive, democratic field, health humanities is "concerned with understanding the human condition of health and illness in order to create knowledgeable and sensitive health care providers, patients, and family caregivers" (3) as they "apply[] scholarship and innovative programming in order to change the world" (4), not only medical education and practice.

Precisely germane to our book is Klugman and Lamb's claim that "health humanities research does not simply reside in an ivory tower" (7).

This statement brings me to an observation I've made over the past couple of decades about the bi-directional trajectories inherent in interdisciplinary fields like the medical humanities (less so in the health humanities, given the working definition above). For the first five or six years that I worked in medical humanities, I did so from the ivory tower, where the starting point was theory: Scholars with little knowledge of – or first-hand experience with – how humanistic dimensions of medicine played out in actual clinical settings provided insightful and potentially helpful theories that, we hoped, would find their way into clinical settings in order to, for one thing, improve the whole enterprise of healthcare. Our goal was – and still is – noble. But in 2002, my perspective shifted during a National Endowment for the Humanities Summer Institute at Penn State College of Medicine. For a month, twenty-five scholars from across the United States gathered to practice our respective "ivory tower" academic passions in the setting of a tertiary-care hospital. Things looked quite different from this side of the table, and I began to understand that theory and practice were sometimes – often, even – far apart. I have always yearned to make a practical difference in the lives of learners and humanity in general, and joining the faculty at Penn State College of Medicine in 2007 gave me the opportunity to work a different way – from a different starting point, one might say. And this necessitated a whole new way of conceptualizing and practicing my disciplinary skills. Let me explain.

Humanities scholars who work in academic medicine can end up in the kind of servile role Klugman and Lamb describe, "aiding" (3) physicians and medical students more than fully utilizing their own training and expertise. To counter the risk of becoming merely a "tool" (3) for physicians and medical students, some humanities scholars go the opposite direction entirely, becoming antagonistic to the very community we hope to engage. In their article "Critical Medical Humanities: Embracing Entanglement, Taking Risks" (2015), Viney, Callard and Woods describe this quandary:

> First, there is a service or utilitarian model, which accommodates but does not actively seek to challenge pre-existing power structures and epistemological divisions of labour within biomedicine, and which claims to "improve the quality of the humane relationship among doctors, clinical professionals and patients" by becoming a "boon companion or supportive friend." ..." In contrast to this servile

> vision of the medical humanities, ... others have defined its work according to its capacity to disrupt, broaden and embellish what are taken to be the overly reductive, materialist and scientistic definitions of human experience promoted by biomedicine ... [thereby functioning as] less a "supportive friend" to biomedicine than a "disruptive teenager." ... This version of medical humanities is hostile, dogged, skeptical, and separable from the medical practices it seeks to target. (3–4)

The former position devalues the wealth of expertise humanities scholars bring to the table and reinforces the very power structure they might critique for the betterment of healthcare. The latter merely alienates people on the front lines of medicine, primarily because practitioners don't have time for what they sometimes view as impractical and presumptuous: A prime weakness in an aggressive stance "is the superiority claimed by those whose critical perspective aims at exposing illusions ..." (5).

To be sure, many of my medical humanities colleagues – including those working in medical institutions – continue carrying out their scholarship largely in the ways they were trained to do; that is, primarily utilizing the methodologies and theoretical paradigms favored in their discreet specialties, some of which are intentionally "disruptive," provocative and confrontational. Robust and often elegant theoretical work comes out of this approach. However, others of us in medical humanities – perhaps especially those working in medical institutions – seek more aligned, even completely intertwined work in which our respective disciplinary training is immersed in medical culture and vice versa. This approach is more along the lines of health humanities as defined above.[1]

To illustrate my point, please permit me an admittedly reductive statement: Whereas ivory tower scholars try to bridge the divide between the humanities and medicine by theorizing, boots-on-the-ground healthcare providers try to bridge this divide by doing. In my experience, within medical culture if something isn't pertinent to the direct care of patients or the direct training of medical students, it simply doesn't gain traction, no matter how appealing and desirable it might be. Materially speaking, this means that scholars who want to make an impact in medicine must

---

1   A note on terminology: Those who teach primarily medical students are technically part of medical humanities even when they also identify as part of health humanities.

discover ways to make their ideas "useful" while also maintaining scholarly integrity. The real challenge for scholars therefore is to find a third way – a *tertium quid*, as it were, akin to the Hegelian dialectic – utilizing one's disciplinary skills robustly while doing so in a way that invites and includes healthcare professionals and trainees who need to "do," who need to see the practicality and applicability of other disciplines.

The "third way" I envision is ably articulated by Viney and colleagues who believe that "the arts, humanities and social sciences are best viewed not as in service or in opposition to the clinical and life sciences, but as productively entangled with a 'biomedical culture'" (2); they therefore argue for a middle ground, one they call "critical medical humanities." As the title of their article indicates, they embrace "entanglement" and "risk" as approaches to "illuminate[] diverse ways of doing medical humanities … [with] critical openness, plurality and cooperation" (3,4). In support of their position, they cite Bruno Latour's definition of the critic (one might use the term "scholar" here) "not as one who debunks, but the one who assembles … not the one who lifts the rugs from under the feet of the naïve believers, but the one who offers the participants arenas in which to gather" (Latour 30). Our book is the embodiment of such "critical humanities."

The Contents of This Book

Breast Cancer Inside Out is meant to be a cross-over book that illuminates breast cancer for academics, practitioners, patients and, indeed, anyone who wants to know more about this disease from multiple perspectives – experiential, biomedical and socio-cultural. To that end and for the sake of variety, the selections here take different forms, including first-person essay, historical overview, scholarly analysis, and original artistic and mixed-media creations.

Although each chapter in this volume focuses on one or two particular aspects of breast cancer – for example, preserving fertility, disclosing diagnosis – the pieces are highly inter-textual; they "speak to one another," thereby providing broader and deeper context than any one by itself might do. I indicate such cross-references within the essays themselves. With regard to disclosing personal information, each author has taken care to respect the privacy of individuals mentioned in the chapters. Some individuals granted express consent to have their names and stories published (e.g., "Communion"); other patients' names and identifying details (those details *not* related to cancer diagnosis and treatment; these all remain actual and accurate) were changed (e.g., "Intimacy and Sexuality in the Context of Breast Cancer"); still others' stories are already public (e.g., "I Promise You Will Feel Better").

Though breast cancer is not, of course, a purely linear experience, certain milestones serve as an arc of its progression – from diagnosis, through various forms of treatment, to death or life that will be forever marked (for bad and often for good as well) by one's cancer experience. Part I loosely traces this journey through the voices of patients and the professionals who care for them.

Beginning with a pre-diagnosis sense that something is not quite right, "When the Patient Knows What the Doctor Does Not (Yet) Know" chronicles a years-long foreboding that culminates in a routine-turned-diagnostic mammogram. Told in alternating voices, a patient and the radiologist who performs the mammogram and core needle biopsy recount their thoughts and impressions as the diagnostic process unfolds. A physician assistant and nurse navigator pick up here to provide "A Step-by-Step Guide through Breast Cancer Diagnosis and Radiation," beginning with the immediate emotional impact of diagnosis and ushering the reader through some of the usual questions and hurdles: decisions about surgeries, chemotherapy and radiation. Especially helpful is the detailed account of precisely what happens in radiation therapy. "Communion" is a breast surgeon's personal reflection about a transformative experience with a young patient and her husband. Illuminating what he thinks and feels during several pivotal moments, including examining the patient for the first time and later removing both of her breasts, this essay reveals keen awareness of the delicate balance between empathy and potential loss of objectivity.

A poet and a plastic surgeon address the issue of reconstructive surgery from their respective viewpoints. "Reconstruction" questions the rightness of an aesthetic that urges us to cover imperfection, and it challenges the reader to "look at an absence straight on." "Gauging Too Much Information" offers excellent insights, through the story of a young mother, into what surgery and recovery look like. An information technology specialist provides "Wisdom from the Trenches" about the common quandaries of whether/how to use the internet; deciding when, how and to whom to disclose one's diagnosis, and speaking up to question a potential mistake. In "Another Catcher in the Rye," a medical oncologist describes cancer care in clinics whose patients have no health insurance. Lack of resources burdens patients, providers and decision-making; but it also creates a different kind of community than one typically finds in private cancer clinics. In this case, the county hospital is a "neighborhood" characterized by warmth and collaboration that, the author argues, can emerge only in an environment where there's no expectation of profit.

In "Reflections on Solidarity," a hospital chaplain shows how one's encounter with breast cancer changes when something that is professional becomes personal. "When Chaos Comes" sheds light on the lesser-known role of a hospitalist, who cares for patients who develop serious complications related to malignancy or treatment. We get a rare look inside the mind and heart of an internist who diagnoses a recurrence of breast cancer in a patient she's never met before and who, despite the doctor's "Best-Laid Plans" and earnest efforts, chooses not to continue medical treatment.

First-person accounts from a palliative care physician and a hospice physician reveal how these specialists are "Always on Your Side," actively contributing to the physical and emotional/existential health of their patients. Debunking the myth that worsening disease and even death are without hope and healing, these stories are evidence of "How Hospice Can Heal" through interventions including a Life Review.

Part I concludes with an interview of a male pastor who received a diagnosis of breast cancer while serving in Uganda. With humor and pragmatism, he shares with readers how it feels to be a man contending with a disease that "seems to be more female" and how he relied on the "Three S's" – song, scriptures, and his fellow breast cancer Soul Sisters – to get him through. Here he echoes a commitment I've seen in almost all people

I've met who have experienced breast cancer: To help others in any way we can – as he puts it, be a good "Steward of Suffering."

The selections in Part II show the importance of prioritizing oneself and one's core values in order to optimize physical and emotional health and preserve self-identity in the face of breast cancer. Relaying stories from his work with "Our Many Teachers," as he calls his patients, an oncology psychologist offers five important reminders of how to enhance mental health – suggesting ways to, among other things, "know what matters most." This concept plays out beautifully in the essay that follows, "All You Need Is Love ... and Research," the account of a medical anthropologist son who deploys his research skills in service of his mother's quest to find a non-aggressive treatment protocol that aligns with her personal convictions.

A researcher in exercise oncology and a nutritionist make convincing arguments that "I Promise You Will Feel Better" if you exercise consistently and think of "Food as Medicine" during and after treatment for cancer. A young couple who are engaged navigate a "Future on Ice" as they work with a fertility clinic to preserve their ability to conceive a child after treatment. This 28-year-old woman tells, with great candor, what it's like to "find ourselves between two worlds. One hour I was among women – bald, thin, dying – and the next, at a fertility clinic with happy couples on the precipice of starting bigger, child-ful lives." Addressing a wider range of concerns around intimate relationships, a sex therapist offers guidance on issues of "Intimacy and Sexuality in the Context of Breast Cancer," including strategies ranging from "redefining sex" to "ways of sexual pleasuring."

Part III is a collection of patients' renderings of their lived experience in various artistic forms. A medical ethicist depicts her reality of being both constant and changed in "Breast Cancer in Six Acts." In this hybrid genre that combines personal narrative and play script, she explores what patient autonomy means and how her professional understanding of the concept is expanded when she becomes a patient interacting with her medical colleagues. In "Breast Cancer Poetry: Voice, Identity, Contingency and Death," a scholar of medical humanities provides rich insight into prevalent themes in poems written in the latter years of the twentieth century and the very early part of the twenty-first century – themes ranging from how patients lose and reclaim "voice"; to communitarian dimensions of breast cancer, including race and ethnicity; and to the breast cancer "marketplace."

A best-selling author portrays – in comic form – two strange events that remind her out of the blue of her past experience with breast cancer and how, paradoxically, such reminders bring beauty "Under the Birdcage," as it were. A comics scholar/medical educator discusses "Breast Cancer Comics in the Classroom and the Clinic," revealing how Marisa Acocella Marchetto's graphic pathography *Cancer Vixen* enables future doctors to understand more clearly the lived experience of the disease and how, ironically, the comic suddenly became quite personal: "Fewer than twenty-four hours after discussing Marchetto's text with my students, I was undergoing many of the procedures – and the emotions – she so memorably depicts in *Cancer Vixen* …. Marchetto was my constant companion throughout … the weeks and months to come" as she underwent chemotherapy, mastectomy and reconstruction.

A curator provides an insightful interpretation of and introduction to *Edges of Light*: *Images of Breast Transformation*, a mixed-media exhibit by a professional photographer and literary scholar-patient. The word-image pairings of this sequence capture various moods, various "moments in time," throughout all stages of treatment. In "The Form," a poet extends questions implicitly raised in the exhibit about one's shifting understanding of bodily form vis-à-vis one's inner sense of identity. Here, she chronicles her own process of "throw[ing] masks out of the car window" in order to "wear the body I've chosen."

As its title indicates, Part IV reveals how meanings of breast cancer evolve over time. An art historian provides close analysis of representative "Milestones in the Depiction of Breasts and Breast Cancer in Art History" from prehistoric to contemporary times; and in "Breast Art," a poet ponders why the female subject of Raphael's painting *La Fornarina* is shown touching her breast. Following the story about his mother's and sister's breast cancer, a surgeon-scientist provides an in-depth "Historical Overview of Breast Cancer and Its Treatments," explaining how the disease has been understood in the Western world since ancient Egypt and how those beliefs have determined treatments. Moving through topics as diverse as humoral medicine; developments in anatomy and pathology (e.g., dissection), technology (e.g., microscope), the surgical environment (e.g., antisepsis and anesthesia) and the laboratory (e.g., radiation); and first-person accounts of mastectomy, this surgeon also describes in explicit detail how he performed radical Halsted mastectomies and how his scientific research culminated in cutting-edge clinical trials for hormonal therapies including tamoxifen and aromatase inhibitors.

In "Radiation Therapy: Evolutions in Treatment, Consultations in Clinic," a radiation oncologist traces the development of his field alongside those of surgery and medical oncology and concludes by showing how he would talk with a patient from the beginning of her treatment into her post-treatment maintenance: how he comes to understand her particular kind of breast cancer, how he explains radiation therapy as she contemplates whether to undergo mastectomy or lumpectomy, and how radiation is utilized therapeutically and palliatively if breast cancer recurs. "Understanding How Breast Cancer Behaves" provides a concise overview of different perspectives on how the disease begins and what happens when it is left untreated – that is, its "natural history" – and discusses evolving data on rates of recurrence, prognosis and survival. A genetics counselor explains the rise of genetic counseling as an important facet of diagnosis and treatment and uses case histories to illustrate why, when and how "Testing for Hereditary Breast Cancer" happens – including some quandaries ironically created by such tests.

A cultural studies scholar looks at "The Marketing of Metastatic Breast Cancer" through an analysis of a prominent television commercial that advertises an oral medication to treat advanced disease. The sometimes troubling ramifications she elucidates are borne out in "The New Normal: Metastatic Breast Cancer Experiences of Survivor Identity," in which a health communication researcher – and MBC patient herself – discusses "ways we MBC patients are making sense of our disease experiences in one online MBC social media support group." The final poem in our book, "Support Group," brings scholarly analysis and social sciences research to a sharp point: the double-edged impact of a patient's regular gathering with fellow patients.

Underscoring a commitment I articulated in the Artists' Statement for the *Edges of Light* exhibit, I say again that "I would do whatever I could, professionally and personally, to help other women and men have a sense of what to expect – and to encourage them – on their own journeys with breast disease." This book is another part of that commitment.

Bibliography

Crawford, Paul, Brian Brown, Charley Baker, Victoria Tischler and Brian Abrams. *Health Humanities*. London: Palgrave Macmillan, 2015.

Klugman, Craig and Erin Gentry Lamb. "Introduction: Raising Health Humanities." *Research Methods in Health Humanities*. Eds. Craig Klugman and Erin Gentry Lamb. Oxford: Oxford UP, 2019. 1–11.

Latour, Bruno. "Why Has Critique Run Out of Steam? From Matters of Fact to Matters of Concern." *Critical Inquiry* 30 (2004): 225–48.

Remen, Rachel Naomi. *Kitchen Table Wisdom: Stories that Heal*. New York: Riverhead, 1996.

Viney, William, Felicity Callard and Angela Woods. "Critical Medical Humanities: Embracing Entanglement, Taking Risks." *Medical Humanities* 41 (2015): 2–7.

PART I

A Trajectory of Breast Cancer:
Diagnosis, Treatment and Beyond

KIMBERLY R. MYERS AND JULIE A. MACK

When the Patient Knows What the Doctor Does Not (Yet) Know

Kimberly

Since I was in my twenties I knew I would be diagnosed with breast cancer. With no family history, no risk factors, no suspicious test results, and therefore no credible reason to anticipate this diagnosis, I nevertheless knew intuitively that I would get breast cancer. And I did.

As a teacher and scholar of medical humanities, I am usually thinking in some way about the nuances of patient-doctor relationships and communication. This professional awareness complicates my identity as a patient, especially because most of my physicians are also my colleagues and sometimes even close personal friends. The inevitable blurring of professional and personal boundaries is difficult for colleagues, whether patient or physician, particularly in the context of a serious diagnosis. What follows is an analytical reflection on the interplay of intuitive and empirical knowing, embedded in the stories of this patient and the radiologist who diagnosed her.

Physicians frequently advise patients, "Listen to your own body; you know it better than anyone." In the actual clinical relationship, though, tensions exist between a patient's intuitive knowledge and a physician's empirical knowledge, and these tensions have very real ramifications. For instance, a central goal of communication in the clinic is that the patient be a "good historian," reporting any and all information that might be relevant to her care. To facilitate this, the physician must cultivate an atmosphere of trust that enables the patient to divulge information that, while potentially embarrassing or awkward, could be critical to whole-person care.

Because of my premonition of breast cancer, over the years my perspective had progressed from sensible concern about breast health, to apprehensiveness about check-ups, to outright fright about anything to do with breast disease. I shuddered at scientific updates on epidemiology that I might encounter in professional journals; personal narratives by patients, or stories in film or television (frequent, given my work with pathographies and my general literature-and-medicine focus); reports on emerging diagnostic or treatment modalities featured on nightly news broadcasts ... and *certainly* the imperative for breast self-exams. Indeed, I finally decided that the burden of stress I experienced once a month at the time of my self-exam outweighed the benefit of potentially discovering a mass early, so I carefully orchestrated annual mammograms and gynecology visits so they would fall roughly six months apart. At least, I reasoned, something or someone (other than me) would be monitoring my body twice a year "before anything might have time to get out of control."

Upon my move from teaching literature in a university to teaching in a college of medicine known for its humanities program, I figured it might be wise to confide in my internist just how dramatically this darkening intuition – and the snowballing anxiety that ensued – was affecting my life. This plan seemed decidedly auspicious since my newly minted internist was a graduate of a program with a strong emphasis on medical humanities and biomedical ethics, and I was one of her first post-residency patients.[1] And after all, over the course of five or six visits in three years, she had always been attentive to the concrete information I had given her. Like any other well-trained physician, she presumably felt empowered to *do* something, to *act*. When I first reported persistent pain in my left breast, for instance, she ordered a diagnostic mammogram. It was normal. So was the next one, a year later. So were the three exams she performed on me, for that matter. But the pain persisted, and my sense of foreboding intensified.

---

[1] This detail, like many others, indicates the privilege I have as an educated patient with exceptional access to medical treatment. Please see Footnote 1 in "Breast Cancer Comics in the Classroom and the Clinic" for a brief statement about implications of such privilege.

"So what does this mean?" I constantly tried to divine, to analyze. Am I imagining things? Am I *creating* things? Is this well-founded intuition or is it some sort of perverse self-fulfilling prophecy? Is it an example of what my well-meaning but woefully oblivious walking buddy said, "You attract what you fear"? (Well, *that's* great.) When medical tests don't validate strong intuition, at what point – and to what extent – does the intuitive patient begin to doubt herself and her perception of her symptoms, especially if her intuition has proved remarkably accurate throughout her life? This is doubly confounding for highly analytical, self-reflective people, and poses an even greater quandary for those who work in health care settings and repeatedly hear frustration and exasperation regarding patients who appear to be malingering.

Not wanting to become a "problem patient" whose symptoms are dismissed by a doctor (Peters et al.), I tried to dismiss my own symptoms and make an uneasy peace with constant cognitive dissonance. "This breast pain must just be a fluke," I repeat in my head, day by day, moment by moment. "Nothing is palpable and nothing is visible on the films." From this vantage point – theoretically mirroring that of any frustrated physician who has dutifully followed up with all the right tests – a vigilant patient's wisdom in "listening to her own body" slowly morphs into shame that she "imagines things." Intuition has become hypochondria, she fears.

Given that patients want and need to be taken seriously, the stakes are high when discussing non-empirical phenomena – even higher, perhaps, when one's doctor is also a colleague. What if the patient is dismissed as neurotic by the very person left to care for her? Fearing that talking about her intuition might affect her physician's opinion of and behavior toward her, to what extent should the patient script a calculated discussion in order to minimize the possibility of dismissiveness or even abandonment? Surely these uncertainties themselves contribute to stress, which is implicated as a contributing factor in a host of disease processes, including breast cancer.

Entangled in this web of concerns, I furtively googled the most clinically detached description I could think of to describe what I was experiencing: "health anxiety." To my surprise, this search yielded links to the DSM (*Diagnostic and Statistical Manual of Mental Disorders*), where I found this condition a "legitimate" diagnosis. Armed with official diagnostic language other than the alternative – and more culturally freighted – term "hypochondriasis," I could come clean with my internist. Perhaps she would respect my dispassionate, straightforward tone as an indication of healthy self-awareness. I would report this information as matter-of-factly as I would present a patient on morning rounds if I were a physician. I had my approach.

Initially, my internist seemed sympathetic to my situation and supported my plan to have mammograms in January and breast exams with her in July. I was gratified that I had withheld the darkest manifestations of my anxiety – she need not know every macabre detail – so that I still had some credibility in the clinical setting. That is, not everything I reported would be disregarded as merely "imagination," a word some use interchangeably with "intuition." This was July, and as usual she found nothing during the physical exam. Six months respite, then, before the onslaught of anxiety surrounding the next imaging test – which was, again, normal. When I saw her in clinic the following July, she asked why I was there, seemingly forgetting our six-month-from-mammogram-to-office-visit plan. When I reminded her, she seemed reluctant to follow through with the breast physical exam and said that in the future she would perform only the tests that were medically indicated, not every test I simply thought I should have. Her tone was condescending, paternalistic, as if she refused to cater to the whims of a hypochondriac and that we needed a little rational rationing to remind us what was what – and who was who. I felt shamed by her.

Assumptions were made and trust was shattered. No longer having an ally and now doubly closeted in my apprehensiveness, I walked into the breast imaging center the following January with an even greater sense of dread than usual. Getting ready that morning, a horde of scenarios careened through my mind: "The next time I make this bed, my whole world could be in shambles"; "When I look into this bathroom mirror again, I could see Cancer Patient"; "This might be the last time I enjoy a cup of coffee without worrying about a tumor in my breast." It went on and on. The morning was cold and rainy. Not a good omen, I thought.

Julie

I wandered down the hallway and looked for the technologist whom I would be working with on my next case. My eyes drifted to the diagnostic waiting room where a face sat perched above a crouched body, shrouded in one of our gowns. The eyes were familiar but the expression was not; the last time I had seen her, I read energetic curiosity in her face. Today her fear confused me.

I walked into the room and spoke her name as a question: "Kimberly?" She looked up at me, her frame looking fragile in a gown, not the woman I remembered. There were others in the waiting room, so I motioned her to the hallway. I asked if she was okay, immediately presuming she was "called back" due to a possible abnormality on her screening test, or that she was there to have a new symptom investigated.

She said, "No, I wasn't called back."

My eyes must have registered confusion. She was in our diagnostic waiting room.

"The left-breast pain I had a couple of years ago has come back." She wrapped her gown closer and apologized. "I'm sorry, this is just a hard test for me. It always has been. I haven't been sleeping."

She does not want to wait for results by phone or by letter. She wants to know now.

I touch her arm, hoping to comfort. "Would you like me to read your study?" For a moment, I see relief in her face and she smiles. "Yes, would you?"

I walk back down the hall and I am unsettled by her fear. The last time I had seen her, she wasn't a patient. She was a professor of literature, energetic, my husband's mentor. Last time she wore a bright jacket, her shoulders broad, and her arms open and waving. The eyes I remembered radiated enthusiasm as she presided over the awards ceremony for submissions to the literary magazine she edited.

I ask one of the technologists to bring the films on Dr. Myers to me when the study is complete. I re-enter the dark reading room and continue on with my daily work. A little later, the technologist returns. The four-view standard images are ready.

My eyes register heterogeneously dense breasts, a mix of greys and whites. A three-dimensional structure flattened into two dimensions. A border catches my eye. "Probably overlap," I tell the technologist. "Can you just take another spot there?" I know this will produce more fear in my patient, but I plan to give her the good news when it is all done. I walk down the hall to let her know that I want an additional image. Overlap of tissue can produce all sorts of odd forms, and another picture will sort it out. She is alone this time in the waiting room, and I am standing. I briefly review what I need. I expect nervousness. The response is panic.

"What did you find? Do you see something?"

Her eyes are wide, her shoulders small. I sit down next to her and begin a longer explanation.

"You have dense breast tissue; overlap of tissue can produce odd shadows on the film. I'm just being careful. If the additional views are normal, we'll be done."

"What if they're not normal? What does that mean?"

Her eyes are wider, her mouth open. I attempt again to calm her. The technologist moves in and takes her into the exam room for the additional views.

The spot view comes back, and I stare at the area. The technologist waits. Was I letting my nerves get the better of me? Had my patient's fear become mine? I walk down the hall for a second opinion from a trusted colleague.

"I know her. She's nervous. Am I overcalling this?"

"Yes."

I pause briefly and contemplate stopping the exam without pursuing additional imaging. Doing nothing feels worse than pursuing the hint of a shadow on the mammogram. I confess to the technologist, "I'm doing this as much to calm my nerves as hers. Humor me and let's put her in ultrasound."

I will feel more confident if I can clear her breast by sonography. But first I have to talk to her again. I take a breath and walk down the hall.

I look again into her fear, and try to explain what an ultrasound can do – that we often see cysts in patients with dense breast tissue.

"Does a cyst indicate malignancy?"

"No, a cyst is just fluid within the normal spectrum of breast physiology."

"Does that predispose me to cancer?"

I try again to comfort, explaining that sonography is just another way to look at the breast. I do not discuss the data on dense breast tissue and elevated cancer risk.

I haven't calmed her down, and her anxiety level disorients me. I explain that we have to contact her physician, as we can't move ahead with additional testing until we have a written order. It will require that she wait. Would she like to come back later? It was a silly question.

I walk by the waiting room several more times on my way to see other patients. It is not typical for me to pay attention to this room, but today I do.

She is reading.

She is tapping.

She is staring.

I call her doctor directly for the order, bypassing the front desk. I can't wait any longer.

The technologist moves her into the ultrasound room and types her data into the machine.

I enter the dark room and see she is quiet, staring at the ceiling, the agitation diminished. I am calm, comfortable in this room with a probe in my hand. I move her gown down and drape a towel over her breast, leaving a portion uncovered. I squirt warm gel on the probe, and place it on her skin. Scattered islands of white glandular tissue separated by bands of grey fatty breast tissue fill the screen, and I am relieved. Her breast tissue is easy to scan, smooth transitions between white and grey, with only inconsistent shadowing from the supporting ligaments. I move the probe down and slightly toward the middle, and an aberration appears on the screen. It is against her chest wall, a small dark splotch, interrupting the normal contour of the tissue. I move the probe away, turn it slightly, and move it back to the area. The splotch persists. I quietly speak to the technologist, "Mark this radial 9:00, 2 cm from the nipple." I make an initial measurement. My patient has turned her gaze from the ceiling. She is staring directly at me, and now her fear is familiar; it makes sense to me, something I witness in most emotionally healthy patients when I find something that needs biopsy.

"What is it? Is it a cyst?

I lift the probe off her skin.

"No, it is not a cyst."

I pause, and phrase my next sentence carefully.

"Kimberly, I don't like the way it looks."

I realize I haven't used many words before she grasps the import of what is going on. More words about what it looks like will not help her understand it any more than she already does.

Her face contorts, her eyes squeeze tight, and she breathes too fast.

I put the probe down, pause, and touch her arm again. I begin the next discussion, a transition to another test. It is the biopsy procedure I later learn she has long been expecting.

Reflections

Julie

I have replayed that day in my mind many times, wondering why I moved to sonography in this patient on that day. I sought a second opinion with a trusted colleague; but even before she had given her opinion that a sonogram was probably not warranted, I had decided to pursue the additional test. On another day, the same findings might not have crossed my threshold of "abnormal" and I, too, would have passed the study as negative. After all, there's no certainty when examining shadows on films for patterns of disease, especially in patients with dense breasts. This is a truth that all radiologists understand and must learn to live with. Nonetheless, on that day, I could not even come to a relative certainty. Sensing that something was off-kilter in Kimberly – even though I could not pinpoint it precisely – caused my mirror neurons to fire early and repeatedly, and my adrenaline rose. Perhaps this synergistic connection and subsequent physiological response enhanced my perception of the subtle finding on the film. Perhaps I just feared missing an important finding. Whatever the process, Kimberly and I now shared the same fear. Something was wrong; something sinister eluded detection.

I sat with Kimberly a few days later as she was waiting for her MRI exam. She looked tired now, but she was calm. We talked a bit about what had happened that day. Remarkably, despite the circumstances of a new cancer diagnosis, she expressed gratitude. She told me she was glad that I had been there that day and that I had moved ahead with additional testing. I too was thankful. Had I not seen Kimberly in the waiting room and connected with her on a subconscious level, I might have seen only dense tissue on her mammogram and missed the early finding that could make a difference in her long-term prognosis.

Kimberly

At some later point in my treatment, Julie asked me whether there was any period of time between her discovering the mass and my receiving the pathology results that I had convinced myself it wasn't cancer. No – not only because Julie is a well-trained, gifted radiologist with years of experience, but also because I immediately recognized this finding as the thing I had known was coming all along. And while I was devastated by the findings, in a curious way it was also something of a relief to finally receive the diagnosis. Perhaps it was because there was no more relentless cognitive dissonance. Or perhaps it was a vindication of sorts that wiped away the awkwardness and distress I had come to feel about knowing something doctors did not yet know.

That said, here's the rub: The mass was in my right breast, not the left where I had felt pain. Although breast cancer is rarely painful, and breast pain is common, my recurring left-breast pain is what warranted a "diagnostic" mammogram (as opposed to a "screening" mammogram); and being in the diagnostic room is what led Julie to see me. In a way, intuition had found a voice considered legitimate in the clinical setting; pain had done its work by triggering the cascade of events that unfolded. What's more, after the initial stages of diagnosis, the pestilential anxiety that had hounded me for decades receded into near quietness.

Though this essay most directly addresses the interplay of intuitive and empirical knowing, it also touches on another way of knowing: knowing people in multiple ways. For example, in the thick of trying to process my diagnosis and the white-hot shock that followed from it, I was also very concerned about Julie. I kept thinking how utterly awful this liminal position must be for her: to have to give this news to a friend, to be saddled with the weight of her professional responsibilities in an otherwise personal relationship. In short, I felt remorse for having (inadvertently, to be sure) put a colleague and friend in this difficult position.

Indeed, writing this essay was itself difficult because it took us out of carefully prescribed professional roles and into murky territory of multiple and simultaneous ways of knowing each other. But it was also wonderfully cathartic and illuminating; in exploring the acts of speaking and listening in a clinical setting we discovered that we recalled the same events, but we remembered the language quite differently. Because the word "cancer" has long been taboo for me when I have been in the position of patient in a clinic, I'm certain that I would never have asked Julie outright if "this is cancer." I would have used all sorts of circumlocutions and euphemisms, as are generally reflected in this essay. But when Julie recounted her memory of that day, she remembered my initial response to her request for extra mammographic views as "Do I have cancer?" It was what I was thinking, and it was what she "heard," but I'm sure those words were never spoken.

The richness of these insights leads us to believe that similar collaboration between patients and physicians would be quite fruitful, fostering better communication and deeper trust, and therefore ultimately more effective clinical relationships. We also believe that, based on the experience we describe here, clinicians should respect intuition – their own and their patients' – even when empirical tests contradict it. Doing so just might save someone's life.

Bibliography

Peters, Sarah, Ian Stanley, Michael Rose and Peter Salmon. "Patients with Medically Unexplained Symptoms: Sources of Patients' Authority and Implications for Demands on Medical Care." *Social Science & Medicine* 46.4–5 (February-March 1998): 559–65.

MARK STOUT AND LYNN FANTOM

A Step-by-Step Guide through Breast Cancer Diagnosis and Radiation

Mark

"Isn't radiation bad for you?"

As a radiation oncology Physician Assistant (PA), I usually cover this question first thing with our new patients to allay fear and begin their education process about upcoming treatment. When radiation is uncontrolled, it is dangerous; but if it is used therapeutically, it can be very effective for safe and long-lasting protection from recurrence or progression of disease. Especially with our breast cancer patients, radiation usually comes late in the treatment process: Our patients have already undergone surgery and possibly chemotherapy. By the time they get to our department, the diagnosis has become more real and the denial phase has usually passed.

Denial is common in the grieving process, whether being diagnosed with a potentially life-threatening breast cancer or losing a loved one. Many women have a mother, grandmother, or aunt who was diagnosed with breast cancer fifty years ago when it really was a death sentence. Women would have disfiguring and debilitating mastectomies (removal of all breast tissue, lymph nodes and, many times, chest wall muscles), then undergo chemotherapy that would cause hair loss, nausea and vomiting. If they received radiation treatment, they had burns, heart or lung complications and other potential lifelong side effects. So when patients hear the terrifying words "You have breast cancer," many of them assume they are destined for a similar fate as their ancestors. Luckily, this is not true – mainly because of the many caring and brave women who have gone before them, participating in clinical trials of new medications or new combinations of chemotherapy treatments, joining new diagnostic test trials in order to personalize treatments, or creating support groups to aid patients and families by providing resources and encouragement. We can now better determine the most effective treatment for each newly diagnosed patient individually rather than using the old shotgun approach of treating everyone with the same treatment when we couldn't determine who would be most responsive to chemotherapy, radiation or anti-estrogen therapy.

But I am getting ahead of myself. Let's go back to that patient who has heard those terrifying words, "You have breast cancer." The diagnosis is most often related to a finding on a routine screening mammogram, unless the person has felt or seen a change in her breast and has come in for an evaluation. The patient is usually alone, without her significant other or family, and she quickly becomes overwhelmed. That is where someone like Lynn, a certified breast care registered nurse, can make all the difference in terms of how this new patient will navigate the next few months or years of treatment. Lynn and I often work as a team, using our respective skills and training to help individual patients.

Lynn

As a nurse coordinator/navigator, I meet women and men who are diagnosed with breast cancer and help them navigate the journey they're about to embark on. When someone is diagnosed with breast cancer, "overwhelming" doesn't seem like a big enough word. Their world is turned upside down, and their first thought is often "Am I going to die?" Some people cry; others are more stoic. They think about their families and how the family members will be affected. When they are first told they have cancer, they usually don't hear anything after that word and only remember about 10 percent of what you tell them. We always recommend they bring someone with them when they come for biopsy results. There is a lot of information to take in and many decisions to make.

I usually explain to the patients that this journey is like a roller coaster ride: There will be ups and downs.

The biopsy is the first step, but then there is more investigation to be done – additional testing, surgery results and treatment recommendations. Depending on the type, size and location of the tumor, patients will undergo either surgery or systemic treatment (hormone therapy or chemotherapy) first. Sometimes systemic therapy is given before surgery to try to shrink the tumor and maybe even make it disappear. The healthcare providers and I are there to help answer questions like these and guide our patients through all the decisions that follow. Breast cancer has become complex, and each plan is individualized. The team of physicians involved in one's care may include a breast surgeon, medical oncologist, radiation oncologist and plastic surgeon.

If surgery is the initial line of treatment, the patient will meet with a breast surgeon early on. Nurse navigators attend these appointments with patients and, if necessary, help explain things in terms the patient can understand. The first major decision is whether to have a lumpectomy (removing the part of the breast with cancer along with some normal tissue) or mastectomy (removal of the entire breast). Many women automatically think mastectomy is the better surgery, as it removes all the breast tissue. This is not true. Lumpectomy followed by radiation is equivalent to mastectomy in terms of effectiveness. The risk of recurrence, locally (in the breast) and distantly (elsewhere in the body), is the same. Some women do benefit from mastectomy, however, especially if they have extensive disease or if they have a genetic mutation that predisposes them to breast cancer. If a patient needs or wants a mastectomy, they then have to decide about reconstruction. Mastectomy is an inherently body-altering surgery that can really impact a patient's self-image. So the decision to remove the breast should not be made quickly. Patients should know that even with a breast cancer diagnosis, there is time to gather information and opinions before making final decisions. I help patients decide what is best for them by educating them and supporting them along the way.

For example, a patient whom I'll call Bethany presented for screening mammogram and it was abnormal; she was subsequently diagnosed with breast cancer. When she received the news, I sat with her and we reviewed what type of cancer she had and what types of treatments were available to her. During our conversation, Bethany mentioned that she had three children at home and wanted more. We discussed why getting pregnant right then would not be a good idea, and I emphasized that she should use protection going forward. She left me that day, went home, did a home pregnancy test … and discovered that she was already pregnant – very early in her first trimester. The first trimester of pregnancy is a crucial time for the development of the baby, so treatment options are very limited during that time. I sat down with Bethany and her family, and we reviewed what the options were, including the risks to her and to her baby. As a mother, she was firmly committed to putting her children's needs before her own. But because she had both young children and an unborn child, this was an excruciatingly difficult decision. Bethany knew her chances of being around to love and care for her three living children were much better if she began treatment soon, so she ultimately decided to terminate her pregnancy and proceed with her treatment plan. Based on my experience with other patients, I thought she might want a memory of this pregnancy, and we discussed having an ultrasound and getting a picture that she could place in a special frame. As I journeyed with her, we had to work through the guilt she felt and how to deal with it.

Reconstruction is a great option with mastectomy, but one needs to know that reconstruction is not like breast augmentation. Reconstruction can involve the use of implants (saline or silicone-based), with or without nipple sparing, or it can involve using one's own tissue (usually from the abdomen, though other areas can be used as well). Again, both of these are big surgeries that require a period of healing. The chest wall is numb after mastectomy, with or without reconstruction. It is important to know that reconstructed breasts will not be the same as natural breasts. The reconstructed breasts do not allow for any sexual stimulation, and they do not feel or look the same. Patients see the scars every day, so every day they are reminded that they had cancer. Once again, there's a lot of information to digest and big decisions to make. A main take-away is that patients must take time to make the decision that is best for them.

One of my younger patients, Gina, had chosen to undergo bilateral mastectomies, but she was really struggling with whether to undergo immediate reconstruction. I showed her a sample of the saline- and silicone-filled implants and let her hold them so she could see and feel what would be going inside her. I also showed her the external prostheses that women wear in their bras if they decide not to undergo reconstruction so that, again, she could get a visual of what that would entail. I suggested that if she were not 100 percent sure, she should not have immediate reconstruction. If she decided later that she would like to have it done, she could and her insurance would cover the surgery. Gina was appreciative and ultimately decided not to have immediate reconstruction. She was very happy with that decision, and she was also happy to know that if she decided to pursue reconstruction later, she could.

One important factor in these deliberations is whether genetics play a role in the cancer. Patients may carry certain genes, passed down from either their mother or father, that predispose them to developing breast cancer. BRCA 1 and BRCA 2 are the most common. I remember a patient – I'll call her Mary – whose mother and sister carried the BRCA mutation. When Mary was diagnosed with breast cancer at age thirty-seven, genetic tests revealed that she, too, had the BRACA mutation. Especially because she was relatively young, Mary was not ready to undergo bilateral mastectomies – though she did so a few years later. Mary's oldest sister eventually went in for testing and found that she was also BRCA positive. The mutation carries an increased risk of ovarian cancer, so the sister went for prophylactic ovary removal but discovered that she already had ovarian cancer. She was treated for this but, unfortunately, a couple of years later was diagnosed with breast cancer and underwent bilateral mastectomies. Wow. Imagine the breadth of emotions for Mary, her mother and her sister – not only for themselves but for one another. Also, the mothers or fathers who passed the gene down feel guilty. Some young patients with a genetic mutation start to consider if they should even have children because they do not want their children to have to deal with potential cancer diagnoses. That is such a big decision to have to make.

Once surgery has been performed, one of the next steps is to figure out what systemic treatment is needed. Does a person need chemotherapy, or can she just take a pill for five to ten years? Chemotherapy is scary; it can involve hair loss, vomiting and feeling extremely tired. Patients think of chemotherapy as poison, but I try to encourage them think of it as the Pac-Man eating the cancer cells or soldiers marching through their blood and going to war with the cancer cells.

Most patients diagnosed with triple-negative breast cancer need chemotherapy because this type of cancer is aggressive and does not respond to anti-estrogen therapy such as tamoxifen or anastrozole. It does, however, respond to chemotherapy. Some breast cancers are HER2/neu positive and require special targeted medicines, such as Herceptin® (trastuzumab) and/or Perjeta® (pertuzumab), which are given in conjunction with chemotherapy. The majority of hormone-positive breast cancers do not require chemotherapy, but some do. So how do you tell which of these patients should have chemotherapy? There is a test called Oncotype DX that can be done on the cancer tissue itself. This test provides a recurrence score: the odds that the cancer will come back somewhere else in the body over the next ten years. The three result categories are low risk, intermediate risk and high risk. It is important to know that these scores are based on the assumption that patients will take endocrine therapy, such as tamoxifen or aromatase inhibitors.

Several chemotherapy regimens can be used in breast cancer, and a medical oncologist will discuss what is best for the patient and her type of cancer. One of the first tough moments after surgery is hearing that chemotherapy is recommended. Usually, the second toughest moment for patients receiving chemotherapy is when they lose their hair, because this is the neon sign that says they have cancer. But some patients take charge and shave their hair off before it starts to fall out. Some patients creatively embrace the journey that they've been forced to take. One of my patients, a graphic designer, was very creative from the beginning to the end of her journey. She sent out a "good-bye to the girls" (breasts) card – it had a picture of her breasts with a bra on – and had a party before her surgery. She had to undergo chemotherapy, so she had another party and let some of her friends shave her head. Two really close girlfriends also shaved their heads at the same time. After that, she would decorate her head! One time, for her mother's birthday, it was decorated as a birthday cake; then as a Christmas ornament (including the hook!) and later, a yellow smiley face. One day she also wore a pink princess hat with "Cancer Sucks" pins all over it. She handed out the pins to other patients and families in the infusion room and tried to make it as fun as it could be. I am sure some people looked at her and thought she was crazy. Why is she making fun? But she needed the humor to help her get through her treatments. She knew she had to do the surgery, chemotherapy and radiation to try and kill the cancer and keep it from coming back, but she also knew she needed to have some enjoyment as well to make things easier. She also had "fun" with her chest. She had undergone bilateral mastectomies, so when it was time for radiation, she would draw on the side that wasn't being treated so that the radiation technicians and physicians would laugh. She drew a crocodile one day, and when she lifted her arm for radiation, it turned into a T-rex. Another time she had drawn a monkey hanging on a banana tree. I was amazed at her ability to make everyone else feel better. So is it wrong to have a laugh and enjoy life while going through cancer treatments? Of course not!

Nurse navigators continue working with their patients even after surgery, chemotherapy and radiation are finished. Some patients have spent the months since their diagnosis in crisis mode. Once they have completed treatments, it is like hitting a brick wall: "Wow, what did I just go through?" "Now what do I do?" "How do I return to who I was before my cancer diagnosis?" Even though this time is just as important emotionally as the earlier phases of diagnosis and treatment, sometimes friends don't call or check-in as often. It is not always the case that the end of treatment means the end of suffering. Other patients seem to do just fine and celebrate the end of treatment. I highly recommend it! Take a trip; cross something off your bucket list! One patient who had undergone bilateral mastectomies, chemotherapy and radiation celebrated by getting beautiful tattoos of flowers and dragonflies over her reconstructed breasts. It helped hide some of the scars from the surgery as well. Tattoos aren't for everyone, but they can help in the emotional healing process.

Survivorship is a big focus of cancer institutes, and it is for me and the healthcare team to support patients throughout what is often a long survivorship. Side effects – both physical and emotional – can last a while. There is almost always a fear of recurrence. And if cancer does come back, that is emotionally difficult as well. We can provide many resources to patients and their caregivers to help them during this time. I try to have patients take one step at a time, one day at a time. People are more than their cancer, and I encourage them to live during their treatments, not let cancer consume their lives. In this way, nurse navigators help the patient and family no matter what part of the journey they're on. We're available to answer questions, help them find and utilize resources (like support groups for patients, children and significant others) and provide overall support.

Mark

By the time I begin working with patients, the breast surgeons have done their best to remove the known breast cancer, and some patients will have undergone several cycles of chemotherapy. They come to our department to learn about the next step in the treatment process: radiation therapy. By now, many have lost their hair, struggle with overwhelming fatigue and feel like they have been living at the hospital because of their many treatments, consults, follow-up visits and, sometimes, complications. Many patients ask, "Why do I need radiation? They said my margins were clear and my cancer was small. Do I really need this?"

So is radiation necessary for all patients? Not always; but since our cancer care is always personalized, we often meet with a patient to review the options and make recommendations. Many times if a woman has had a mastectomy, she will not need radiation unless there is nodal involvement. We provide treatment to minimize the risk of disease progression. Once we have determined that our prospective patient needs to be evaluated for radiation treatment, the first step is for her to go through the consultation process with one of our doctors or physician assistants to gather information about her particular breast cancer diagnosis and past health history, and to undergo a physical exam to determine her status for possible treatment. (See also the essay by Dr. Henry Wagner elsewhere in this book.) We must always consider the health of the patient, and sometimes we don't offer radiation if it might complicate future care. Another concern might be a past history of previous radiation treatment for another type of cancer of the chest area like lung cancer or Hodgkins lymphoma. This could lead to radiation doses that would exceed acceptable amounts. We also need to take into account other issues that might cause us to consider utilizing briefer periods of treatment or newer techniques to avoid prolonged trips to the hospital for radiation. If a patient is demented, living in an assisted living environment or is of advanced age, for example, we might consider shorter treatments that would provide coverage but minimize the psychosocial challenges that regular schedules would present.

During the initial consultation, we explain the details of treatment to the patient and lay out a timeline of activities for the radiation process. Many of our patients will not have needed chemotherapy, so we see them soon after they have undergone surgery. We want to make sure that they are healing well and that enough time has passed so we can safely begin the next phase of treatment, the CAT scan simulation.

This is our time to get an accurate picture of the affected breast for planning purposes so we can then develop the radiation plan. The simulation usually takes about an hour and involves changing into a hospital gown and having a CAT scan of the affected breast, usually with arms elevated above the head. Sometimes a special bag will be made to fit the individual patient specifically, and it will then be used for each treatment. This is a vacuum bag – somewhat similar to a bean bag – that will conform to one's body. This step is essential since radiation involves "fractions," which means small doses of radiation given daily to the same area. We need to be consistent with these daily fractions, so a bag that can help put the patient in the same body position on the treatment table is ideal. The pictures we take and the measurements we calculate help the radiation therapists to be consistent with the daily treatments.

Another part of this simulation process is the making of a small dot tattoo of India ink in the mid chest as well as the sides of the chest. These are used daily as markers with our laser lines to orient the patient when she is set up on the treatment machines. The lasers allow us to be very accurate so our treatments will not vary from day to day. Although the dot tattoos will remain after treatment, they aren't very noticeable; they look like tiny blue freckles or moles. Receiving radiation is not painful, but for those patients who have shoulder issues, the arm position can be a challenge and we work with them to find a comfortable position.

Sometimes this planning process creates a whole new issue: Sometimes this non-diagnostic picture becomes diagnostic – when, for example, a lesion is discovered in the lung. Several of our patients have had to hold off on treatment for their breast cancer because we first have to treat the lung cancer that we found in our planning process. Ironically, having breast cancer for these patients might have saved their lives!

After the CAT scan simulation, it's usually seven to ten days before the actual treatment begins. During this break, the radiation oncologist goes through a process called "contouring," during which she outlines the area or areas that the radiation beams need to cover during the treatment. The radiation oncologist then works closely with staff members called "dosimetrists" who develop the precise radiation treatment by utilizing computer processes to determine the angle and amount of radiation. This planning stage often includes several recalculations to ensure accuracy – especially so that the radiation will not adversely affect nearby organs such as the heart, lungs or spinal cord. Once a final plan has been completed and approved by our physicists as being appropriate and accurate, the patient will then return to have a block check or "dry run" as we affectionately call it. The patient is placed on the treatment machine while our radiation oncologist observes to make sure that the plan that looks great on the computer will work on the actual patient. Once that has been verified, the actual daily treatments begin.

The daily treatments, known as "fractions," are necessary to give the amount of radiation that will be effective in destroying any remaining cancer cells but not harm healthy tissue. I describe this process to my patients as similar to climbing stairs: We can get to the desired dose safely, one step at a time. If we tried to give the whole dose in one treatment, it would be harmful to diseased tissue but also very destructive to healthy tissue as well. The dose remains the same every day until the end of treatment, but then we might want to give a little extra radiation to the area where the tumor was initially found, called "the tumor bed." If a recurrence were to happen, this is typically the place it would be found, so we give a few more treatments just to that area.

As our patients go through treatment, each week they will have what is called an "on treatment visit." This is a weekly meeting with their radiation oncologist to review progress and any side effects, and to make sure things are going well. (Obviously if there is a problem during treatment that doesn't fall on the treatment day, we see the patient for evaluation immediately.) The radiation therapists are constantly watching for adverse changes, and they will quickly contact our nurses or doctors to evaluate the patient if there is a concern.

So what does radiation treatment feel like? Many people assume that it will feel like they're being zapped with a ray gun or a stun gun, but there is absolutely no pain involved. The treatment process merely involves the need to lie still on the treatment table once the therapists have placed a person in the proper position, using the exact measurements that were calculated for the initial CAT scan simulation. This positioning may take a few of the fifteen minutes typically designated for each treatment. The red laser lines will make sure a person is straight horizontally and vertically, just as she was for her simulation. This is where the dot tattoos come into play, as they are markers for placement. Once a person is positioned, the therapists will leave the room and close the door behind them. The patient isn't really alone, though. In the treatment booth the therapists can see and hear her, so if she has any type of problem, they can quickly open the treatment room door and come in to help. At times the therapists might get some CAT scan pictures of the person's placement to make sure that she is truly lined up accurately. Then the treatment will begin. The patient's part in this is now easy.

The treatment machine, or "linac" (linear accelerator), will move around the patient to certain points and stop as the radiation beam is produced. The fact that this is completely painless confuses many patients, and they wonder if the therapists have actually turned on the machine. Rest assured, the treatment is given. Patients typically tell me that for the first few weeks they feel fine – like the treatment is a piece of cake. But the fractions for breast cancer treatment can last from one to six weeks. Most patients receiving six weeks of treatment will eventually feel some fatigue and may experience redness and dryness of the skin, like a sunburn – possibly even with some blistering. The reason that the skin can burn is that radiation created from the linac is similar to the sun's rays that lead to sunburns. To combat these skin problems we always recommend that our patients use some type of over-the-counter moisturizer or, occasionally, prescription medications specially made for radiation side effects. If patients religiously apply the moisturizer two times a day – right after treatment and after a bath or shower – skin irritations are usually mild. We advise patients not to apply moisturizers right before treatment to avoid complications such as increased reaction of the skin, similar to the old practice of using baby oil many years ago to "improve" or speed up a suntan like basting a butterball turkey!

Skin reactions can vary widely. I had a patient of Irish descent who was very fair-skinned, and I was concerned that she was going to burn very badly. On the other hand, I had a dark-skinned African American woman who I thought would breeze through her treatment. Instead, each of these patients turned out the exact opposite of what I had expected. The fair-skinned lady came through her treatment with no significant skin changes, while the dark-skinned lady had dramatic skin changes with moist "desquamation," skin breakdown and increased pain. Because of these two experiences, I tell my patients that everyone's reaction to treatment is different.

Even if someone gets skin burns, they will quickly disappear over a few weeks after treatment is complete. However, there is a strange phenomenon that occurs for most patients that can be baffling. Many patients will tell me that they make it to the end of treatment relatively clear of skin irritations, glad that they got by without any serious problems. But then, over seven to ten days after they complete treatment, their skin will blister and become sore, as if they are still getting daily treatment. The skin may darken, like a weird suntan, in a square pattern over the chest area; but this too will slowly fade with time. It's just the cumulative effect of the radiation and is not an indication of any problem. To avoid continuing dryness issues, we recommend that patients use moisturizers after bath or shower and SPF 30 sunscreen if they go to the beach or have sun exposure. At all costs, we want to avoid burning the area again.

So the treatment is done, the skin has cleared from the redness, now what? As Lynn explained, our breast care team will continue to follow the patient with visits to make sure she remains cancer free. I typically see our breast patients one month after they complete treatment to make sure the acute side effects that we described above are clearing, and also to answer any questions about the treatment process. I find that many patients had been overwhelmed by the initial diagnosis and had just shown up as directed and gone through the treatments as planned without really understanding why they had their specific treatment. I feel that a review of their breast cancer markers, estrogen and progesterone sensitivity, HER2 status, nodal involvement, Oncotype score and other important factors that determined their treatment is important to help put their disease into perspective. Many patients can now deal with the information (that can understandably overwhelm any of us) in a more logical, less emotional way.

Radiation can be a wonderful tool in the fight against breast cancer. It is not your grandmother's radiation treatment that caused terrible side effects and lifelong challenges. Like all things medical, there have been great improvements in the dosing, precision and effectiveness over the years; and the future will only get better.

GORDON L. KAUFFMAN, JR.

Communion

She strikes me as a strong woman when I first meet her in my clinic, a tall, composed brunette whose green eyes are glazed from fear and apprehension. Her attire perfectly matches her professional bearing. She is wearing a lightly cabled white turtle neck sweater, calf-length patterned skirt, navy blazer and expensive shoes that accentuate the subdued reds in her skirt. Her husband is physically attractive, too. He is well built and is wearing chino trousers, a bright striped button-down shirt with no tie and matching tan loafers. The mousse in his hair provides the strength for the ends to stand straight up. His brown eyes are clearer than hers but his fingers are persistently fidgeting.

Immediately, I am engaged with this couple.

In the small examination room we exchange introductions. I sense that they are deeply in love with each other, but under the circumstances, the visible signs of that love are muted. They do not hold hands; they rarely look each other in the eye. Her speech is slower and more subdued than his, and he is quick to amplify on the history I am taking from her. Her voice remains strong, without cracking.

They have been married for four years and decided to wait until she finished her doctoral degree before starting a family. She received her degree two months ago, and has just accepted a position in the business office of a firm that designs contemporary women's sportswear. What a perfect opportunity for this sophisticated 31-year-old woman, I think. Her husband has successfully developed his own business and carries himself as though he is in control of the situation.

But life has a way of interrupting dreams. The lump she found in her right breast is cancer, potentially spreading throughout her body and killing her. Perhaps it is my physician's knowledge of what she – starting a career, in love, emotionally strong – is about to face that generates an unusually strong bond between us.

I wonder how large I will find the tumor to be and whether or not I will feel enlarged lymph nodes in her right axilla, and I experience anxiety as I begin examining her. The tumor feels to be about two inches in diameter. I know that she is carefully assessing my facial expression. I must maintain a neutral expression regardless of my findings. My gaze focusses on my fingers. She knows from surfing the Internet that it will be encouraging if I cannot feel any enlarged lymph nodes. I am relieved that the tumor is mobile and there are no detectable lymph nodes, perhaps the only bit of positive news that that she has received in several days.

I know that neither she nor her husband will retain much of my explanation during this first meeting. Where does a physician begin and end these discussions? Although I often have these "difficult discussions," each one is always stressful for everyone involved. As we talk, she is outwardly more inquisitive than he is. Her physician had called her with the diagnosis, based on a core biopsy, a few days ago. It was a shock to both of them. She seems familiar with some of the terms I use and is attentive to my description of the short- and long-term risks and benefits of different treatment modalities. Her anxiety wanes; in fact, I sense the slip of a smile on her lips occasionally, when the discussion becomes slightly lighter. His countenance, however, falls throughout the discussion. I know that he is oblivious to specific points. When she looks at him, it is obvious to her that his outward appearance reflects more than stoicism; he is terrified. His fidgeting has given way to a numbed state. Their questions focus on a single concern: Will she survive?

I touch her shoulder and look at him: "She will," I tell him. If I told them I was not sure, they could lose hope, a critical component of emotional and perhaps physical survival. When I see my face reflected in the mirror every morning, I want to see an empathetic person. But, I wonder if I have been completely honest. Balancing honesty and hope is difficult. At the end of our first visit I am an empathetic realist. There will be time for further honesty as test results unfold. Our subsequent visits will be frequent and intense.

The vectors in any dialogue are bi-directional, but the only vector obvious to them is the one directed at her survival. They do not perceive those that are very real to me. I feel hope not only for her healing but also for life together, that it will be filled with joy, excitement, adventure and humor. As I look at them I reflect on the sense of uneasiness that I periodically experienced at their age: Would I be a caring and competent surgeon, a supportive husband and a father whom my children would be proud of; or might I resort to holding my professional life above these other goals, at the expense of my family?

Following a week of reflection on the panoply of therapeutic options, she has chosen chemotherapy before surgery, hoping for a measurable reduction in tumor size that will allow for less cosmetically maiming surgery. They are reassured that I support their hope that at the end of this nightmare she will have a reasonable self-image. At their age, appearance makes a difference; as age leaves its tracks, perhaps soul intimacy matters more. Now, however, is not the time for this discussion.

She is stronger today; her statements are resolute. Her voice reflects acceptance of the situation, and her face appears softer. I candidly talk about the discomfort and pain that she will likely experience during chemotherapy. She will accept the paleness of anemia, gut-wrenching dry heaves, and baldness, hoping for a response that may not occur. I am aware of how her inner strength and personal determination inspire me. She is contemplating pain, disfigurement, even death with a level of courage that I am not sure I could muster. How would I respond if I were prescribed chemotherapy with its potential for peripheral neuropathy or cardiac dysfunction, either of which could end my identity as a surgeon? Would I be as courageous as she is? Would I be as supportive of my wife as her husband clearly is of her? There are too many questions, few legitimate answers.

A month later I see her at the mid-point of chemotherapy. Her eyes reveal apprehension about whether or not I will see an obvious response on her breast MRI or find on clinical examination. Her demeanor is more melancholy than usual. Her husband still fidgets. How burdensome must be this ambiguity of not knowing whether the cancer has responded to treatment. The ravages of chemotherapy's terrain can be appreciated only by those who have actually walked it; only she knows that truth. I compliment her on the pastel turban that accentuates her brunette eyebrows that have been spared. She understands my feeble attempts to appreciate what occurs when foreign fluids invade her veins in the infusion room.

Ready to move to the business at hand, I acknowledge that any confidence she has in me is based on mutual candor, and I assure her that I'll tell her what I see on the MRI and feel on physical examination. We view the MRI together. Apprehension begins to give way to confidence as simultaneously we see that the tumor is measurably smaller. As I help her to the examination table, she anticipates that my physical findings will be congruent with the MRI, and I sense only a modicum of apprehension as I begin the exam. The tumor is clearly half the size that it was when I first examined her and there are still no palpable lymph nodes in her axilla. We share a sense of relief as I tell her what I have found. When she sits up, I feel the urge to give them both a hug. I feel more confident in my response to the question of her survival, now. Yes, she *will*, I think. This is a moment of joy for all three of us. Her husband's eyes are smiling and he has stopped fidgeting. The enemy is retreating, at least for now.

Two weeks later, in the evening darkness of the office and tired from an unusually strenuous day of operating, I read an email from them. She has attached professional photographs of herself, with a message: "Thanks for being there." Her face is serene, her smile bright, her dimples mischievous. Some photos show her husband holding her and smiling, but still with a hint of apprehension.

I wonder what happens at their home. Does she ever drop her guard and share her anguish with him? He with her? Does he hold her head when she vomits? Do they eat dinner together? Breakfast? Do they think about what chemotherapy is doing to their chances of having a child? Are there intimate times in the midst of this turmoil and ambiguity? Does either of them have one hour in the day free from thinking about the future?

As I reflect on these questions, I realize how delicate the balance is between empathy and loss of objectivity. My work continually forces me to face the stark fragility of life and, on reflection, my own mortality. Do I possess the strength of character exhibited by these two young people? Do I treat my wife with sensitivity, or is my capacity for kindness, flexibility and love drained, leaving nothing for her? When I am at home, do

I hear my wife when she tells me what she needs? Am I conscious of her unspoken needs? Preoccupation with patients has often stolen our quality time. I am either engaged or I am not. There is no middle ground. Physical presence is not synonymous with engagement.

Ten days later I find a "post it" on the back of my office chair indicating that she requests that I call her at home that evening. Knowing that a young woman who develops breast cancer may be harboring a mutated breast cancer gene, I had encouraged her to meet with our genetics counselor. When I hear her voice, I can tell that she has been crying. The molecular analysis has confirmed that she carries the mutated BRCA1 gene, which places her other breast and both of her ovaries at significant risk for malignancy. Her husband takes the phone when she can no longer continue. With a stronger voice than hers, he tells me that they both are aware that we have to modify out treatment plans. Additional risks and cosmetic consequences of bilateral mastectomy with reconstruction and, later, bilateral prophylactic oophorectomy must now be addressed by a woman who has yet to experience the pain and fulfillment of giving birth. I wonder how much more grim news any of us can endure.

At her clinic visit just before surgery, she is surprisingly calm. Her husband is fully engaged. This recent blow seems to have jolted them into a matter-of-fact mind set. I show them photographs of the various forms of breast reconstruction. Her breasts would no longer be perfectly natural, but I try to reassure her that reconstruction is cosmetically acceptable to most women. She is taking one sure-footed step at a time, while I imagine the surgery. My exhilaration at the tumor's response to chemotherapy has been overshadowed by my need to do a more deforming procedure – in addition to what chemotherapy has done to her ovaries which will be removed, too. They will not have the luxury of time to begin a family, but feeling sorry for herself has never been worth her time. Survival is her ultimate goal. I admire her intensity and fearlessness, and almost as if by osmosis, I, too, am stronger at the end of that visit.

The morning of surgery she appears more apprehensive than the last time I saw her. This is the day when she will perhaps, in her own mind, become less a woman. She is quiet, and I suspect that she is thinking of the risk of death during surgery, of postoperative physical and emotional pain, and of the cosmetic outcome. I hold her hand. She asks me to pray with her, and I do. Together we move to the starkly bright and cold operating room in which no object, other than my eyes, are familiar to her. The circulating nurse asks her the prerequisite questions: name, date of birth, allergies, who is in the waiting room? She begins to cry as she answers, trying to hold back audible sobs. Carefully, I ensure her modesty as she moves to the table. After I pull up my mask, I smile with my eyes. The smile she returns makes us both feel secure; we'll go through this together. She seems at least superficially composed as her hand no longer squeezes mine.

Laying the knife on her skin I am anxious about what I will encounter. I remove three sentinel lymph nodes that are of normal size and consistency. Good! I now send them to the pathologist to give me an indication of whether or not tumor cells are seen on the slide. When the pathologist, over the speaker phone, indicates that no tumor cells are seen, everyone cheers. I am uplifted at what the pathologist has just told us, yet saddened at the thought of removing both breasts from this young woman who is so young. So that I remain focused, I brush these feelings aside.

When the cancerous breast is removed through the small incisions, I feel carefully to assess the proximity of the tumor to the margins. The malignant mass that has disrupted the lives of these two wonderful people is deep within the substance of the breast, giving me confidence that under the microscope the pathologist will confirm that the margins are adequate. Then, I remove the normal breast for prophylaxis. As I place into cold pans the two globes of unformed fat, I wonder that our society attaches such significance to female breasts. When I finish, her torso is exposed from umbilicus to neck, and her chest is entirely flat. Only the redundancy of the preserved breast skin and the two incisions through which the breasts were removed evidence what has just occurred. I wonder for a moment if there is an expression of relief on her side of the ether screen, too.

The reconstruction is now in the hands of the reconstructive surgeon.

I head straight to the family waiting room to speak with her husband. He is pacing fast, his countenance sullen and his lips quivering. When our eyes first make contact across the room, I smile. There is no exchange of words, yet I sense immediate relief in his face. His body relaxes. Knowing that the woman he loves is alive lifts his spirits. The hand I shake is clammy and thankful. We sit together on adjacent chairs in the overcrowded waiting room. When I tell him that the initial evaluation of the lymph nodes is favorable and that the reconstruction is as fine as any I have seen, he is revitalized. Tears appear in both of our eyes as he thanks me.

Their picture is on the Christmas card they send the next year. He is muscular, clean-cut, well dressed in a Hawaiian short-sleeved shirt, smiling, and embracing her neck. His lover and he have finally been released from the torment they have endured for months. She is as stunning as ever in a flowing gauze patterned dress, exposing a modest natural cleavage. Relief at living through the year is evident in her strong green eyes. Her short hair is stylish and amplifies her contagious smile. She appears soft and secure in his arms.

I ponder their future. I do not know how long it will take for them to come to grips with this bitter intrusion that has disrupted their lives so unexpectedly. I know only that their love for each other – and of life – far surpasses what it was before her diagnosis.

LISA KATZ

Reconstruction

You say I should rebuild
with a sack of plastic, or
one part of the body
replaces another.

A woman might love
a man without a leg.
They can have children.
And men whose legs
don't work
make children
with women who climb on.
Sometimes a child disappears
like a lost limb.

Couldn't we have
a different aesthetic,
asymmetrical,
Japanese,
because of the war,
because islands get invaded.

Couldn't we
admire the ruined, the torn, the perfect
error, because the weaver
skips a row
for the sake of humility,
because your love
needs a few stitches?

Reconstruction

See the scar,
the flat plain on my chest.
Connect the dots.
You won't get many chances
to look at an absence straight on.

JOHN D. POTOCHNY

Gauging Too Much Information: Discussing a Young Mother's Options for Reconstructive Surgery

I opened clinic door number one to find a very young woman who looked more like a child than a mother. Her hopeful dark brown eyes were fixed upon me as I entered the room. An older woman with similar features and a nervous appearing young man with a blank stare solemnly accompanied her. At her foot was a baby, a few months old, asleep in an infant seat, covered in a pink knitted blanket. The young woman was not much older than my own college-age daughter, yet the lines across her forehead revealed that the stress from her diagnosis had robbed her of several years of her youth. Neoadjuvant chemotherapy – medicine given before surgery for breast cancer – had also taken away all the hair from her head, including her eyebrows. Because she was diagnosed during her third trimester, no more time could be wasted attempting to shrink the cancer that had been growing within her left breast during pregnancy.

Before I meet a patient, I am reminded of the need for respect, support and warmth. I smiled when I entered the room, sanitized my hands and extended my right hand to my young patient, Melinda, as I introduced myself. I acknowledged the man sitting next to her and the middle-aged woman next to them, who offered that she was the young woman's mother, and I thanked them all for making the ninety-mile trip to see me that afternoon.

"What is your baby's name?" I asked.

"Brooke," Melinda replied.

"She is beautiful! She has your eyes," I said. I couldn't help but think how I might react if I were instead this young woman's father, seated where they sat, looking at me. I summarized what I knew about her recent diagnosis of invasive ductal carcinoma, noting from her medical history that she had two aunts and one cousin who had also been diagnosed with breast cancer before the age of forty. Her mother stated that they were awaiting the results of genetic tests to determine if Melinda also had the BRCA gene which predisposes one to breast cancer.

This visit was pre-arranged to accommodate their long journey and maximize her opportunity to meet with several consultants on the same day. Earlier, she had met with a breast oncology surgeon to outline her options for surgery. Most people don't associate plastic surgeons with cancer treatment, but she understood that I would work to minimize the visible impact of breast cancer.[1] Since she still had to complete chemotherapy, there would be yet another round of scans the following week to determine whether her cancer had shrunk, then a meeting with an oncologist, and perhaps a radiation oncology specialist – all this before she would undergo any form of surgery. This gave her time to consider her options. I would be presenting a lot of information in a short amount of time, so I had to take care not to overwhelm her at this initial visit. No 24-year-old woman should have to confront the complexities of cancer at this stage of life, when she needs to be focusing on how to be a mom for her baby daughter.

Today, all she needs to know is that no matter what treatment she chooses to rid her body of the malignancy – either lumpectomy or mastectomy – I can replace what is removed of her breast and provide her with symmetry. What she doesn't need to know today is that I cannot erase scars or give her breasts that will feel like her natural ones. She doesn't need to know today that she will likely need multiple surgeries in the future to counter the effects of aging scar tissue or perhaps to exchange a failed breast prosthesis. I must introduce her options with measured restraint to help her navigate all the choices and dispel any myths and misinformation she might have read on the internet or heard from friends and family.

Melinda was not naive. One of her aunts had breasts created from skin and fat from her lower abdomen; another aunt and a cousin had silicone breast implants for their reconstructions. So I begin by explaining all the forms of reconstruction that are available to her; some will require more recovery than others. She is a solid "C" cup and likes that her breasts had increased in size with the birth of her daughter.

---

[1] Not all women elect to have reconstructive surgery. Please see "Reconstruction" and "The Form," by poet Lisa Katz, and "Milestones in the Depiction of Breasts and Breast Cancer," by art historian Siobhan Conaty elsewhere in this book.

But she hasn't found breastfeeding easy, so she pumps and supplements with formula, using a bottle to feed baby Brooke. The fact that she is supplementing is an especially good thing in her case because Brooke will be more accustomed to formula than she might otherwise have been after Melinda's surgery.

At the start of this hour-long consultation, Melinda already understands the differences between autologous breast reconstruction (constructed from one's own tissue), tissue expanders and permanent breast implants. She knows a girlfriend who had breast enhancement with implants and heard something on a recent newscast about breast implant-associated lymphoma. I explain that there is no one-size-fits-all best breast reconstruction, but I will help her to decide what is right for her. Using abdominal skin and fat to create a breast is a great option, but it requires a longer recovery and several days in the hospital. She could always have that done at a later time, when Brooke is older. Using "permanent" breast implants will require only one night in the hospital, but breast implants don't last forever and will likely need to be replaced someday. If I cannot place a permanent implant immediately following her mastectomy and must use an expander first, then there would be additional clinic visits during which saline would be injected in order to slowly and fully expand her chest muscles and breast skin. She would need to travel weekly to one of our clinics over a one- or two-month period to undergo this tissue expansion and then undergo a second operation to exchange the expanders for the permanent implants.

Just then, Brooke began to cry. It was time for her to eat, and the young man sprang to action. Recognizing the need for Melinda and her mother to complete this consultation uninterrupted so that they could ask their questions, he swiftly lifted the delicate child, took a baby bottle from a diaper bag backpack, and headed for the waiting room.

After Melinda's partner had left the exam room, I turned to her just as a tear ran down her cheek. I reflexively reached for a facial tissue box on the counter and handed it to her as her mother pulled closer and held her hand.

"I know this is a lot of information for you today and it can be overwhelming. Please know that you don't need to make any decisions today. My staff and I are available to answer any questions that you and your family have after you leave." I waited for that to sink in, then said, "Before you go home, is there anything else you would like to ask?"

Their silence meant either that they were overwhelmed with too much information or that I had anticipated and answered questions to their satisfaction. Usually, it is the former. Most people grasp only a fraction of what they are presented under the duress of a visit to see a surgeon for a cancer diagnosis. Who knows what she really heard?

This visit was TMI for Melinda, so I suggested we meet again in two weeks. By then, her genetic tests and repeat staging scans would be completed, so we would be able to form a concrete plan. In the meantime, she and her family will grapple with the gravity of what they heard today.

Consent to undergo surgery

Melinda returned alone for her preoperative visit two weeks later. Her hopeful dark brown eyes revealed a new resolve to fight to win, like there was no other option. They said, "Cancer, I'm gonna kick your ass." Instead of throwing in the towel and retreating when she learned that she carried a genetic mutation that places her at 90 percent lifetime risk for breast cancer, she had made the decision to fight for her life. She planned to have both of her breasts removed because she never wanted to go through this nightmare again. She still had a wedding to plan with her partner, and Brooke needed a mother to raise her. Melinda knew what hard work it would be. As a former state swimming champion in high school, she was familiar with physical pain from endurance and weight training. And, hell, she'd just finished chemotherapy. But now she had two real reasons to win: her daughter and the man she planned to marry.

Surgery is not benign. Although these operations are part of my weekly routine, there is no such thing as a minor surgery to rid the body of breast cancer and create two new breasts. I owe her an explanation of what could go wrong and what to expect during recovery. The act of surgery is an assault on the body. Blood could be lost, requiring a transfusion; an infection might occur; permanent scars will remain, perhaps even become constant painful reminders of her ordeal. Unique to mastectomy reconstructions are also emotional scars from loss of self-image and perceived femininity after her breasts are removed.

Respecting surgical risks took me years to comprehend, but I must help her gain understanding in a single half-hour appointment. How do you best summarize risks like reconstruction failures, blood clots or bleeding – even very rare events that can occur, such as implant-associated lymphoma or death? Some of my colleagues might tell her that bad things can happen to anyone on any day: We could be in a car accident and emerge critically injured – or worse; serious complications from surgery are less frequent than that. While this may be true, such a paternalistic approach minimizes the potential specific risks and could possibly even undermine her real expectations. What she needs to know is that her new breasts will be similar to each other but will not be like her natural breasts. She will likely need some further surgery in the future, perhaps some minor tweaks or maybe major revisions. And, yes, although bad things could happen, my team and I would be there to take care of her in that rare event. Although I strive to set and exceed expectations, at the end of thirty minutes I wonder whether I have truly achieved informed consent.

Under the knife

The day of her operation has arrived. "Good morning," I say, addressing her, her fiancé and her mother. It is 7 a.m., and the crowded preoperative holding area is already bustling with activity as nurses register patients and confirm their identities by names, birth dates and planned procedures. The nurses start intravenous lines and complete surgical checklists to ensure the correct operation is being performed on the correct body part of the correct patient. The scene vaguely resembles an airport gate during check in, before the first flight out in the morning. Gowned patients wearing ID wristbands substitute for ticketed travelers, and anesthesia staff taxi stretchers in line toward the operating rooms. I pull the cubicle curtain closed for some privacy as I draw my blueprint on her breasts with a marking pen. This purple ink template will direct her breast surgeon where to cut, and the lines will soon become precursors to healing scars. With that, her surgical checklist is complete and, after a kiss from her partner and a prayer with her mother, Melinda soon finds herself in the line of stretchers heading to the operating rooms where she will sleep.

Two hours had passed before I entered the operating room to begin her reconstructions. Both of her breasts, along with several lymph nodes from the side with cancer, had to be removed by her breast surgeon before I could assess the pair of empty envelopes of skin and fat. One breast had contained her cancer; the other breast contained a risk to incubate another cancer in the future because of her genetic predisposition. Preliminary frozen section evaluation – thinly sliced frozen samples of her lymph nodes – showed no cancer, which meant that, as far as science could tell us, there was no additional cancer in her body. Good news!

Women tend to be more satisfied with the results of reconstruction when they can keep their nipples. Fortunately, Melinda had had an excellent response to preoperative chemotherapy, and her breast surgeon was able to preserve hers. The thickness and circulation to the skin flaps were adequate to allow me to place her tissue expanders above her pectoralis muscles and begin the process of creating two matching mounds that would soon resemble breasts. Because her muscles remain in place, when the temporary tissue expanders are removed and replaced with more permanent breast implants in several months, lifting and caring for baby Brooke should be less cumbersome for her. Not all patients are candidates for total skin- and nipple-sparing mastectomies or placement of implants above their muscles. Skin-to-skin, the time from my colleague's surgical incision to my placement of drains and final sutures, took a total of five hours. For her part, Melinda would remember only being asked by the anesthesiologist to pick out a good dream and to take some deep breaths, before she woke in the recovery room.

Recovery

Recovery from breast cancer doesn't end when a patient wakes up after surgery; it really just begins. I locate her family in the surgical waiting room one floor below the operating room. It is a bright open space lacking privacy, lit partly by a wall of windows and two monitors – one projecting the local news, the other displaying patient arrivals to the recovery room. Several couches, chairs and a few tables are occupied by other families as passers-by browse the gift shop where a life-sized inflatable Little Mermaid, Ariel, is positioned next to a piano man who plays the happy calypso tune "Under the Sea." The smells from a nearby Starbuck's kiosk permeate the room while some people check their phones or stare at computers, and still others have fallen asleep while waiting for updates about their loved ones. After learning that no additional cancer was seen in her lymph nodes and that her first stage of reconstruction went well, both her mother and fiancé express gratitude and relief. I go on to explain the likely scenario of her recovery from surgery, and that she will require another hour to fully awaken before they may visit with her.

That evening I checked Melinda one final time before leaving the hospital for the night. She was sore but comforted to have her fiancé and baby Brooke camped beside her. A quick look at her bandages and drains told me everything was fine, and I left her to rest alongside her family. I've learned that visiting with patients before I leave the hospital to answer any questions they or their family might have – and to ensure that no unexpected bleeding or other complications exist – allows everyone a better night's sleep.

With each passing week since her operation, Melinda grew more accepting of her "new normal" human-engineered breasts. Once the remaining surgical drain was removed, she even smiled and allowed a warm congratulatory hug from our nurse. It is a milestone that every breast reconstruction patient anxiously awaits.

Today we begin her expansions. Anticipating pain from the needle stick, Melinda welcomed the deadened sensation of her chest skin as intravenous saline was injected into her tissue expanders. "Will these babies float?" she asked. Caught a little off guard, I realized she wanted to begin swimming again. "Yes, but you're on the bench until a full month has passed from your surgery to keep the risk of infection low." Usually the first two to four weeks after an operation will reveal any smoldering infection. We had one more week to go before I felt comfortable lifting all of Melinda's restrictions.

Before long, her expansions were complete and her once shapeless chest now filled her clothes so that no stranger would awkwardly stare. The only signs that hinted to her battle with cancer were the slightly red and raised scars across her new breast mounds. Even her hair had grown back and that, with some added color, gave the buxom brunette an air of confidence. The former high school swimming champ was regaining her swagger and ready to begin training again. She was also ready to set a date to remove the stiff baby-sitter expanders and replace them with softer silicone gel-filled implants, the kind that wouldn't push her fiancé or Brooke away when she embraced them. So we set the date, and she told me she'd also set the date for her wedding in three months. Both of us had some work to do to get her ready to wear her wedding dress.

Two months later the day had finally arrived. Her second surgery would be a breeze. Taking out her stiff tissue expanders and replacing them would take less than half the time of her first operation, and she would feel very little pain. She would even be home in time to feed Brooke dinner. The big stuff was done and she was on the final lap now, heading for the finish line. This surgery would allow her to restart her life as a newly wed mother – the life she had dreamed about until cancer had interrupted her. By mid-morning she was comfortably resting in the recovery room. Mission accomplished.

In two weeks, Melinda would see me for the last time before shopping for her wedding dress.

KATE JOLLIE

Flashpoints: Wisdom from the Trenches

Using the Internet (or Not)

They say that knowledge is power … which I believe is true. But "knowledge" can also be conflicting, unmanageable, confusing, overwhelming and downright wrong! It's important to have access to information for its own sake, of course, but information without the supporting context can be a disaster.

I received my diagnosis by phone while I was at work, and I went numb. It didn't matter that I had found a lump on the right side of my upper torso a few days before. It didn't matter that after being seen by my primary care physician's associate, an Advanced Practice Registered Nurse (APRN), a new mammogram and ultrasound showed a significantly inflamed lymph node on my right side, as well as a mass deep in the tissue of my right breast that was not palpable. It didn't matter that a needle biopsy of the lump on my right side had been ordered. I had already decided it couldn't possibly be cancer. I was healthy and happy in my work and relationship with my boyfriend, and I had never had any type of serious medical issue or family history of breast cancer. Despite being told by the APRN that it was very important to confirm what was going on and that cancer was a possibility, I had already decided it couldn't be happening to me.

When the APRN scheduled my biopsy, she asked if I had any questions. She let me know she would be happy to answer anything and if she didn't know the answer, she would find out. She encouraged me to get the information I felt I needed, but to do so from a trusted source – because misinformation is worse than no information at all. She suggested that I start looking at the American Cancer Society (ACS) website. When I got home that night, I went on the Internet to research "breast cancer." I entered the words in the search engine and my screen exploded with information, links, user groups, and pop-up ads. On and on. It was overwhelming. I focused in on the American Cancer Society site, but it was still overwhelming. My fears were staring me in the face, but I still didn't want to believe this was going to apply to me.

After an hour of reading, I was more afraid and more convinced that if I indeed had cancer, I was destined to die much younger than I had expected and would go through a great deal of difficulty. Since that thought completely blew my mind and I hadn't yet had an initial biopsy to determine my diagnosis, I decided to *try* to start at the beginning and focus only on the information on the ACS site that dealt with initial diagnosis. The ACS provides a pamphlet that shows how to read the pathology report that is created as a result of the biopsy. It's written in laymen's terms and is designed to help you understand which areas of the report are most important and the types of questions you should ask of the technicians and physicians with whom you are working. This was all I could handle that night. I printed the document, shut down my computer, read the document again and put it in my folder – in what would affectionately become known as "my cancer bag."

I decided early on that I was going to limit my investigation to only the information that pertained to me. I was not going to read every possible scenario and subscribe to every possible support group or blog, as I felt it would not help me and could, in fact, actually harm me. I wanted to know the information that pertained to the exact type of breast cancer I had and the treatment options available to me. I appreciate that there are many people who are, in fact, helped by being immersed in the broader world of cancer once they are diagnosed: Perhaps they feel like a part of a community of people who are going through something similar and therefore experience a great sense of support by being involved. I am glad that there are places where they can gather information and that it helps them deal with an overwhelming situation. For me, though, horror stories by others going through treatments – "my friend's favorite aunt" or "my next-door neighbor's mother-in-law" or anything similar – would be, well, *horrible*. I guess I got a little selfish, you might say. But I agree with my APRN: Be careful of the source of the information you take in. Look first and foremost at the trusted, professional information about the specifics of your situation. There is indeed strength in the knowledge that will enable you to make some of the most important decisions in your life. Information is invaluable – and so is its reliability.

As for me, I tried to focus on the type of information that could be gleaned from the testing and how that would help my team put my treatment plan together. I functioned almost as an observer instead of a participant, which allowed me to stay focused on the present instead of becoming fearful of the future. Compartmentalizing is a wonderful thing – sometimes!

Deciding Whom to Tell and When

Telling anyone about your cancer diagnosis is a personal decision. I don't believe for a second that there is a right or wrong decision. Everyone who is faced with the diagnosis of this, or any other serious condition, has the right to determine who can be trusted with such private knowledge. The Friday morning I received the call at work I was blown away – although I shouldn't have been. The surgeon who did the needle biopsy of the lump on my right side advised me that I had breast cancer and that he had scheduled me for three ultrasound tests later that day. He said he would call me late in the day with the initial findings.

After I got the call, I ended a meeting I was in. I phoned my boyfriend to let him know about the diagnosis and testing, and we agreed to meet back at my house that afternoon. I went to my manager's office and asked to speak with her for a minute. She was not aware that any of this had been going on. I blurted out my news, told her I had to leave for the day to have the tests and let her know I'd be back to work on Monday. Then I just stood there. We were both stunned and both crying. After a few minutes, I dried my face, grabbed my stuff and was out the door. All I focused on was the next two hours: getting to the location for the scans, having the tests, then getting home and hugging my boyfriend. I didn't think about why the tests were being ordered and certainly didn't think about the impact of the results. I was just following orders.

In the first few days – in fact for the first few weeks – I told only my boyfriend, my two closest friends and my manager. There was a lot going on for the different members of my immediate family at the time, and I didn't want to get them upset until I had a much better understanding of my situation. I definitely didn't want to tell anyone else at work, as I had just taken a new position in the organization and had recently become the manager of a forty-five-person team that was going through a reorganization. They didn't need any more stress.

In the next few weeks I met with my care team. My medical oncologist coordinated the recommendations of my overall care program, based on the staging of my specific cancer: chemotherapy first, then surgery, then radiation. My boyfriend and I met with my surgical oncologist, radiation oncologist, medical oncologist and oncology nurse to make sure we had a clear understanding of the treatment options, the risks involved with all aspects of treatment and the state of my overall health.

It took four weeks to complete all of the additional testing that was needed to determine the extent of the cancer in my body, confirm my ability to withstand treatment, select the treatment options and establish the treatment schedule. It was at that time that I decided to tell my father and his wife, as well as my sister and her family. This process of informing people was more complicated than it might otherwise have been because my sister was scheduled for a very involved surgery, and I was supposed to help her family during her recovery – at the same time I was scheduled to begin sixteen weeks of chemotherapy and guide my new team at work. Additionally, my mother, who lived near my sister in a different state, was in the early stages of dementia. After talking with her physician, I decided not to tell her about my diagnosis and treatment in order to avoid any additional stress for her.

I also held a meeting with my new team at work to let them know what was going to happen for the next six months or so. After chemotherapy and surgery, I would undergo seven weeks of radiation, five days a week. My colleagues gave me the amazing gift of unbridled support. Fortunately, I was able to manage the side effects of treatment and continued working throughout sixteen weeks of chemotherapy (except for two days off during every two-week cycle) and seven weeks of radiation. And I was out of the office for three weeks following surgery.

I was extremely fortunate to live in a place and time where this type of care was available to me and to have a dedicated support system of medical professionals, an intimate partner, friends and, ultimately, family and co-workers to get me through the most difficult time of my life. While receiving treatment, I heard of others at the cancer center whose families would be unable or unwilling to help. I also thanked God every day that I had insurance coverage and a job that provided some flexibility in terms of when and where I could work. There are places in our country, in our workplaces, in our society where a serious medical condition will severely jeopardize a person's professional life, and I knew people who were trying to keep their condition secret for fear of being fired. Such secrecy is incredibly stressful and can therefore worsen disease and compromise healing.

The bottom line is that each person has to determine whom they tell, what details they share and when to confide information about personal health.

Double-Checking and Speaking Up

Being a strong advocate for yourself, your health and your life is critical. My real understanding of this fact started after I first discovered the lump on my side and my primary care physician's office told me it would be weeks before I could see her. They could get me in to see her APRN associate, however, and she taught me a lot about advocacy. In the first few days of this journey I was overwhelmed, and she guided me. She made sure I understood what the initial biopsy could tell me or not tell me and that additional testing would ultimately need to be done in order to understand the whole picture. She also made every effort to ensure that I understood what my surgical options might be. Later, when the first surgeon I met with basically offered me a very quick decision regarding surgical alternatives before the total picture was understood, she pointed out that I could chose a different surgeon. And I did – one of many very good decisions!

After my needle biopsy, when I went in for further tests, the technician said, "Okay, you're here for chest and abdominal scans, right?" I replied that I thought they had mentioned pelvic scans as well, but when she checked the order, those had not, in fact, been included.

"Are you sure?" she asked.

"Yes," I replied, more sure of myself.

She told me to hang tight while she called the surgeon's office. When she returned, she told me that I was right: They wanted the pelvic ultrasound too, and the order had been written incorrectly. She told me I was right to double-check what was being done and to *always* question and, when necessary, challenge to make sure the services I was receiving were the services I was supposed to receive. Empathetic and professional, she stressed that being your own best advocate is critical. As a result, I am much more comfortable making sure I am advocating for my own best needs in all areas of my life, and I encourage my friends and family to do the same.

KEVIN B. KNOPF

Another Catcher in the Rye: Oncology Care at the County Hospital

Dina was a scared young woman who came to our clinic about a rapidly growing breast mass. Thirty-two years old with long black hair, she is single, poor and has a child. The biopsy has come back as a triple-negative breast cancer. Our breast surgeon sits with her and calms her, holds her hand, spends an hour with her. After Dina's first chemotherapy treatment, her cancer shrinks and she relaxes some; by the end of her chemotherapy, the mass has disappeared. She smiles more; the nurses in the infusion clinic smile when she comes in. And now, a year out, she is in remission and likely cured. Today in clinic her hair is back but not yet long enough for dreadlocks.

After sixteen years in private practice, I shifted back to the public sector – at the county hospital. This decision harkens back to 1988, when I wrote a college term paper on "How Hospitals Can Stay Financially Viable While Caring for the Poorest Patients." The answers varied – from a very profitable hospital (we cater to the rich; we have no emergency room; we seek out well-insured patients), to Boston City Hospital (we get our budget, spend it as best as we can; after that we're in the red), to a mixed hospital where the CEO seemed to suffer greatly from trying to find a solution to this vexing problem. He reminded me of American cancer care in general: nervous, conflicted, undecided, tending toward overtreatment of the wealthy and undertreating the poor – a problem not just in America but in the rest of the world. Later, I studied Public Health and spent a few years researching health economics before embarking on this strange new world of cancer care in twenty-first-century America.

Types of Breast Cancer and Treatment Options

My spare time is spent reading papers on cell biology, cancer clinical trials and statistics, trying to understand how better to treat our patients. We now divide breast cancer roughly into four subtypes based on receptors to molecules we find in the nucleus of the cancer cell (estrogen receptor, progesterone receptor) or on the cancer cell membrane (epidermal growth factor receptor #2 [EGFR2], aka HER2). In the four subtypes that follow "+" means "positive" (i.e., something is present), and "–" means "negative" (i.e., something is absent):

Luminal A: estrogen-receptor and progesterone-receptor highly positive (Estrogen receptor and progesterone receptor are scored from 0 to 100 percent expression. The higher the expression, the more likely to respond to anti-estrogen therapy – and the better the prognosis.)

Luminal B: breast cancer that is HER2 negative, and either estrogen-receptor positive or progesterone-receptor positive

HER2+: any breast cancer that expresses HER2 on its cell membranes

Triple negative: expresses neither estrogen nor progesterone receptors nor HER2 receptors

When deciding what treatment to recommend, we consider several factors: the grade of the tumor (low, intermediate, high), the size, the number of lymph nodes involved, the age of the patient, a biological parameter called the Ki67 (what percent of cells are actively dividing at a given point in time) and the patient's overall health and desire for aggressive care. We also consider how the tumor grew: Whether it was picked up on a mammogram (uncommon at the county hospital), seemed to grow overnight and the patient felt it (more common), or had been growing for a while but the patient was too frightened to mention it until now.

We used to believe breast cancer grew linearly from one cell to many – with metastatic potential increasing as the tumor grew larger – but this is a gross oversimplification. Breast cancer growth, at least the estrogen-receptor-positive kind, may actually best be modeled as non-linear dynamics (chaos theory), which explains why it can go into remission for years or even a decade before returning. I've read about chaos theory and now need to spend more time reading Professor Michael Baum's books[1] again to get a better sense of this ... when I have "free time."

Based on the biology (above), hundreds of clinical trials and the patient's preferences, we recommend surgery – either a lumpectomy (better when possible, as the surgery is less extensive and the cosmetic result is better) or a mastectomy – possibly with one or more of the following: chemotherapy before surgery (called "neoadjuvant therapy"), chemotherapy after surgery (called "adjuvant therapy"), and/or hormone therapy (aromatase inhibitors, sometimes with a targeted antibody called trastuzimab as well). We offer these treatments all in the hopes of preventing metastatic disease – which we can treat but not cure.

Our Clinic, Our Patients

Our clinic is very modest: linoleum floors, no paintings on the walls, small windows to let light in. Functional. Sparse. Minimalist. No named hallways or buildings, no plaques, no refreshments, no wigs for our patients who lose their hair from chemotherapy. In short, we look quite different from private oncology offices and clinics. Our chemotherapy suite is urban and gritty, yet clean and efficient. It feels different from hospitals in wealthier places. Some other things are different too. The staff, physicians and nurses are diverse, multicultural. And the pace is more frenetic.

---

1   See Bibliography.

The greatest difference in our clinic is the patients themselves – not biologically that I can tell, but coming from a life of poverty and hard knocks. In the US healthcare system there are the haves and have-nots, and socioeconomic status has enormous implications for access to care – and often, health outcomes. We tend to see more breast cancer patients with aggressive, locally advanced disease than patients with "screen-detected," smaller cancers. More than half our patients come in with rapidly growing cancers that need chemotherapy before they're small enough to operate on. Yet somehow the patients – once we can see them – end up with the same quality medical care I've seen at the grand palaces of cancer care, private hospitals all over the U.S. that are extremely profitable.

In some ways our situation may actually be better for the patient, in that we have no financial incentive to overtreat. To be sure, "overtreating" is not always the result of physician greed (a common misconception). It's just that physicians are often measured by and rewarded for how much money they bring to their employer. Even the "not-for-profit" hospitals in America all strive to run in the black as much as possible. Apart from institutions that function purely as charity providers of cancer care, most hospitals and medical systems are inherently interested in maximizing revenue. The business of America is, after all, business.

On a macroeconomic scale we are now in trouble. In the U.S. more than fifty cents of every dollar spent on health care is diverted for profit, and more than half of all women with metastatic (incurable) breast cancer in America are being actively pursued by debt collectors as they undergo treatment and struggle in myriad other ways with their situation. Forty-two percent of newly diagnosed cancer patients end up bankrupt within a few years of diagnosis. These realities compound the tragedy of breast cancer.

> *A decade ago Nicki came in with a breast cancer. She was with her husband, scared and in her early thirties. I have a picture of her from two or three years ago hanging on my wall. She's smiling, pregnant; and I understand that she gave up her position as a corporate attorney to practice public interest law. She works on global warming. Sometimes I glance at her photo when other patients aren't doing well – to remind myself that it's the total results that count.*

Our Providers

For the providers, our clinic is a warm, collaborative experience with a rhythm and camaraderie not felt that often in medicine in 2020. Without the constant need for profit, all the physicians are cooperative rather than competitive. It's kind of a throwback to an earlier era of health care in America. We still have lunch together. We're not judged solely by how many patients we see a day, how many tests we order, or our "productivity" to the organization. Instead, we're evaluated by how well we take care of our patients.

We have Dr. Laura K, the young, dedicated and gifted breast surgeon – perhaps the best I've ever met. She is an incredibly kind, patient and devoted woman who has spent her career – starting in medical school – caring for the poor. Seeing her in clinic makes me believe again in humanity. We have a breast cancer navigator – "Zed Lightning" we call her (or sometimes just "Zed") – who grew up in this neighborhood and knows everything about it. She is incredibly kind and compassionate and does what she can. We now have two oncologists (usually) – myself and Dr. F – talking back and forth to the surgeon and figuring out our recommendations.

> Toni is a jazz singer and pianist, a former model, whose breast cancer was advanced with four positive nodes. Now a few years out from chemotherapy, surgery and radiation. Now a fan and teacher of tango dancing.

This year we have been working on efficiency – getting patients seen as quickly as possible and getting their treatment going as soon as we can. All of us who care for breast cancer patients make a point of being in clinic at the same time. Our infusion center is down the hall so we can see patients there when they come in for chemo. We sit in clinic as doctors, nurses, cancer navigators, and others and try to find the "best" of all possible treatments for our patients with breast cancer. What we offer can actually do only two beneficial things for our patients: (1) improve how long they live (their overall survival) and (2) improve their quality of life. We could also harm patients if we're not careful, either individually or collectively; and the fundamental principle of medicine is "first do no harm." It's a careful balancing act to always do the right thing by a patient – exactly as we would wish to be treated if we were in her shoes. Helping our patients understand what we're doing and why we're recommending a treatment course and helping them chose what feels right to them is our daily job.

Why would anyone become an oncologist?

"I don't like work – no man does – but I like what is in the work – the chance to find yourself. You own reality – for yourself not for others – what no other man can ever know. They can only see the mere show, and never can tell what it really means." (Joseph Conrad, *Heart of Darkness*)

> When I was a medical student, my mom was diagnosed with breast cancer and I went with her to see her medical oncologist. Of course I was anxious and nervous and heard only every fourth word or so. When he said he thought she had a 90% cure rate, I thought, "Hmm, that's not a bad job, curing women of breast cancer."

It was the chance to improve a patient's quality of life that in part led me to oncology. When I was a medical student on a surgery rotation, we had a woman in her fifties – kind, bright, attractive, well-educated and admitted with the hope that her metastatic colon cancer was operable so that she might still have a chance at cure. I spoke with her and performed a physical exam to "present" her to my team the night before surgery. I remember the moment during the operation when I saw the picture on the ultrasound machine: too many cancer nodules in her liver to remove; it had already spread too widely to do anything to save her. I realized in that moment that she had less than a year to live. After the operation I spent a great deal of time talking with her and learned that her husband had shunned her when she was diagnosed with cancer. Over time that evening, she seemed to feel a little better. I think I was making her feel better just by listening to her stories – on a service, no less, where we traditionally believed that "to cut is to cure." It's one of the amazing things in health care how much you can "heal" a patient without affecting the underlying disease – just by being kind and compassionate, by being another human who understands how hard it is to get through this life. Even in the twenty-first century, "doctor as healer" is still a viable concept. As George Eliot wrote in her novel *Middlemarch*, "What do we live for, if it is not to make life less difficult for each other?"

I also like the high stakes we have in clinical oncology. I likely have the wrong temperament for making small modifications to a patient's overall disease course, and I'm too klutzy to be a surgeon although I love the definitive nature of problem-solving they enjoy. In the oncology clinic we have daily fights with life and death. When there are victories, they are big ones; and when there are losses, they are sad. And yet for our patients we can't cure, our role doesn't diminish; helping them focus on what's possible and live each day to its utmost is something we can do. We explain the options for a patient to choose, and we provide guidance and advice. We stay with them throughout their journey, no matter how dire the situation.

> *I saw Shannon at the hospital, coughing and complaining of back pain. Her breast cancer had returned. Twenty years ago she was the greatest surgical resident I had met: a former ballet dancer for the NYC Ballet, brilliant, kind, genuine – who then trained in pediatric surgery, rising to the top of her field, only to be diagnosed with breast cancer seven years ago. And now it has returned. She doesn't see me as a patient, but when I run into her I can sense how she is doing. She is quiet about her struggles, continuing work for now. Shannon reminds me of Dr. W, an oncologist at Harvard – a hero of mine, of all of us – who passed away at age fifty-two from breast cancer; and my medical school classmate who passed away at thirty-two from the same disease. It leaves me asking, "What does this any of this mean?"*

The triumphs: all the patients that were cured, some against strong odds. My first patient in private practice, a lovely woman with a bad breast cancer, still emails me from time to time. We got her through some rough chemotherapy – four cycles of doxorubicin and cyclophosphamide and twelve weeks of paclitaxel – and things veered back to normal. She bought me a green tie with four-leaf clovers on it I wear it every St Patrick's day and think of her, hoping her life is now happy. Most breast cancer patients are cured, and it's gratifying to help them through this process, see them get back to their regular lives – jobs, marriages, travels.

The tragic: – all the patients whose lives ended despite our best efforts. I can see several breast cancer patients in my mind, vivacious and full of life, who passed away under my watch. I can hear their voices and see their faces, and I become sad all over again: young women with aggressive cancers that appear out of nowhere, or women whose cancers weren't supposed to return but did.

> *I had a patient who was kind and wonderful and worked as a dietician at my hospital. She received aggressive treatment up front, yet the cancer recurred a few years later. Her husband always read interesting novels when he came in to the office with her for every treatment. I walked by her office for two years after she passed away, four years after my institution laid her off while she was battling her cancer during another "reduction in work force." I saw her husband last week in a grocery store near my home and he thanked me and I felt sad all over again at seeing him and knowing the suffering he had endured. I hope he has been able to move on and rebuild his life and wanted to ask him. But today my wife is with me and I can't introduce her to him because of patient confidentiality.*

> *When my wife was diagnosed with breast cancer, I took her to see a medical oncologist I know well who is now practicing in my town. My former resident, Barbara, has matured as a kind oncologist. She was a blessing in the middle of a tragedy; she was there for me. Even though I've treated thousands of breast cancer patients, I could never have imagined how hard it is to go through chemotherapy until I lived with my wife through diagnosis, losing her hair, feeling exhausted and facing her mortality day to day.*

The more tragic: my current gig at the county hospital – patients who are down on their luck economically. Some started out well and have fallen on hard times – lost jobs, lost careers, went through bad divorces, fell into drug or alcohol addiction. Many are immigrants moving to the US for a better life. Some are doctors themselves who moved to the US to be near their children but can't afford health insurance.

> *Lori is always smiling in clinic and usually wears rock-and-roll T-shirts: Hendrix, Led Zeppelin, RUSH. She's almost done with her year of chemotherapy and Herceptin and has now moved to a small town six hours away. She wants to "get back on the dating market," to move forward. Now in remission, she comes to follow-up appointments every three months.*

This is the hardest job I've ever had. The patients are very sick; their lives are hard; resources are not plentiful. Our patients don't just have breast cancer; they have other illnesses and many times a problematic social life. Most of the mothers are single. Some patients are homeless. Perhaps there is something in the environment that makes these women predisposed to aggressive cancers. At wealthy hospitals and medical centers it's mostly ductal carcinoma *in situ* and stage I or II breast cancer. Dr. K and I always wonder.

Theodicy: Seeing this sadness – death from breast cancer, the ravages of poverty – how can we explain the suffering in the world? I keep returning to the Bible to two specific sections: Ecclesiastes and Job. I've long lost my view of God as all-powerful and all-knowing. Another oncologist friend who studied philosophy in college suggested reading Spinoza, and his interpretation of God seems to make the most sense to me. Perhaps the world is really composed only of chance and physics after all.

Tragedy of another sort: I knew a beautiful young, gifted breast surgeon, Dr. A. She and I became good friends and I loved sharing patients with her. But she was young and a bit naïve and was bullied by the senior breast surgeon she worked with and by the other women in her office. The senior breast surgeon knew that she could make money – to support her two children who hadn't seemed to find their career paths and still lived at home – by seeing more patients with breast cancer. So she would take the breast cancer patients off Dr. A's schedule and leave her with benign breast disease, which is less lucrative. Dr. A grew more despondent over time and started drinking more. One night she was called in to the ER, but she was slurring her words, and her partner had her fired. She lost her license and her practice – travelled a bit, got pregnant by a good-for-nothing guy who moved her far away. All that kindness and all that talent wasted. If I could change the world, I'd give her a medical license and bring her to work with me because she was a fantastic doctor.

Other doctors will often say, "I could never do what you do." But it's not hard. We oncologists balance the tragic with the triumph, and overall there are more triumphs than tragedies in any given month. W (and men) are cured of breast cancer with our modern medical techniques. And I love the vibe of being in clinic with Zed Lightning and Dr. K and now Dr. F, seeing patients who would otherwise fall through the cracks. I sometimes imagine myself as another catcher in the rye.

Bibliography

Baum, Michael. *Breast Beating*. Tunbridge Wells: Anshan Publishers, 2010.
———. *The History and Mystery of Breast Cancer*. Newcastle upon Tyne: Cambridge Scholars Publishing, 2019.

DAVID CARNISH

Reflections on Solidarity

Solidarity is a unity in feeling or in action where there is either a common interest or mutual support. Solidarity is hard to find these days. From the Kiwanis club to the local worship center, the sense of community belonging and common purpose – of solidarity – is often absent. As a healthcare chaplain for twenty-nine years – serving, at various times, as a staff chaplain and certified pastoral educator working in mental health, pediatrics, hospice, critical care and oncology for both community and academic medical centers – I have observed a decline in solidarity, even as healthcare spoke of well-being, holistic care and, more lately, person-centered care.

When I introduced myself to my first supervisor, the CEO of a large Level I academic urban hospital, he said, "You are here to remind the rest of us of our humanity and our common bonds in life and death." For many people, I serve as a representative of and resource for access to the divine. To others, I am part of the health team that contributes to the holistic care of persons. It is my job to cultivate solidarity. Solidarity with individual patients as they live out their own stories, experiences, values, and meaning. Solidarity with other healthcare professionals as they process how their profession invigorates them and wears them down. Solidarity in research that aims to improve the social conditions that impact the well-being of persons from all walks of life. In other words, the chaplain is a "conspirator" who commits to journey with another person into the deep places of life (Tillich 53).

Like other professionals, the chaplain utilizes a special skill set and body of knowledge. An effective chaplain must understand a range of religions, rites, rituals and symbols, and must, above all, embody cultural humility. A larger part of the professional chaplain's role is his ability to utilize and listen for theological, religious and philosophical language.

Theologian Charlie Winquist called this language the "language of desire" (ix). Desire is different from expectation. Whereas expectation is riddled with notions of privilege and sets us up for disappointment, desire is the stuff of theology, focusing on yearning, longing of life for life (ix). While working with many people over the years who are in the throes of crisis, trauma and death, I have learned that most of their stories are about longing and desire. Chaplains intentionally join a person at the source of her greatest desires and longings. This is a sacred privilege.

I remember one of the first breast cancer patients I met who taught me to listen and gave me glimpses of the importance of solidarity. Anna was 25 years old, the same age I was. She was scheduled to have a mastectomy, followed by chemotherapy and/or radiation. Anna was terrified. But her greatest fear was not the immediate surgery or other treatments that were looming on the horizon. Her worst fear was rooted in her longing for a companion. Could any man love a woman with only one breast – much less marry her? What about the children she dreamed to have, to breast-feed, to nurture? I listened to her anguish. I felt her defeat and anger. Her body reverberated a muted stillness from the violent diagnosis of breast cancer. Silence was in every deep place, and her hopes for a future fell into an abyss. Never again would she be the same.

I might have approached Anna with sympathy, a process of "feeling with" the other that would lead me to focus on my own experiences of similar events as I considered her situation. Sympathetically, I was also 25 years old. I was unmarried. I wanted children. I understood all these desires we had in common. But sympathy would necessarily shift focus to my own pain; as such, sympathy would not lead to solidarity. Alternatively, I might have approached Anna with empathy, making efforts to understand her thoughts, perceptions and experiences. I could say things like "Tell me more about that" or "That sounds painful." I would feel her pain her and maintain some distance. But neither sympathy nor empathy seemed quite right.

Pastoral Care and Counseling scholar David Augsburger proposed another way for a chaplain to meet the person where she is suffering: "interpathy" (29). Interpathy is an intentional cognitive and affective envisioning of the other's thoughts and feelings, non-judgmentally accepting truths that might seem foreign – from another culture, worldview and way of knowing the world. Interpathy is akin to the "suspension of disbelief" we need to enjoy a movie like *Star Wars* or *Harry Potter and the Sorcerer's Stone*. When disbelief is suspended, the viewer is one with the story, no matter how foreign, spectacular or illogical that story might be. Rather than assume that Anna and I are similar (i.e., sympathy's path), I enter her world, accepting her reality at face value, hearing her carefully, remaining fully present to her, being one with her. This approach dovetails with work of French philosopher Emmanuel Levinas, who argues that otherness and difference – not similarity – are the keys to building rapport, relationship and support. I have a responsibility toward the other because, while the other person is separate from my life, she is also sharing life with me at the same time. Making the leap to suspend one's own assumptions and worldview means jumping headlong into experiencing how life is lived by the other person. Love occurs in the epiphany of meeting the other. Otherness and difference were my path to solidarity with Anna, a framework that encouraged her to communicate desire, longing and love – her vital depth.

 I learned to be with Anna by listening for her hunger. Political activist and mystic of World War II, Simone Weil believed that we live on bread and desire – a longing to be satisfied, complete, fulfilled (Weil 62). Weil lived her own life in the threshold between the religious and the secular. Her mysticism showed me that I needed to attend to Anna in the threshold between life and death. "Attending" is Weil's word for emptying of self. I had to empty myself to receive and become immersed in Anna's truth. Anything else is my agenda, my hope, my creative attempt, my ego.

 Imagine entering a hospital room where you meet a stranger. In your mind, you have so many things you need to hear from them and so many things you want to tell them about. The situation is awkward. Now imagine going in to that room and letting go of all of that. You turn to the person and you present yourself as hungry and wait. Presume nothing. Hold no certainty. Suspend judgment. Her life is in front of me. I have to take it in and appreciate it. This is what Anna taught me. Yes, she was crushed. Yes, life threw her. But pity was not what she needed. I listened, and Anna helped me understand a reality of breast cancer in the vibrancy of one person who held desire, longing and love simultaneously. She wanted only to know if I could be with her and, by being with her, acknowledge her hunger for a more intimate knowledge that leads to a deeper love of life (Anselm 53). My hungry, attending presence with her was solidarity.

Many years after meeting Anna, I found myself in a completely different relationship with breast cancer, solidarity and desire. My wife, Deborah, and I had moved across the country to a new state, new city, and new apartment with our 3-year-old son and our 13-year-old dog. The weekend prior to my beginning a new job – the very day we were unpacking – our dog, Lady, was hovering close to Deborah and attending very carefully to her. Lady was my loyal companion and usually stayed close to me. But not this day. After we'd been working a few hours, Deborah called out to me from another room. When I went to check on her, I discovered she was bleeding from her nipple. I had a bad feeling the moment she told me what was happening with her body.

Time collapsed. It was no longer linear at all. I went with Deborah to her appointment days after the bleeding began. The nurse called her back. In the breast cancer waiting room, bodies retreat into themselves and build a private little hell of timelessness. I sat in the space that the English-speaking world calls the "waiting room." I saw the bodies of other spouses, partners, friends, mothers, daughters and sons. There wasn't a trace of solidarity to be had in that room. The room was filled with silence. Each person was terrified in place and all alone. I imagined Deborah's private hell, too, running the gauntlet of biopsy, x-rays, robing and disrobing over and over again.

I felt like I was in a train station, a modern nowhere land, a liminal space where people converge as they arrive from x and depart for y. No one actually lives here. From my vantage point, we folk in the waiting room were waiting for permission to move. We had no idea where to go, although arguably anywhere would have been better than here – anywhere, that is, except the other side of the door, where our loved one was waiting to see the doctor. For an eternity, the receptionist and nurses did not call out. The waiting room remained a silent void. Here and now, I could not have conjured my professional chaplain skills even if I'd wanted to.

When Deborah finally emerged from the other side of the door, her nurse motioned for me and said to her, "We need to see you on Friday, and please bring somebody with you." I had been around hospitals enough to know what the nurse was conveying without speaking directly: "I have bad news." Rather than tell us then, she ushered us to the exit and wished us a good weekend: "Go have dinner, go out on a date, have fun." What happened instead was three sleepless nights of tossing and turning, three days of dread. I was plagued by the story playing over and over in my head: *This could be it. I have brought my wife up here to die. My son and I will live on. He won't remember much of his mom. What am I going to do? How am I going to do it?* Some Christian people would say that these thoughts indicate a lack of faith. Ah, the quick and unfair judgments we sometimes make!

That three-day-later meeting came. It was as I had known before: My wife had breast cancer. What happened after that is fuzzy at best. I remember being in the room with her. Endless questions were met with answers and sympathetic eyes. She was an object of pity and something that energy would be poured into in order to "fix." Neither of us remembers a thing anyone said that day. She had just learned she had cancer, and the train was already calling us to board, bound for treatment options. I believe a common sentiment goes something like "Let them get their feelings out, and then we can get to rational conversation." But our feelings are the path to the real conversation! How did we feel? Angry. Deborah was angry. I was angry. She had been betrayed. All the images of my wife going to have her yearly breast exam flashed through my mind. For the past few years she had told them something didn't feel right. Nothing "showed up" on the scans, so they did not listen. Certain that they had the "facts," they explained away her physical sensations as "atypical symptoms."

Even though the cancer was only on the left side, Deborah opted for a bilateral mastectomy with no reconstruction. The medical team was perplexed by this decision. Had they only listened to her they would have heard that she wanted to see the scar so that she could grieve and come to embody a new life. She wanted the scar to teach our son that a woman is more than parts of her body.

On tax day that year, we went to the hospital for the operation. This was after she had returned to the clinic so a stranger could take photographs of her breasts in case she wanted reconstruction later on. I sat there and watched as the young woman took photos of her. Feeling great tenderness for my wife, I saw in mind's eye flashes of intimate moments: her breastfeeding our son, her naked beauty. Then it hit me. Soon I would not touch her body in same way. Soon I would not see her the same. Deborah grieved losing her breasts, but more than that, she wanted us to have another child. If she had elected to undergo chemotherapy or radiation instead of mastectomy, the odds of another healthy pregnancy would have decreased. Although there would be no going back after her mastectomy, I also felt relief in knowing that the surgery gave us the chance – a really good chance – that she would live and that we would grow our family.

Post-surgery memories are like individual snapshots. I remember during this time bringing Deborah home and walking her up the three flights of stairs to our apartment. She was having a very hard time breathing, and I remember feeling sheer terror. I recall the first shower she had after surgery and hearing her say that, on many levels, the recuperation phase was worse than she had anticipated: She felt a sense of death about her – that the walls of our home closed in on her while she recovered. Once, our young son glanced at her, lifted up his shirt and asked innocently, "Mommy what are these pink things I have, and where are yours?" One afternoon at church, in an attempt to provide comfort and solidarity, a member offered Deborah flowers from the altar to take home. Mindful that pink is the color of hope and memory for breast cancer research and survivors, the person offered her the pink flowers instead of the yellow ones. Ironically, Deborah's favorite color is yellow; it is her sign of hope and recovery.

Two years later, on Father's Day, we found out that we were expecting our second child. The joy of being parents again, however, paradoxically led to other griefs. Deborah had breastfed our first child, but she would not be able to breastfeed our second. I thought back to the lactation nurse's teaching us how to help a newborn "latch" and, now, we would need to teach our second child to bottle feed. In both instances, though, I witnessed my wife hold our boys dearly. And I noticed throughout all the grief Deborah's desire and longing; her essential faith in being a good mother was not diminished. The contradictions of grief, loss, love and longing became the poetry of her life as a mother and as a woman.

Any journey with breast cancer is on-going, and years later, we live with the possibility that Deborah will have a recurrence. We are not alone with these fears, of course. Each day we and others like us carry our burdens much like *bastaixos*, the historical characters in the 2006 novel *Cathedral of the Sea*, by Ildefonso Falcones. The *bastaixos* of fourteenth-century Barcelona were Spanish laborers who carried heavy stones on their backs and cut them into form in order to build the Santa Maria del Mar cathedral. Most of the *bastaixos* never lived to see their work completed, but their work itself was a daily devotion. In many ways, the work of chaplains, too, is like that: joining a person at a particular moment in time, doing some heavy lifting and often not being present to see how things turn out. We stay hungry. Longing, we attend. What I've learned is that this heavy lifting requires practice and dedication in order to build up the muscles of compassion and presence that enable us to join with others on their journey toward healing. The work itself is a privilege.

Bibliography

Anselm, Saint. *Proslogium; Monologium; An Appendix in Behalf of the Fool by Gaunilon; and Cur Deus Homo*. Trans. Sidney Norton Dean. La Salle, Illinois: Open Court, 1951.
Augsberger, David. *Pastoral Counseling Across Cultures*. Philadelphia: Westminster Press, 1986.
Tillich, Paul. *The Shaking of the Foundations*. New York: Scribner's Sons, 1948.
Weil, Simone. Waiting for God. New York: Harper Collins, 1966.
Winquist, Charles. *Desiring Theology*. Chicago: University of Chicago Press, 1995.

IAN R. ROSS

When Chaos Comes: The Role of a Hospitalist

A shrill beeping startled me awake. I had just sat down to rest my eyes after finishing my eighth admission of the night. It was 4:00 a.m., and no more than fifteen minutes had passed before the ER was calling me again. I squinted as my vision came into focus, allowing me to read the message waiting for me on my pager: *new admission. 62-year-old female with metastatic breast cancer presenting with fever.*

I knew who it was before I even returned the call. Her name was Denise, and she was a well-known patient at my hospital. She had been diagnosed with breast cancer years ago. Despite treatment with surgery, radiation, and chemotherapy, her disease had continued to progress. She eventually developed diffuse metastatic involvement of her central nervous system, also known as leptomeningeal carcinomatosis. Patients with this condition typically pass away in a matter of weeks without treatment. Clinical trials have shown that the patient's prognosis "improves" to about six to eight months after the most aggressive forms of therapy.

Denise had clearly either not read these studies or didn't care about what they had to say, because she was still very much alive over two years after receiving this terminal diagnosis. She was on fifth-line treatment for her malignancy and suffered numerous complications from both her disease and its treatment, including severe infections, profound dehydration, and swelling of the brain. As a result, she was hospitalized at least monthly to treat these complications. My colleagues and I frequently cared for her during these hospitalizations, and she was universally respected and revered by us for her unmatched tenacity.

I rose from my seat after reviewing her chart and guided my arms one at a time through the sleeves of my long white coat. My footsteps echoed through the empty halls as I walked toward the ER, stethoscope bouncing off my hip with each step as it sat coiled in my right front pocket.

I came upon the ER exam room where Denise was being housed. It was dark, but even so I could make out her unmistakable silhouette. Most patients with metastatic cancer appear to be halfway between this world and the next: ravaged, with sunken eyes, wasted muscles, and paper-thin skin barely able to conceal the underlying bones. But Denise appeared largely untouched, still physically imposing with broad shoulders and weighing well over 200 pounds. It was almost as if death himself were too afraid to start a fight with her. In fact, the only visible sign of her extensive war with cancer was her mostly bald head, a consequence of her many chemotherapy treatments. Somehow, this feature made her appear even more formidable.

"Hello, Ms. Denise, you might remember that I am Dr. Ross, a hospitalist in Internal Medicine. I will be admitting you to the hospital tonight. I work with your oncologist to provide your care here."

The first person most people meet when they receive a diagnosis of cancer is an oncologist. Outpatient oncology offices are often luxurious, outfitted with marble floors and mahogany book shelves. Staff are kind and compassionate and greet you with a warm smile. Relaxing music plays softly in the background. The whole experience is appropriately designed to be calming, a counterbalance to the trauma of receiving a diagnosis of cancer.

Most people don't realize that their oncologist will not be caring for them if they develop serious complications related to malignancy or treatment. That's where I come in. I'm a hospitalist, which means that the linoleum floors and cramped exam rooms of the inpatient setting are my full-time "office." My outfit of choice is typically aqua-colored scrubs, and I may be sporting a 5 o' clock shadow that is just long enough for you to question if I have actually been home in the last few days.

I'm an organizer of chaos; my job is to get you through the roughest times of your life and back home in better condition to continue the treatment for your cancer. I have not completed a fellowship in oncology, but I am specially trained to deal with life-threatening complications that can arise during the course of your treatment. The oncologist, who decided what is next in your treatment, is typically not involved in the inpatient care for your complications. I can touch base with him or her in a quick email or phone call, but for the most part, hospitalists like me are in charge of the day-to-day decisions and intricacies of inpatient care. It's not that your oncologist doesn't want to be involved; it is simply too demanding for him or her to simultaneously coordinate care for many outpatients as well as patients who are hospitalized. This addition of another doctor to the care team is often a shock for some people, but Denise was an experienced pro.

"Yes, I remember you, Dr. Ross," she said as she softly chuckled. "Leave a nice voicemail for my oncologist to let him know I've checked into my home-away-from-home again."

Denise was being admitted with the diagnosis of neutropenic fever. This is a medical condition where the immune system is so compromised by the effects of chemotherapy that the body starts developing infection even to the "good bacteria" that typically cohabitate benignly with us. The body also becomes susceptible to infections by other pathogens, such as fungi, viruses, or invasive bacteria. Treatment consists of broad-spectrum, powerful antibiotics to keep the infections at bay until the immune system recovers. Often, we need to "boost" the immune system's recovery with special medication. The diagnosis of neutropenic fever can range from a mild illness that is treated in an outpatient setting, to a life-threatening crisis that requires hospitalization.

Unfortunately, Denise's course was the latter. Despite an extensive battery of lab testing, microbiological cultures, imaging studies, diagnostic procedures, and aggressive treatment for her symptoms, she continued to have fever, severe rigors, and intermittent confusion for several days. Denise was one of the strongest people I had ever met, but I thought this might be the clinical complication that would finally overcome her. As a hospitalist, I often care for patients who are living their final days, and I serve as a guide through that process. This involves discussions about their goals of care, where I mainly help patients understand the effects further treatment can have on their bodies, and discuss prognoses and realistic outcomes of further treatments. Many times, our conversations focus on quality versus quantity of life. In circumstances such as Denise's, I often see the heavy price that invasive procedures and harsh treatments exact on patients without meaningfully prolonging their life. I encourage these patients to consider how they might live their last days in dignity and peace.

It was with this heavy heart that I brought up reconsidering goals of care with Denise. It was not the first time I had discussed this with her, as she had frequently been on the precipice of death during previous hospitalizations. Before now, she had always adamantly refused to consider a transition to hospice care, and this time was no different. Denise wasn't rude about her disagreement with me, but a mere glance into her eyes told me that she was still brimming with determination and fight.

Denise's goal was clear: to cling to every thread of life still within her grasp, no matter the cost. I didn't understand her choice. Her life over the past year had been spent more often than not in the hospital, where she'd been subjected to sharp needles, beeping monitors, and the side effects of harsh medications. I had actually seen her more times in the past year than her own outpatient oncologist. I didn't understand how that quality of life could be meaningful for anyone, but ultimately this was the way she had decided to continue her journey, and I respected her choice. My goal was to do whatever I could to help her have the best quality of life possible. In the end, she and I worked together to organize the chaos of her present condition, and she recovered from her infection. She was discharged home and was well enough to undergo further treatment for her metastatic breast cancer. As I expected, she was admitted again several times over the following weeks and ultimately passed away nearly two and a half years after her initial terminal diagnosis.

Denise has remained seared into my memory in the years since her death. I think about her often when my patients, grappling with their own imminent mortality, choose to pursue an uncomfortable life of obstacles rather than a peaceful death. I sometimes disagree with their choices, but I firmly stand with them as a partner in their struggle. And I smile, as I recall the times Denise repeatedly delivered an uppercut to death's jaw, as she laughed in his face.

ELIANA V. HEMPEL

Best-Laid Plans: When Follow-Up Fails

As is common for a first-year internal medicine resident, I was spending much of my time in clinic establishing care with patients I would have the privilege to care for during the next three years of my training. This Wednesday was no exception. The only unusual aspect of my 9:00 a.m. appointment was that this patient had absolutely no medical records in our health system. In the past few months, I had become accustomed to meticulously reviewing the electronic medical record to learn as much as I could about my patients. I felt like a detective in one of my favorite mystery novels as I tried to glean as much as I could about their past medical history while also reading between the lines to pick up tidbits about their personality and attitudes from my colleagues' prior documentation. I'd start to imagine what they looked like from the detailed notes on their physical examinations. I'd learn about their interests, hobbies and beloved travel destinations from their social history. I'd get a sense for their approach to their healthcare by reading of their acceptance of the proposed next steps in the assessment and plan. By the time I met them at our first appointment, it almost felt like I was meeting up with an old acquaintance rather than a stranger. This time, though, I was utterly blinded by the lack of prior clues. I felt a mixture of excitement and apprehension as I rapped my knuckles on exam room 15, where my next patient waited.

Ida perched on a blue vinyl chair next to the computer in our exam room. She was sitting literally on the edge of her seat. Her scuffed white sneakers shifted as her thin frame, clothed in a white turtleneck and frayed red sweater, rocked back and forth. Her pale, bony hands twisted together ceaselessly. In sharp contrast, her sister, who I would later learn was named Ingrid, sat ramrod straight in her neat-as-a-pin prim white sweater set. As different in personality as they were in appearance, Ingrid projected an air of confidence and strength, while it was clear to me that Ida could not have been more nervous. I gulped, hopefully noiselessly, and sat down on my rolling stool.

Not yet comfortable or used to introducing myself as a doctor, I stumbled through my initial greeting. "Good morning, Ida. I'm Eliana – er, I mean, Dr. Hempel. It's nice to meet you." She quickly responded, "No offence to you, doc, but I just really don't like hospitals, so can we make this quick?" With a refrain that would become incredibly familiar, Ingrid interrupted and said, "Now, Ida, let the doctor do her job."

I felt a small swell of pride and gratitude toward Ingrid in hearing her refer to me as "the doctor." Despite having worked toward this point in my life since the age of four, I was still in a state of disbelief that I was finally getting to care for patients. As a young female doctor, I was also pleasantly surprised by her tone of respect. Lately, I had been told that I was too young to be a resident, too pretty to be smart and that it just plain wasn't possible for me to be The Doctor. Thus, this moment of acknowledgement of my role in that one unembellished word made my day.

Over the next thirty minutes, I learned that there were no records in our system because Ida hadn't seen a physician in twenty years. Her distaste for the medical system had only grown ten-fold throughout the past few years as she'd cared for her husband, who had recently died of cirrhosis. I also learned that Ingrid was Ida's somewhat disapproving sister who, after a career spent in the age of nursing defined by starched white caps, had finally convinced Ida to take care of her own health. It was clear that their relationship was somewhat strained, but the obvious affection between them was evident. Ida, reticent to provide any information, answered in mainly yesses and nos. So it was Ingrid who provided me with the details of Ida's history of breast cancer, diagnosed in her late forties and treated with a mastectomy and radiation. It was Ingrid who ignored Ida's annoyance with being "ratted out" and divulged that Ida had not returned for any of her scheduled follow-up visits and mammograms. And it was Ingrid who shared that Ida was still smoking at least one pack of cigarettes per day. Finally, after cajoling, joking, smoothing ruffled feathers, and mediating between two iron-willed women, I managed to get most of the information I needed. Though Ida had not seen a physician in a long time and was out of date for many of her screening tests, she had no complaints and seemed reasonably healthy. The death of her husband had left her stunned, and her anxiety was palpably uncontrolled; but I felt fairly confident that if I could only earn her trust, I might be able to help.

One of my mentors taught me early on that as a primary care physician, my job is to know my patients fully. This means identifying them not only by their medical problems, but as whole people with interests, hopes, dreams, and lives outside the exam room. This means understanding their own personal brand of normal and respecting their decisions even when they do not align with my own personal values. This also means practicing the dying art of the comprehensive physical exam. My mentor explained to me that there may be no one else looking at the aging skin of their sun-damaged backs susceptible to melanoma, no one else listening to the whooshes of their straining hearts that no longer perform their vital duty normally, no one else feeling the elusive lumps and bumps that are early indicators of abnormal cells starting to ravage the body. She taught me that in order to do this, at least once a year, I needed to ask my patients to don those fashionable gowns and take the time to look for the subtle signs of something amiss. So, despite much grumbling and grousing, I convinced Ida to let me do a comprehensive exam.

Her sclera, the whites of her eyes, were reassuringly ecru, and her cornflower blue irises surrounded responsive pupils. Her heart lub-dubbed in a wonderfully normal rhythm. Her lungs demonstrated the crackly sounds that belied her years of smoking. Her bowel sounds rumbled away, indicating a stomach that was ready for a meal. Throughout the examination, Ida tittered nervously about this and that. I tried to be thorough, but also mindful of Ida's obvious desire to escape my presence. Finally, I realized that I could put it off no longer. Because of her history of breast cancer, I had to do a breast exam.

The utility of a screening breast examination by primary care physicians has been called into question (American College of Obstetricians and Gynecologists; Fenton, et al.; Oeffinger, et al.). Some professional societies suggest that primary care physicians are no longer adept at feeling for the subtle changes in breast tissue that reveal an underlying cancer. But as I awkwardly pressed the pads of my fingers on the tissue of her previously healthy left breast, even I, a newly minted, inexperienced physician, immediately knew something was wrong. A firm, round area of abnormal tissue, pushed back against my hand. I desperately tried to keep my inner horror from showing on my pallid face as I continued my examination by feeling in her underarms for the telltale almond-shaped bulges that would indicate that her cancer had spread to her lymph nodes. My spirits continued to sink as I palpated more than one unmoving mass in her left armpit.

With my heart hammering in my chest, I frantically ran through the file folders of information I learned in medical school looking for the file marked "How to Give Bad News." Despite being trained by lectures, practice with standardized patients, and observations of other skilled providers, I felt unprepared to tell this lovely, scared person I'd never met before that her cancer had returned. I battled indignation. How could she, after having survived breast cancer, have given up on all of her screenings? How did she not notice the obvious alarm bells her body was sending her? How could so much hardship befall one, kind person?

I've frequently been asked by non-medical friends how I deal with the emotions that come with caring for patients, often at some of the worst times in their lives. As a medical student, I used to think that those emotions needed to be separated from patient care. That acknowledging how I felt about my patients, or even that my patients and my job sparked feelings at all, was somehow a failure. I thought from my misguided interpretation of some of our medical school teaching, that those emotions needed to be bottled up and processed in some completely separate space and time. Yet, as I have grown as a young physician and gained life experience from my own personal tragedies, I have realized the errors of my old ideas of a physician's emotional connection to her work – though, of course, there are times in a physician's career when emotions cannot get in the way. During those critical moments when urgent, life-saving decisions are being made, calm, clear thinking is paramount. However, there are also times when, in my opinion, it is not only acceptable but essential to share a small piece of ourselves with our patients. This may be by discussing a shared experience, divulging our own fears or uncertainty, or just by demonstrating, in some small way, that we too are crushed by the bad news we are giving.

Even in the forty-five minutes I'd spent with Ida, I had already developed a connection with her. I felt grateful for the small amount of trust she had placed in me. Cognizant of her fears and anxiety, and her desire to engage with the healthcare system as little as possible, I felt incredibly dismayed at my news during our very first visit. I also feared that the way I delivered this news could have an impact on Ida's next steps. A misstep here could contribute to Ida's decision to retreat and not seek any further treatment, but a careful approach might encourage her to at least hear about the possible next steps.

I understood all of this because I had walked a similar path with my own father. While I was a first-year medical student, my beloved father was diagnosed with oral cancer. My dad, a hard-working, tough former merchant marine, was much like Ida. Despite having lots of medical family members, he too had a discomfort with the medical system that caused him to avoid it at all costs. I remember being surprised that even in the face of cancer, he was reticent to pursue the recommended treatments. When we talked about why he felt that way, we did not go past the surface to talk about his fears of pain, treatment failure, social isolation, and ultimately, death. We did, however, talk about how the way his doctors delivered news and treatment options made him angry, how he sometimes felt bullied by doctors who presented only one approach, and how a lack of compassion could make even a simple treatment, like a medication for high blood pressure, seem unpalatable. Although I knew my father's experience was relevant in this moment, I wasn't sure whether any of it was appropriate for me to share with Ida. Would talking about my father connect us through some form of shared understanding, or would it shift the focus of this encounter from my patient to me? Knowing my next actions were crucial, but not knowing how to maneuver this delicate conversation, I left the room to seek the counsel of my supervising physician.

I did not know it at the time, but my patient and I were both terribly lucky that day. My supervising physician was a wise mentor, a women's health expert, and most importantly, a wonderfully empathetic human being. Though I'm confident that she saw the dread in my eyes as I recounted Ida's history and my exam findings, she encouraged me by displaying only confidence in my ability to do this, one of the hardest of a physician's tasks, with skill. She reminded me that even though our relationship was short-lived, I was the healthcare provider who had developed the most rapport with Ida in the past twenty years. She gave me the courage to try to communicate this bad news with kindness.

When faced with giving bad news, I think physicians try to anticipate all the possible reactions. Will there be matter-of-fact questions about next steps, prognosis and complications of treatment? Will there be a hysterical breakdown marked by wrenching sobs? Will there be shocked disbelief? Will there be anger and hostility toward the unfortunate messenger? With Ida's jumpiness and Ingrid's practicality, I expected Ida to break down and Ingrid to sensibly ask about a treatment plan. Now, years later, I have learned to suspend expectations and prepare for anything. Even patients I have known extremely well have reacted in wholly unexpected ways when faced with immense challenges. Ida and Ingrid started to teach me this lesson on that Wednesday, as it was, in fact, Ingrid who broke down and began to cry, and Ida, who calmly accepted my grim words.

Ida quickly shared that she wanted to be conservative in her treatment. Remembering my dad's retreat in the face of what he perceived as a high-handed approach, I tried to be careful to respect Ida's wishes and present the options as non-judgmentally as possible. We negotiated about the most prudent next steps and settled on a mammogram and a consultation with an oncologist, but none of the other tests, screenings or vaccines that were indicated for someone of her age. I tried to encourage her that although I would no longer be the primary physician making recommendations about the treatment regarding her cancer diagnosis, I would do my best to walk with her every step of the way. One hour and fifteen minutes after I had, with trepidation, entered exam room 15, Ida stopped me before I left. She said, "Doc, thanks for not being pushy. I was really scared to come to the office today, but I'm glad you're going to take care of me. You made something really hard easier by being you, and by letting me be me."

Not surprisingly, Ida's mammogram and subsequent breast biopsy confirmed a second instance of breast cancer. Ida was scheduled for a mastectomy and lymph node dissection. I had the chance to speak with her on the day before her surgery. She was, of course, hesitant about moving forward, even in the last hours before her scheduled procedure. I answered whatever questions I could and told her I'd be sending positive thoughts her way since I, as her primary care physician, could do little else. The surgery was successful, but the pathology yielded yet another bombshell. The lymph nodes showed a second, different kind of cancer. Though I wasn't the provider who shared this bad news with Ida, she and I did commiserate about the injustice of her diagnoses at our next visit.

As a primary care physician, I sometimes feel a little bit helpless when faced with a diagnosis of cancer. I am rarely the one to pursue the next steps in testing, and never the one to propose treatment options. Often patients ask to follow up with me less regularly because of the frequency of their appointments with oncology. I try to follow along in the medical record. Still, it is never the same as being able to see my patients in person, and I'm often struck by the marked change in their appearance during our intermittent but highly anticipated visits. I do my best to monitor for complications of the disease or treatment, to coordinate their care amongst the various specialists involved and to provide informational and emotional support for patients and families. As much as is possible, I share in the sorrows of poor biopsy results and the joys of benign follow-up PET scans. But it is challenging to find the balance between serving my patients and merely adding to the burden of their already burdensome care plans. That balance was especially tricky with Ida. Thankfully, despite the alarm bells that clanged in my ears as I palpated what I thought was a recurrence of metastatic breast cancer, Ida was treated for both cancers with chemotherapy and radiation and initially did fairly well.

Over the years, Ida returned to her old practice of avoiding the medical establishment. She would miss or cancel appointments with me frequently, saying she didn't need me and that she'd just be wasting my time. I'd call to check up on her and urge her to come and see me, but on the rare occasions when she'd answer the phone, she'd insist she was okay. It was only through reviewing my oncology colleague's notes that I learned that her cancer had again reared its ugly head. Even then, when she would come in for a visit, she'd decline a full physical exam and encourage me to do my job as quickly as possible. As she went in and out of treatment for her cancers, she often came to see me only when her symptoms got severe enough to crack through her resilient exterior. I was thrilled when somewhere along the way, Ingrid, who had continued to care for Ida throughout her illness, requested that I take over as her own primary care physician.

When she would come in like clockwork for her own check-ups, I'd hear updates about Ida. I continued to try to make a point of calling Ida every few months or checking in after a follow-up appointment with another doctor, but as the years went on and my own practice got busier, Ida's lack of responsiveness wore me down, and our calls and visits became less and less frequent.

I only heard of Ida's passing only because Ingrid's son called to tell me he was worried about his mother and how she was coping with Ida's death. I was devastated. I was shocked that Ida, one of my first patients ever, was gone, but even more so, that I hadn't even known how ill she'd become. I was saddened to realize that I had not kept my promise of walking with her every step of the way and that I never got to tell her how much she taught me. I hope that in sharing her story – and the many ways in which she taught me the parts of medicine that can't be learned in medical school – I can somehow make up for not consistently connecting with her. So, Ida, thank you for giving me the privilege of taking care of you. You made something really hard easier by letting me be me, and by being you.

Bibliography

American College of Obstetricians and Gynecologists. "Breast Cancer Risk Assessment and Screening in Average-Risk Women." *ACOG Clinical Practice Bulletin* 179 (July 2017). <https://www.acog.org/clinical/clinical-guidance/practice-bulletin/articles/2017/07/breast-cancer-risk-assessment-and-screening-in-average-risk-women>. Accessed July 6, 2020.

Fenton, J. J., M. B. Barton, A. M. Geiger, et al. "Screening Clinical Breast Examination: How Often Does It Miss Lethal Breast Cancer?" *Journal of the National Cancer Institute Monographs* 35 (November 1, 2005): 67–71.

Fenton, J. J., S. J. Rolnick, E. L. Harris, et al. "Specificity of Clinical Breast Examination in Community Practice." *Journal of General Internal Medicine* 22.3 (2007): 332–37.

Oeffinger, K. C., E. T. Fontham, R. Etzioni, et al. "Breast Cancer Screening for Women at Average Risk: 2015 Guideline Update from the American Cancer Society." *JAMA* 314.15 (October 20, 2015): 1599–1614.

JEFFREY M. KOWALESKI

Always on Your Side: What All Patients Should Know about Palliative Care

Lindsey, a good friend of my wife, called me recently. Well, she called my wife ... but she really needed to talk to me. Lindsey is well-educated, well-read and quite health literate, but she was terrified because her oncologist referred her to palliative care for her breast cancer.

"I don't understand, Jeff. Am I dying?"

Her situation is not unique, unfortunately. Despite descriptions of palliative care in books like Dr. Atul Gawande's *Being Mortal* and Dr. Paul Kalanithi's *When Breath Becomes Air*, this medical specialty remains a black box to patients, families and, sometimes, even healthcare providers. What's worse is that it's a black box wrapped in taboo and stigma. Perhaps because of this mystery and fear, some institutions' palliative care groups don't even refer to themselves as such – "Supportive Oncology" is a common substitute – so a breast cancer patient with needs that an existing oncology team cannot manage might not even be aware that he or she is being referred to us.

It says a lot, I think, that my first task as a palliative care Fellow (a physician who is training in an area of specialization) was to learn how to explain my field to patients and families. Cardiologists don't have to do this. Neither do orthopedic surgeons, psychiatrists, dermatologists or most other specialists. Palliative care is inherently different, and people tend to fear us. Maybe every other week, a family stares at me blankly – and warily – after I introduce myself, my field and my role in their care, even when they obviously need my help.

I can't remember the exact words I used to explain palliative care to Lindsey, or to anyone else in her situation, but the gist is always the same:

- We're another layer of support for folks with serious illness – at any point in the course of their disease and treatment.
- We try to take care of everyone in the room, not just the patient.
- Sometimes we help people navigate the healthcare system and make decisions. Sometimes we help plan. Sometimes we help with difficult-to-control symptoms. But no matter what, we try to maximize quality of life.
- The palliative care team doesn't take over. We're another part of a patient's team, collaborating and coordinating to maximize the person's well-being.

To clarify these points further, I usually invite patients and families to watch a two-minute YouTube video, "Palliative Care: YOU Are a BRIDGE"[1] with me.

You'll notice that nowhere in my description are the words "end of life," "dying," or "hospice." I'm not intentionally avoiding those words; they just don't belong in my introduction to a service that people are often already nervous about. It is true that hospice and palliative care are related. The official medical specialty certification and physician fellowship training are called "Hospice and Palliative Medicine," and both hospice and palliative care utilize interdisciplinary teams to care for the "whole patient" – that is a person's physical, emotional, psychosocial and spiritual needs. Only when someone's disease progresses to the point where the goals of care become purely comfort-based do I refer my patients to hospice.

---

1 (<https://www.youtube.com/watch?v=IDHhg76tMHc> Accessed August 18, 2019)

How Palliative Care Works

In terminal illness such as metastatic breast cancer, it is **not** an "either/or" situation between standard medical care (primary goal = prolonging life) and Palliative Care (primary goal = maximizing quality of life):

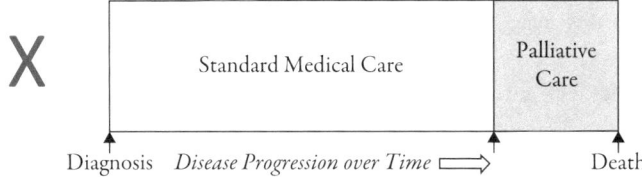

Rather, Palliative Care works alongside an oncology team as disease and symptom burden worsen, and, when the time is right, refers to Hospice (where Palliative Care may or not continue to follow):

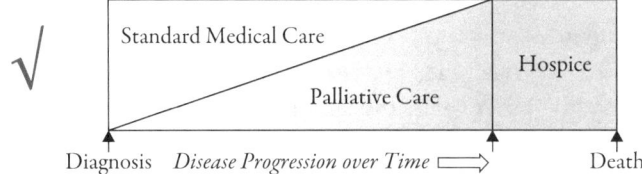

"This sounds great and all, Jeff, but I'm still not sure what it is you actually do ... or where."

Palliative care is primarily delivered in the hospital. That's where the crises occur, where patients face crippling emotional distress, where families may need to make a heart-breaking decision. Hospice, on the other hand, is rarely delivered in the hospital.

Let me give you an example. I recently helped take care of a Spanish-speaking woman in her 50s with triple-negative breast cancer, who had been referred to our team for an incredibly painful pathologic fracture (a break resulting from cancer having spread to the bones) of both her femur and pelvis. Maria was a complex patient to care for. She had received radiation therapy, the first-line option in this situation, but her terrible pain persisted. Her team then considered other potentially helpful interventions, including orthopedic surgery; but the specialists felt the risks outweighed the benefits. Thus, an aggressive pain medication regimen, my team's domain, was the only remaining option for her. But these, too, didn't help, and, in fact, likely contributed to the sleepiness and hallucinations she experienced. To make matters worse, Maria and her husband didn't understand – or were unable to confront – the bigger picture of her progressing cancer. Given her constant physical distress, it would be inappropriate for us, or any other team for that matter, to engage Maria and her husband in the existential issues at hand.

With some persuasion, the hospitalist and I were able to arrange for a pain-block procedure and a reevaluation for surgery. Mercifully, the block provided relief, and Maria finally slept. After she'd had some pain-free rest, I, armed with patience, a chair and a remote video interpreter, was able to dig deep. Exploring the person in front of me, I learned much about her life, her perspective on her disease, and her hopes moving forward. She very clearly understood the severity of her situation, but she was hopeful, praying for more time with her little grandkids. Family was the priority. Two weeks after my team first met this woman, I finally completed a comprehensive palliative care assessment. Our rapport-building discussion would pay dividends again and again as the course of her disease evolved.

> *"Geez, Jeff, I haven't been admitted, my cancer's not in my bones, and I just started new therapy. I still don't understand why my doc sent me to your clinic."*

Again, fair question. In the most basic sense, a physician refers a patient to palliative care because the patient has unmet needs or because the referring physician would like help with an aspect of patient care like Advance Care Planning. Referral allows establishment of a longitudinal relationship with our interdisciplinary team. Depending on the institution, a patient may meet with an RN, a social worker, and/or a chaplain in addition to her palliative care doctor. Together, and over time, we will help mediate breast cancer's impact on the emotional, social, and spiritual dimensions of life.

Furthermore, palliative care physicians regularly identify and address non-pain symptoms that often fly under the oncologist's radar. Insomnia, shortness of breath, constipation, lack of appetite, fatigue, nausea, anxiety and depression are all very common in people with cancer. Often, just being able to talk about these issues – let alone receive therapeutic relief – can be cathartic. I can't promise any given symptom will disappear, but I can promise that as a palliative care clinician I will listen to you, support you, and do everything I can to help you.

Let me tell you about another patient as a way to show what palliative care can look like. This second patient was an African-American woman in her late 40s. My team and I first met her in the hospital where she had been admitted with pain in her left breast, chest, and arm. I increased her long- and short-acting oral morphine regimen to allow her some relief from constant pain. A nine out of ten rating on a ten-point pain scale might not sound good to you or me, but to Roberta, this was a "blessing." Now "in the door" for opioid management, my interdisciplinary team went to work on the rest of her suffering.

Despite recently becoming unable to lift her arm, Roberta couldn't see that her disease was worsening, and she flatly did not believe she would die from cancer. Roberta was existentially stuck, and she was socially stuck, too. We never saw her husband, someone she described as "distancing himself" during her four-week-long admission. She had only her mom, and her mom had other family members to care for, too; plus, her mom lived five states away. Despite the fact that her family was not physically and/or emotionally able to care for her, Roberta adamantly insisted on being discharged home.

I can't imagine being in her situation ... but we tried. We – the social worker, chaplain and I – we sat with her. Our listening to her, patiently and without judgment, was critical. We explored her fears and her hopes and helped her process the distress and suffering that she was experiencing. And, working with her mother, who was acting health care power of attorney, we made the best post-hospital plan we could for Roberta, all the while respecting her autonomy. Even so, I didn't feel like we did enough for her. It didn't feel like I earned the "thank you" she always offered at the end of each encounter. I wish we – and by that I mean the entire healthcare system – could have done more for her.

"Man, Jeff, palliative care sounds like draining work, but it sounds like you really help people and their families. With everything you've told me, I feel like 'supportive oncology' might be a better name for your service."

Maybe so. "Supportive oncology" certainly carries less stigma than "palliative care." Furthermore, the term highlights our inclusion as part of a comprehensive cancer team and our primary role as supportive. Something said to a pediatric palliative care colleague is worth sharing here: "Palliative care is always on the side of the patient and family." This is a telling statement. In the hospital, in clinic, or on the phone, we provide empathy, validation, and guidance. It's not that surprising, then, that when something happens at home, many of our patients call us first, before calling the primary specialist (the oncologist, for instance) who is managing their condition, They are comfortable that we know what matters to them on a personal level. And they trust us.

GEORGE R. SIMMS

How Hospice Can Heal

I am a hospice physician. I care for patients for whom everything has been done, but to no lasting avail. Cure is no longer possible. They have all fought the good fight and are in the last stage of their journey. What they need now is comfort, care and closure.

I consider it a privilege to care for dying patients. As grim as it appears, walking with men, women and children through the valley of the shadow of death has been the most fulfilling part of my professional career. When a patient knows she has only a limited time to live, everything changes. Life is now defined by two realities: (1) Nothing more can be done to alter the course of her disease, and (2) the moment will soon come when she will be separated from those she loves. Faced with this reality, she must chart a new course. For this she will need help.

Over the years I have developed a philosophy that I discuss with every patient. First, there are no curative "fixes" left. It is what it is, and we are where we are. Second, there is a lot we can do together to make life bearable – and hopefully meaningful. And third, I can alleviate your pain and other distressing symptoms, which will hopefully free you up to explore what you would like to do in this last chapter of your life. I am persuaded that this last stage in your journey – as painful as it is physically, emotionally and spiritually – can be the most fruitful time of your life.

Helen was referred to me by her oncologist with a diagnosis of metastatic breast cancer. She was 52 years old and had been on chemotherapy for two years. Despite a positive initial response, the treatment was no longer working and she was getting worse. Reluctantly the oncologist felt it was time for hospice. By the time Helen and her husband, Ken, got to my office, anger, fear and desperation had set in. I saw fear in Ken's eyes and despair in Helen's. They were an intelligent, happily married couple who never thought such devastation would befall them. They had worked hard, played by the rules and deeply resented their fate. Ken was angry with God and feared the unknown. Helen said she was resigned to her fate, but admitted that she felt God had betrayed her. Looking in her eyes, I thought of a line from Hamlet: "A countenance more in sorrow than in anger."

Hospice is not a one-man show. In addition to my role as medical director, there is a team of trained professionals – social workers, nurses, chaplains, therapists, nutritionists – all capable of meeting the various needs of the patient and family. And so it was that a series of family conferences was set up with Helen and Ken to chart a course that would best meet their needs. Helen's metastatic bone pain was a major hurdle to overcome. But over the next several days and weeks, with a regimen of various narcotic and non-narcotic pain medications, she began to feel better and was able to begin the arduous journey of looking back on her life and deciding what she needed to bring closure to.

The concept of "looking back" is what we call a Life Review. It is a slow, gentle review of each stage of one's life to identify what and to whom one needs to bring closure. We all carry baggage from the past – some of it positive, some of it negative. Some memories are precious and need to be remembered as highlights of our journey. Others are painful and bring us a grief that sometimes persists and becomes an unbearable burden. At the end of life, one needs to draw up a balance sheet of unresolved conflicts and, where possible, find ways to bring closure in order to die in peace. For Helen, the battle was not with Ken, but with God. She had been raised in a conservative faith tradition that taught that God would reward those who were obedient and punish those who weren't. If evil befell you, it was probably your fault. Cancer was evil and hence a godly punishment. Helen's problem was that she was befallen by a form of "punishment" she felt she didn't deserve – hence her despair and sense of betrayal.

Ken was not filled with despair. He was filled with anger and fear. Anger at God for taking his wife, and fear of having to raise their two teenage daughters by himself and to begin life as a widower.

Over the next few months Helen felt much better – so much so that she and Ken contemplated taking a trip to Yellowstone National Park. Each year they had celebrated their anniversary by going to Yellowstone, and they very much wanted to do this one last time. Arrangements were made amidst great excitement. But five days before their departure, Helen suddenly lost movement in both legs. The cancer had spread to her spine, causing compression of the spinal cord and paralysis of her legs. Radiation therapy was begun; it reduced the pain, but she never regained the full use of her legs. This was a bitter disappointment and set the stage for a rapid decline in her condition. The cancer quickly invaded her vital organs, and she required more pain medication, which made it difficult for her to stay awake. Yet there was something different about her response to this devastating turn of events. Something had softened inside her. Her eyes had lost their pain and sadness, and it was almost as if she had moved from resignation to acceptance. Still, somehow she couldn't let go.

Ken could not let Helen go. He had been a fighter all his life. Fighting to the bitter end was the only way he knew how to live. He had been raised in poverty and learned early on that fighting was the only way to survive. It was this fighting instinct that made him a successful businessman, a stern but loving father, and a devoted husband.

One morning as Helen lay only partly conscious, I took Ken aside and told him that his beloved was afraid to leave him by himself, and that was why she was suffering. I told Ken that because he loved her so deeply, the best gift he could give her would be to release her from her suffering. As painful as this would be for him, this would be his supreme sacrifice of love for Helen. Ken wept, but he went to her bedside, leaned in closely, put his arms around her, told her how much he loved her and gave her permission to leave him. He whispered that he would always miss her, but that he'd be okay. Within five minutes Helen stopped breathing.

This is the mission of hospice: to walk with our patients (and their families) through the valley of the shadow of death. It is a dark and lonely path from which there is no return – and, to be sure, some people do not reach the kind of acceptance that Helen and Ken experienced, despite the earnest efforts of a hospice team. Yet we strive to make the burden lighter for every person. For Helen and Ken the way was made easier. Though we could not cure her cancer, we were able to make their last weeks and months together bearable – and in a mysterious way, blessed. To die in peace, dignity and love is to die a good death.

MARK L. HUNNICUTT

A Steward of Suffering: One Man's Story of Breast Cancer

An interview with Mark Hunnicutt

K: Hey, Mark!

M: Hey, Kimberly. How are you doing?

K: I am just fine. How are you?

M: I'm great, doing great.

K: Good! Mark, just to be clear, I just want to make sure that you're okay that I'm recording this.

M: Oh, yeah, sure. Definitely!

K: Okay! Your piece in this book is going to be unique on a lot of levels. Uh, you're the only patient who is male who's talking about this. I can't even begin to tell you how important that's going to be for the readers. Thank you so much.

M: You're welcome.

K: You also have a distinct perspective as a minister. There is spirituality elsewhere in the book but not as foregrounded as yours, so I think that's super important. I was also thinking it would be so neat if we could use the transcription of our conversation as the essay. What do you think?

M: Oh, yeah, yeah. Definitely. Yes.

K: I think that would be cool for the readers to feel as though they're listening to a conversation, which is different from reading an essay. This would also be a unique dimension to the book.

M: Yeah, I'm perfectly fine with that. That'd be great.

K: Okay! Well, just in general are you doing, are you doing okay? Is your medicine still working?

M: Yes. Doing great, feeling really good.

K: Good! I don't know how anybody manages to feel great in this heat, but I'm so glad that you are. [both laugh]

M: Yes, Ma'am.

K: So, um, Mark, how did it feel to you to be diagnosed with a disease that most often occurs in women?

M: Um, almost comical.

K: Hmm.

M: So like, like "Really, God?"

K: Yeah ...

M: It seems to be that in my life, a Hollywood script writer couldn't write a script, you know, that would .... It just seems, uh, foreign and far-fetched. So, you know, you just have to sit back and kind of grin.

K: Yeah, can you talk a little bit more about that – like if it were a script, it would be far-fetched. Can you give me kind of an overview of how it happened and what -

M: Yeah, you know, being involved in – so I had leukemia as a kid, and then I started helping people, uh, through diagnosis and through tragedy and, uh, 'cause I had a big spirit of empathy and was able to do that, you know, as a survivor.

K: Yeah –

M: – you know, as a cancer veteran.

K: Yeah.

M: And then, uh, you know, some years later, was diagnosed with male breast cancer, and it was like, "Wait a minute, God, I'm the one that *helps* people with diagnoses. I'm not the one that gets this diagnosis again."

K: Yeah ...

M: So I'm like, "This is my second time. If you'd like to be a little more – uh, spread it out a little more – I'm fine with that. I don't want to be selfish!"

K: [laughs] Yeah.

M: And then, uh, the diagnosis was male breast cancer. And I'm not trying to be cute or, you know, crass here, but my wife asked me, said, "Would you rather have testicular cancer or breast cancer?" And I said testicular cancer. You know that's totally male. The breast cancer seems to be more female. And, um, the reactions I get when I say I have breast cancer .... you know, it's uh, it's a platform to tell my story because people lean in, people go "Really?"

K: Yeah.

M: And they tend to listen more.

K: Why did you feel that it would have been better for you to have testicular cancer? I mean, I understand that, but what – how – can you help me understand?

M: Yeah, as a man – you know, breast cancer is a woman's world.

K: Yeah.

M: And, you know, when I went to my breast care navigator,[1] uh, it was a girl that was actually at our wedding ceremony; she's a kid in my church. And that was totally a God thing: I walk in there, and she's the one who's going to walk me through this.

K: Wow.

M: And anatomically correct. You know pictures of women and breast cancer. [laughs] This picture – one side of the body you get to see through with all the veins, and the other side was just

---

1 Please see Lynn Fantom's discussion of her role as nurse navigator in "A Step-by-Step Guide through Breast Cancer Diagnosis and Radiation" elsewhere in this book.

the outside. And, um, you know, she goes, "I'm sorry we don't have a man to, um, show you." The breast cancer center, you know, it had women's pictures with their testimonies and their ads were pink and everything.

I remember going in for a mammogram and there's three women sitting there with little smocks on, waiting their turn. And I go in there and sit down, and there's an elderly lady in my church, and she leaned – she looked over at me and she goes, "Hey, Pastor Mark!" [laughs] "Hello! What are you here for?"

And I said, "I'm getting a mammogram."

And she's all "What?!"

So, yeah, it's a woman's world. So every October, when it's Breast Cancer Awareness month, I mean by the end of the month, I've spoken at so many Relay for Life rallies and women's groups and red hats societies, I feel like at the end of that month I need to get a four-wheel drive and chew some tobacco and shoot a shotgun."

[both laugh]

K: That's great! And then here I come, asking you to do it once again for a book!

M: Which is fine, I mean which is totally fine. That's what I'm ... I mean, you and me probably wouldn't be talking if I had testicular cancer.

K: Yeah, that's, yeah, that's true. It is.

M: One of my favorite things is, uh, at women's rallies for breast cancer. They, um, the organizers usually don't tell them they're having a male come speaking about survivorship for breast cancer. So I get up there, and I say, "I bet you're wondering what I'm doing here." And then I say that I was diagnosed with male breast cancer, and I pause, and I say, "Ladies, my eyes up here. Look up here!" [both laugh] It kind of, it breaks the ice.

K: Yeah, you know isn't that funny? Um, I mean, I can't imagine it from your perspective, but I do know that whenever I tell somebody I've had breast cancer, the first thing they do is look at my chest [laughs], and I really want to say kind of what you said. I really want to say, "Okay, just go ahead. Look at my chest. I know you're doing it, and you know you want to do it. I'll just stand here." You know, it's, I think it's awkward for everybody.

You know, I really, I've never heard, Mark, anybody use the term "cancer veteran," and I like that so much. I kind of like that a lot better than "survivor." It just – yeah.

M: Right.

K: Well, uh, could I ask what your symptoms were and how you were diagnosed?

M: I was, uh, just going hard, doing ministry and caring for people, and I got a lump on my right chest. It felt like a bone spur – really hard.

K: Yeah.

M: Nipples a little abnormal, right one a little different than my left one. And I noticed it about six weeks before I actually went to the doctor. You know, the last thing on my mind was that it was breast cancer.

K: Sure.

M: Um, so when I went to the doctor, there was no pain, there was – it was just that, that lump. And, um, he looked at that and he said, "Hmm." He said, "I'm going to refer you to a surgical oncologist, um, to get a biopsy of this to see what it is." And I said, "What, what do you think it is?" And he said, "I – I'm not sure, you know."

K: Yeah.

M: So when I went to the oncologist, he was a little more, you know, gave me that kind of look. You know, they don't tell you anything before it comes back. So he said, "It does look suspicious. Uh, you know, it may or may not be cancer." And so then I had my surgical biopsy on Thursday, and then I got on a plane to go to Africa Sunday.

K: Oh. Wow.

M: I was on the mission field, serving, uh, Kiringa, Uganda, and I finally got through to him- he got through to me. The cell service there was a little wonky. It was a Thursday, and we just got back from serving and caring for people and were kind of getting ready for supper, and he finally called – finally got through – and said, "Yeah, it's invasive ductal carcinoma." And my, my wife and I are like "Ah. Okay," you know. And then [he said], "Hey, I'll call you back tomorrow with the protocol – some options, what's going on." So we went from there.

K: Wow. How did it feel, Mark, being so far away from normal life and getting that news when you, you know, kind of untethered from everything you knew?

M: It could not have been in a better place. Because, um, I think with suffering, any kind of suffering with bad news, your tendency is to turn inward and to think of yourself and how's this going to affect me and is it gonna hurt? And we were on the mission field, and so we had a schedule, you know, get up that day and help people, and so I just kept that schedule. You know, and so it helped me focus, get things in the right perspective. And, um, I honestly don't think it could have happened in a better place. If I'd have been here [home], I think people would have – it would have been a little more pity, you know, "Oops, I'm sorry," you know, and those, those brain pathways that were created early – that hey, I'm going to serve through this, I'm gonna encourage people through this. And, uh, the Bible says in the book of Proverbs, "He that wants to be refreshed, needs to refresh others." And a lot of time when we get diagnosed we turn inwards. We forget about other people, and we wonder why we're so sorrowful. I mean, there's so much grief and depression. And you know, hey, get your head up. It's not over, you know. It's not over. If you're still breathing, I mean, if your heart's still beating, you still got a purpose.

K: Yeah.

M: So, yeah you still got a purpose.

Steward of Suffering: One Man's Story of Breast Cancer

K: Yeah, that, that is, um, wow, that is powerful. And that's been my experience too, by the way. I – but I've never heard anybody talk about it the way you just did, Mark, that when you get something like that, you tend to turn inward but, yeah. Absolutely. And I think you're right. One of the things I've noticed in, you know, just talking with other people with breast cancer is that a lot of us really, really want to do something with this lousy thing that we've been given. And that's the, that's the absolute reason for this book.

M: Right.

K: You know, it's just do *something* with this and keep serving.

M: And see, society doesn't want to talk about disease. They don't want to talk about death. And the only thing – the world's getting more divided, and the world's getting more – there's different narratives. But we all have something in common, every single person, every single language, every single country: We all are gonna face tragedy, we're all gonna face trials, and eventually *every*body is gonna face death.

K: Yeah.

M: And it's the one thing we *should* be talking about. I think it would unite us, but we, we don't talk about it.

K: Yeah.

M: And especially – it's just amazing to me that it's coming. There's no doubt it's coming, but we don't want to talk about it.

K: Yeah.

M: But talking about it is healthy.

K: Yeah, I do too, and did you find – I've never been to Africa, um, did you find – this is kind of off the path, but I'm just interested in your story here – that people in Africa are more able to talk about death and are more receptive?

M: Yes. They are because it happens more frequently. It happens to younger people. And they – it's a part of life, like, um, like a birthday or like an anniversary, or, um, there's more normalcy to it. So they do talk about it.

K: Yeah.

M: And they don't name – the part of Africa that we were in, they don't name their kids till they're two because the infant mortality rate is so high. So on the second birthday, they'll give the kid a name because they guess they're gonna make it. You know, they don't grieve like we grieve. It's, uh, kind of beautiful, really. It sounds kind of morbid, but I get it: It's a part of life.

K: Yeah, I don't think that's morbid at all. I can understand exactly what you mean. Part of the stuff that I do is with advance care planning and, um, people are terrified to even hear that term. And for me it's just practical. Like why wouldn't you want to plan?

M: Right. Yeah.

K: Um, did you find it harder to get information about male breast cancer or about just cancer in general because you are a man?

M: You know, I thought I would, but I found out – so of course you know this too – but breast cancer, when you've got one case, you've got one case.

K: Absolutely.

M: I mean, it can be the same diagnosis, but the way it's – all the idiosyncrasies of the diagnosis, where it came from, and even how people handle it, uh, is just different. But there's not much difference between men and women when it comes to the diagnosis.

K: Uh huh.

M: So I got a lot – I called them my Soul Sisters. I couldn't find a man that had breast cancer, so there's about three ladies that just rallied around me and just, uh, just helped me with the basics, with nausea – how to deal with nausea, how to deal with constipation.

K: Yeah.

M: How to deal with the thought-life, how to deal with a lot of things. So they were my Soul Sisters. And what I say to people is "I got some Soul Sisters, I got a song, and I got some scripture." And between those three things, I would always rely on those.

K: How wonderful! What do you mean by your "song"? Is it your story? Is that –

M: No, I just – there's two or three songs that meant a lot to me. Music, you know, changes everything.

K: Yeah! What were they, Mark?

M: Uh, there was one in particular that was, uh, oh my goodness. I'll have to find it and send it to you. I can't believe I can't remember the song! I was flying over the Rift Valley in a plane and it came on, and it was, uh – golly bum. Man alive! [both laugh]

K: It's okay. [both laugh]

M: But that's – then another song would come. So I'd rotate between those three things when I started feeling bad … "Even when my life is spinning, you're the rock I stand on …". I'll have to find it for you.

K: Okay. That's amazing. You were flying over the *where* when you heard it?

M: The Rift Valley, between Uganda and Kenya. It's just a beautiful rift in the earth and it's cool thing.

K: Wow. Um, so you said the surgeon told you it was ductal carcinoma. Was it *in situ* or was it, uh –

M: Invasive.

K: Yeah, so that was my diagnosis too.

M: Okay.

K: But when I heard that, I thought oh my gosh, that means it's spread. And of course it *doesn't* mean that, but that's one of the things, even kind of being in a medical environment, that language can really mess you up. Um …

M: Uh huh.

K: Did you, did you go, uh, did they stage it?

M: Yes. It was Stage 2 and when they did a lymph node dissection, it had spread to my lymph nodes so it became Stage 3 B.

K: Okay.

M: Then I had a mastectomy and then some time later I had a lymph node dissection. They removed all the lymph nodes from my right arm.

K: Wow, and and, um, actually when I was at your church I saw you have the compression sleeve.

M: Yes, Ma'am.

K: Yeah, um ...

M: That's my [?]. [laughs]

K: [laughs] That's your what? [both laugh]

M: My friend.

K: Oh, your friend!

M: Yeah. [both laugh]

K: Did you – so you had the surgery. Did you have chemotherapy or radiation?

M: Um hmm. I had sixteen weeks of chemotherapy and six weeks of radiation.

K: Wow. What was that like? I'm not going to keep you on the phone forever, Mark, but I'm just fascinated –

M: No, you're fine. You're fine .... Um, chemo was, um, was hell. I mean, it was, it was bad.

K: Yeah.

M: And that's what I try to tell people. 'Cause I'm a, I'm a realist. I'm very optimistic about life, but I'm also a realist. I think if you go into it knowing what you're facing – don't lie to people. It's – I mean, chemo is a little better than it used to be. But still it just plays with your mind.

K: Yes.

M: It causes fatigue. And fatigue, if you've never experienced it, it doesn't matter how much you nap.

K: Absolutely.

M: You're still fatigued when you wake up.

K: Yeah.

M: You know, so you know, all the little nuances of how to deal with nausea. Some people don't get nausea with the same chemo, same protocol but they don't get nauseated. Some people get extremely nauseated. Some people have a large reaction to it. It's just you gotta be ready.

K: Yeah. Did you have any one thing or two things that happened that were kind of unexpected?

M: Yeah, so the Neulasta®. So I had leukemia, like I said, when I was younger. So they didn't want to see that repeat itself. So they did a lot to try to protect my bone marrow. So the Neulasta was a way they did that. It makes your bones ache really bad. So I kind of expected nausea because I had leukemia before and had radiation and chemo. But the Neulasta: There's really, there's really nothing like a bone ache. It's like a headache that's different throughout your whole body. It's kind of weird.

K: Yeah, I had Neulasta and was fortunate in the sense that the only place I really ached a lot was my lower back. But I couldn't really walk very much. It was a whammy.

M: Yeah.

K: What was – I did not have radiation. What was radiation like?

M: Easier than chemo. It was grinding, though 'cause you went the same time every day five days a week for six weeks.

K: [groan]

M: [chuckles] So I guess I would tell people to spread it around. It's easier for them to say Tuesday at 10 – you know, every day at 10, Monday, Wednesday through Friday. I'd spread it around some so it's not so ... It's like Groundhog Day. I mean, it just got ...

it's grueling, and then you're fatigued. So I, I'd do one in the morning, one in the evening, you know. That kind of thing. It's harder to plan that way, but I would spend some time on the front end trying to plan that than trying to do the same time every day.

K: Uh huh.

M: [chuckles] And it takes longer to drive there and get prepped than it does to get the radiation. Then you put your clothes back on and say, "What just happened?"

K: Yeah. Well, can you speak a little about how this impacted your work and your family and your social life? I mean, I didn't have a social life at that point. I just, I just didn't have any energy. Did you find that to be the case, or …

M: Yeah, it just affected … You know, some days, um, I didn't feel like … I'm a pretty good … So I would give myself a day. You know, I'd look to feel miserable for a day. If I didn't feel like being around people, if I was irritable, okay, today I'm not gonna be around people. And I would say, "Tomorrow, I'm going here. I'm doing this no matter how I feel." Because you're not hurting your body. You know, the Neulasta, the pain in your legs – if you get up and move, you're not causing long-term hurt. It hurt – it hurts you but you're not causing that, so … So some days I'd do a day and try to be home the next day, and then the next day I'd say, "Okay, I'm going to get up and there's going to be another day." And I'm going to get up the next day. So I wouldn't, I wouldn't try to say, "I feel bad" and I'd just say, "Well, I'd feel bad forever." You know, so I'd say, "I'm going to give myself today, and I'm going to close the door. Nobody bothering me. Cut the phone off. But tomorrow, I'm going to try to get back in the – in the picture." So we made no plans. So without any plans there wasn't any pressure about making it or not making it. We were kind of more impromptu – when I say "we," my wife and I …

K: Yeah.

Steward of Suffering: One Man's Story of Breast Cancer

M: ... if we were there. So workwise, they'd say, "Do what you need to do; we got it," which I'm eternally grateful for.

K: Absolutely.

M: And family, same deal. Um, you know, they'd come by and if I didn't want to see them, Cheryl would tell them, "Hey, thanks for coming by, but he's in there pouting."

K: [laughs]

M: ... and he's closed the door today ...

K: Yeah.

M: And some days I'd greet them in the driveway. We'd go for drives and other things.

K: That's great. Um, do you have kids, Mark?

M: No Ma'am. We have three cats!

K: Well, we have two!

[both laugh]

M: Great!

K: I don't have kids either, and you know, that – I'm really glad for that, actually, at this point because, um, I don't know if you were offered it, but I was offered genetic counseling and I said, "Well, why would I even need genetic counseling ...

M: ... Right

K: ... 'cause I don't have any kids, and I'm – I'm glad to know that I don't run the risk of passing that gene on, you know?

M: Yeah.

K: Yeah. Um, well I guess just my last thing is, is there anything else that you think might help somebody? You've just been a gold mine. Like I'm so excited that this is recorded because there are so many nuggets of pure gold in here that I, I wouldn't have missed it ...

M: ... thank you ...

K: ...like the three Ss: the Soul Sisters, the song and the scriptures. You know, just these things, I'm just smiling right now.... So in that vein, do you think anything else that you might have as a perspective to help people either physically or mentally? I know the spiritual part you've written about already, um ... What other thoughts do you have?

M: Yeah, the real thing is that, uh, negative thoughts, it'll flood you if you let it, so that's what I mean by try to stick to a routine, try to tell yourself who you are. So what I try to do just in life is, okay, I'm not going to base a thought on the last two months or the next two months. Because you know, we all go through valleys and hard times and trials and, I mean, look at the Big Picture. Back up and look and see yourself the way God does and the way people that love you do. And I'd say a negative thought would be anything contrary to that. So it may be different for other people, but don't see yourself – don't paint the picture of yourself that's contrary to what God sees you as, what your people that love you see you as.

K: Yeah.

M: And walk in that picture. Don't walk in the past that "Oh gosh I'm depressed. I'm not gonna to make it. I'm ugly. I've lost my hair." You know, see yourself the way God sees you and other people see you.

K: Yeah.

M: And you know, we tend to isolate ourselves, and that's the most dangerous thing you can do. And there are several people that I've talked to who didn't want anybody to know. Their spouse knows, but they don't want their kids to know or anybody else to know. And I would just caution against that *big time*. That's dangerous. Isolating yourself is dangerous.

K: Yeah.

M: So Africa again. A lion picks off the wildebeest that's isolated. [chuckles] You're lion meat.

K: Yeah, yeah.

M: Get in the middle of the herd!

K: And you know, it adds so much to your suffering to have to lie – you know, "cover" all the time, you know?

M: Right.

K: Oh, Mark, thank you so much for this. This is just wonderful. Oh, and just one more last question, I promise. Where do you see your life going right now after this whole thing? The reason I ask that is that I think after you come face to face with your mortality, it has to change you.

M: Right.

K: So how do you construe that? That's an existential question, I guess.

M: Well, yeah. One in four people – the latest statistic, I don't know where I read it – one in four people will face cancer of some sort, some time. Three in four people will have someone in their family or a close loved one that faces it. So I want to steward my suffering well, and I want to use it as a platform to say, "Hey, you're not a statistic. This disease doesn't define you. Um, and the Bible says – I think it's Second Corinthians 1:4 – we have been cared for so that we can care for others.

K: Wow.

M: So my medical team, my family, my friends really did a good job caring for me, and so I want to spend the rest of my life equipping people, one in four people that will be diagnosed with cancer and the three in four that will be caregivers – you know, how do you do that well? How do you do that well? And so, I've just spent my life doing that ... and it seems to, you know, I'll get emotional when I read your story and what you wrote down that will be in a book because you don't think about that when you're laying there getting chemo ... [chuckles]

K: Absolutely, yeah.

M: But "God, I wouldn't volunteer for this, but if You want to set me up to have a platform to where I can teach and care ... and maybe something I say can encourage someone else, you know, for a day, then so be it. So be it."

K: Wow. "A steward of suffering." That is just profound. In fact, that might be – that might be a great title for your essay.

M: Yeah!

K: What do you think?!

M: That's good [laughs] that's good.

K: Okay, Mark, again, many, many thanks for your time ... God bless you. Bye-bye!

M: God bless you.

PART II

Enhancing Your Health by Honoring Your Self

MICHAEL HAYES

Our Many Teachers: Wisdom for Psychological Health during Breast Cancer

Pausing, Nancy glanced away. Curious, I wondered what might surface next. Moments later she looked back at me and said, "You know, life is terminal." Wow, after twenty-eight years of practice as a clinical psychologist, another pearl of wisdom was offered up in a private moment between me and a patient in the midst of treatment for advanced breast cancer. Like many others throughout my career, she taught me a valuable lesson. One that I could not have asked for or anticipated. One, like so many others, that surfaces during a human-to-human encounter where I am called to be in a place of awareness, fully open to listen and to see deeply into the truth of another's direct, lived experience. In so many ways it is a sacred opportunity to simply be present and to serve others in a time of need.

A beloved and wise mentor, Dr. Barbara de Lateur, shared a quotation attributed to the Buddha: "*Those who need to learn patience are sent many teachers; those who have patience are sent very few.*" The wisdom conveyed here is manifest in my experience serving those diagnosed with cancer. Each of us has much to learn. When we are able to view what "is" through the prism of the Buddha's wisdom, being diagnosed and treated for breast cancer can be experienced, in a certain way, as one of our many teachers – as an opportunity to learn and grow. This truth surfaces time and again with each patient who becomes my teacher.

Imagining what might have led you to this book, I turn now to share a few of the many lessons offered and received, lessons that illuminate with awe and wonder what appears as the realities of breast cancer. Life, death, and all that lies in between are laid bare.

Tuning In to How You Think

Bonnie: A few months before she was diagnosed with breast cancer, Bonnie took the plunge and bought herself a recumbent bicycle – something important she had wanted to do for herself for quite some time. However, in the wake of diagnosis and treatment, Bonnie's dreams of riding this bicycle faded and disappeared as dealing with breast cancer gave rise to a period of significant depression. Bonnie stopped doing many of the things that had previously been important to her, including taking care of her house and going out with friends for lunch or to shop.

I proposed to Bonnie that we work together using cognitive-behavioral therapy (CBT), an evidence-based form of psychotherapy that focuses on the role of automatic thoughts, expectations, and core beliefs in shaping how one reacts or responds to events as they unfold in one's life. One of our early treatment goals was to demystify the cognitive-behavioral model through psychoeducation – in effect, pulling back the velvet curtain for Bonnie to see and understand the basic elements of the cognitive model and how CBT works. I used the white board positioned on my office wall to illustrate the model and its core components, and together, we rolled up our sleeves to tackle her depression over the course of several months.

One day along the way Bonnie said, "You know, this stinkin' thinkin' is the pits." I wasn't quite certain I had heard her correctly and asked, "What did you just say?" She responded, "You know, the dark, negative thoughts that get me down. It's stinkin' thinkin'." In thinking about how she'd been thinking, Bonnie had identified a major pitfall for herself. Just like the ability of a bunch of rotten eggs to sour one's stomach, stinkin' thinkin' tends to lead the mind and body down the rabbit hole into a pit of depression.

By way of example, a prominent thought that kept surfacing as Bonnie described her experience of depression was "I can't." Pausing, I reflected, "Hmm, I notice a particular thought keeps coming up again and again when you talk about feeling depressed. I'm curious if you notice it too." Bonnie looked at me with a puzzled expression and said, "What thought is that?" I responded, "Can't." Bonnie probed, "What do you mean?" and

I replied, "I wonder if it is true – actually true – when you tell yourself, 'I can't.' " In her own defense, Bonnie asserted that it felt that way, and this insight led to our carefully investigating the interrelationships among her thoughts, feelings, and actions (or inaction), looking for concrete evidence to either support or challenge the veracity of specific thoughts and feelings that were fueling depression. At a certain point Bonnie pointed out, "You know, I didn't realize I was telling myself – really convincing myself – some things that were not really true at all. Well, what do you know?!"

Bit by bit, Bonnie began to chip away at her stinkin' thoughts. At the same time, we worked to effect small, successive increments of change in her behavior, such as clearing her sink of dirty dishes and relocating her bicycle from the covered porch into her living room, then just simply sitting on her bicycle once each day. Gradually Bonnie displayed growing motivation to actually ride her bicycle, and eventually she shared, smiling widely, that she took her first short ride in the driveway. Much like Dory in *Finding Nemo*, I cheered Bonnie on: "Just keep pedaling!"

Asking for Help

Kitty: As I sat across from Kitty following her diagnosis, she described a life dedicated to taking care of her husband, daughter and grandson, as well as having, out of financial necessity, to work into what she imagined would be her retirement years. She came across as someone with boundless energy, yet I gathered that at the end of each day there was little, if any, left in the tank for Kitty to give to herself. She commented that the surgeon told her that she would not be able to drive or lift more than five pounds for a period of time following surgery, and then she looked at me and asked, "How does he think I'm going to be able to do that?" She was serious. She was the chief doer and sole helper in her world. Her husband was in ill health and spent most of his day sitting in the recliner due to chronic, poorly managed pain. His auto garage, which they had hoped might secure a comfortable retirement, failed to be a success.

I gathered Kitty harbored feelings of resentment toward her husband as a result of not pulling his weight financially and, therefore, leaving them in a position where they simply could not afford for her to no longer work. Their daughter and her son, whom Kitty adored, lived with Kitty and her husband. The daughter was employed full-time in a local health system, which often required working beyond the normal workday; and the grandson was in high school and attended the local vocational-tech program. It was a busy life.

As the pieces of her life circumstances came into focus, I said to Kitty, "You know, it's okay to ask for help." The expression of incredulity on Kitty's face said it all ... as if I were an alien creature with twelve heads. She responded in a matter-of-fact manner, "I've never asked anybody for help. I just don't do that." I wasn't inclined to roll over and play dead; instead, I poked and prodded a bit further, thinking surely there was a time or occasion where she had asked someone for help. Nope. Not a one. Quite literally, Kitty could not recall a single instance when she'd asked someone for help. That said, she did confess that her neighbor, a lovely young woman, had asked her on a few occasions whether Kitty might like anything from the grocery store. Kitty informed me she had always said no, even if there might have been something she needed from the store. I pushed back, asserting it is okay to ask for help and adding that following surgery to remove the cancerous growth in her breast it would be necessary for her to have help. I went so far as to suggest that Kitty needed a button proclaiming, "It's Okay to Ask for Help!" Then, I had a bunch of them made with the attribution, "inspired by Kitty."

Kitty accepted the button and, following surgery, for the first time in her life, accepted her neighbor's offer of assistance. The next time we met, she described this happening and said, "Ya know, it actually felt kind of good. I always thought I'd feel bad, but that wasn't the case. And I think she felt good too. She seemed really happy to help me." We celebrated this new learning, and Kitty became a true advocate for allowing others to help. On occasion she'd comment with pride about meeting someone who was wearing one of her buttons, beaming from ear to ear. For me, Kitty symbolizes the ways in which so many women have been socialized as caregivers – often at their own expense. They give and give to others, and in the process, they tend to neglect their own wants and needs in service of ensuring that everyone else's needs are met. Over time, this pattern of selflessness can lead women to feel physically and emotionally bankrupt and perhaps more susceptible to falling ill.

As Kitty recovered from breast surgery and completed daily radiation therapy over the course of six weeks, her supervisor at the deli went on medical leave. The store manager approached Kitty, asking if she'd be willing to cover while the deli manager was out. Characteristically, Kitty said she'd take on the added responsibility even though she privately confessed to me that she didn't want to do it. She simply felt that saying no was not an option. This heralded an opportunity for me to say, "You know, it's okay to say no." This time around, Kitty simply grinned and said, "But I never say no." What she really meant was that in her mind saying no is not an option. With a wry smile, I said to Kitty that she needed another button – one that said, "It's Okay to Say NO!" And so I had a second batch of buttons made, once again with the attribution, "inspired by Kitty." As with asking for help, Kitty would find it an uphill battle to marshal the courage to say no when doing so would be wise and in her best interests. Eventually, and with a fair amount of support, Kitty did, though. She was clearly outside her comfort zone, yet – it was equally clear – she gained something in the process of saying no that came as a complete surprise. She recognized a budding sense of self and self-worth in honoring a personal limit – something that was totally foreign to her prior life experience. It felt good. And while saying no continued to feel unnatural, I witnessed Kitty gain confidence in doing so when it was called for.

Knowing What Matters Most

Lydia: Seated across from me next to the arm of the sofa, Lydia was in her mid-70s and appeared quite fit. She had recently been diagnosed with an early-stage breast cancer. Her surgeon met with her and her husband, a long-tenured engineering professor, to review her diagnosis and outline the recommended treatment plan: lumpectomy followed by radiation and possibly chemotherapy, depending on whether there was any lymph node involvement. She mentioned that her surgeon and husband were both in agreement that she should simply begin the process. I sensed some hesitancy in her voice and caught a flash of emotion in the corner of her eye. I paused, then asked, "But what do you think?" Lydia responded, "That doesn't seem to really matter. They both think it's the right thing to do." I wasn't convinced. In fact, I had a feeling there was a great deal more to this story. I said, "I care about what you think and how you feel about what's being proposed. And I'm hoping that in here we can focus on what matters most to you."

Lydia proceeded to share that she was most concerned about whether she would be able to continue to play tennis. I came to understand that playing tennis was not simply a pastime for her; rather, playing tennis was core to Lydia's identity and something that provided her with a sense of purpose and meaning. As it turns out, she had been playing tennis regularly – nearly daily and sometimes two to three times a day for more than thirty years! Life without tennis was unimaginable, and she feared that undergoing surgery might sideline her permanently. Further, she added, "My mother is 104 years old, and I don't want to live to be that old." She was a faithful daughter, and visiting her mother at the nursing home several times each week brought her face-to-face with the sobering reality of one's inevitable physical decline with advancing age. She was clear in asserting that she didn't want any part of that, which, in turn, appeared to steel her conviction to play on as long as she possibly could.

When I asked what her surgeon and husband said in response to her concern about the impact breast surgery might have on her ability to play tennis, she indicated they didn't seem really interested, didn't seem to hear her concern. To her, they seemed intent on scheduling surgery to get it over with as quickly as possible. Given her diagnosis with an early-stage cancer, I suggested that there might be time to step back and make space to ensure her thoughts, feelings, values and priorities were given full consideration before moving ahead. Prior to that moment, it was as if Lydia had been invisible. Being seen. Being heard. Making an effort to honor and respect her and her wishes was a game-changer. She gave me permission to speak with her surgeon and to advocate for a brief pause so that she could weigh her options. Also, Lydia wanted him and her husband to understand that an ability to play tennis would impact her quality of life significantly.

Her surgeon had absolutely no idea how central tennis was in Lydia's life. Waiting a week or two would likely make no difference in either the risks or outcomes of surgery, and he was fully supportive of her wish to delay surgery until she was ready. A week later Lydia decided to go ahead. She underwent lumpectomy on Friday, and on the following Monday, she was back on the court playing tennis with her doubles partner. (Of note, knowing when it's okay to return to normal activities, including sports, is an important consideration each patient should discuss with her doctor before resuming such activities.) Lydia remarked that serving was a bit tricky and that she therefore had to serve underhanded for a week or two while her incision was healing. Weeks later, Lydia shared with me that her medical oncologist was awestruck by her ability to tolerate chemotherapy with few side effects. With a wry grin, she remarked, "He doesn't know I'm a serious athlete. Apparently, I don't look like one." It was not lost on me that Lydia's baseline conditioning was on par with women several decades younger.

Sharing Your Feelings

Donna and Jerry: Donna and Jerry attended a couples' retreat for breast cancer survivors and their partners in the fall of 2014. They planned to attend the retreat the year before but, just as they were set to leave home, their son developed acute appendicitis and had to undergo emergency surgery. Their son was doing fine a year later, and they were both excited to participate in the weekend's activities.

Late Saturday morning, just before a break for lunch, I led a group discussion that included all five male partners and a few additional members of the retreat staff. We began the discussion with the following prompt: "Of all that lies ahead, what concerns you most?" Without their partners present, the men – except Jerry – began to reveal the experience of their wives' diagnosis and treatment for breast cancer. Common threads emerged, including a concerted effort – almost without exception – among the men to mask and conceal their own distress, a maneuver clearly intended to protect their wives from any added worry. Talking about their own feelings seemed not only burdensome to their loved ones but also a waste of time. After all, the point was to "fix it" and "get back to normal."

At a certain point as the sharing progressed, I turned to Jerry and said, "I need to say something to you." Glancing around the group, I continued: "I am about to break every rule that psychologists are supposed to follow, and I'll probably be thrown out of the profession, but you need to hear it just like I did when my college cross-country coach said it to me." I paused. Everyone looked on. And then I said, "Jerry, you need to get your head out of your ass." It's worth noting here that Jerry is built like a man's man, big and burly. I, on the other hand, am tall and lanky with a scrawny upper body. There's no doubt Jerry could mop the floor with me if he wanted to. Stunned, Jerry just looked at me silently with shock and disbelief. Everyone else looked on, awaiting Jerry's reaction. He opened his mouth and said, "Wow, I can't believe you just said that. But ya know, I think you're right. Maybe I do need to tell Donna how I've been feeling. I just didn't want her to worry about me and how I'm doing."

Sometimes we have to crack a few eggs, and Jerry presented the chance to break open an important myth – that by suffering silently, a person is protecting his partner. Meanwhile, the partner senses and misinterprets the silence as distancing, being emotionally unavailable. The women suffer in silence too, withholding fears about how they may be unable to satisfy their partners sexually and about deep feelings of guilt and shame that go with that fear. Speaking the truth of your feelings is a way to honor your partner and your relationship.

Living in the Living Room

Anne: Anne was diagnosed with metastatic disease, and when we first met, she remarked that her doctor told her she might have three years to live. She smiled, then added that three years had come and gone about a year ago. She said, "Guess I am already living on borrowed time." She was acutely attuned to the status of her disease, which she regularly measured during each chemo cycle with cancer blood marker levels and scans she had every three months or so. In a very real sense, she was waiting for the other shoe to drop.

Anne described what was most meaningful: her husband, children and grandchildren. A few of her "live long enough to see" milestones had been achieved in the prior four years, and she was finding it necessary to keep readjusting the line markers and end zone of her life. Now she hoped to live long enough to see her grandson graduate from high school in the coming year. Meanwhile, the rigors of treatment and the onslaught of side effects were a harbinger of a foreshortened future.

One day Anne sat on the sofa with a big smile. She shared that her oncologist decided to give her a chemo holiday. The cancer markers in her blood had been stable over the past several months, and he knew the toll that treatment was taking on Anne. So over the next few months, Anne was "living." She went to Atlantic City with her husband to gamble, one of life's pleasures that she had placed on hold. Using a scooter, she also attended a local fall street festival, an annual community highlight that she had foregone for the past few years. Each time we met during the chemo holiday, Anne's energy and spirits soared.

And then Anne had another PET scan, followed a few days later by an appointment with her oncologist. When we met the following week, there was a dramatic difference in Anne's demeanor. She began to cry. As the words formed, Anne shared that she needed to start chemo again; her cancer markers were increasing and her most recent PET scan showed disease progression. She said, "I'm dying again." We sat in silence as the weight of her assertion washed over us. Eventually I said, "I'm curious. Thinking back to the moment before you walked into the appointment with your oncologist and the moment you left that appointment, what changed?" I noticed a quizzical expression surface on Anne's face as she reflected on this question; then she responded, "Really, nothing was different ... I didn't feel different in my body." She continued, "The only thing different was that he told me I needed to resume chemo. I guess I went from thinking that I'm living to thinking that I'm dying. You know, I never noticed that before."

The discussion that followed gave birth to a metaphor that resonated with Anne: spending time in the "living room" or the "dying room." Wisely, she recognized that it made sense from time to time, like when awaiting blood work or PET scan results, to visit the dying room; however, she wanted to make every effort to spend as much time as possible – like during the recent chemo holiday – in the living room. She came to appreciate a not-so-subtle choice that had eluded her consciousness before contemplating the question I'd posed: She could lean into living instead of dwelling on dying. After that day, it was as if a mental switch had flipped, one that propelled her to plant herself – as much and as often as she could – squarely on the sofa in her "living room." Live on, Anne!

A number of my many teachers, each with her unique experience of breast cancer, give voice to its hidden gifts – often in strikingly similar terms. Gifts. Wait, what? Yes, gifts. And chief among them is the special gift of perspective and seeing one's self, others, the world and what matters in one's life with a fresh set of eyes. In short, life is both precious and terminal. Each one of us will die, and what may matter most is whether and how fully we live life, from moment to moment. Just as it is. No Matter What.

DEBRA REX GEORGE AND DANIEL R. GEORGE

All You Need Is Love ... and Research: A Mother-Son Team Navigate a Non-Aggressive Approach to Breast Cancer

Deb

It is 1963. I am 11-years-old. I am staying with my grandmother to help her as she receives medical care. She has been diagnosed with breast cancer a few months earlier. My dad is moving our family back to his hometown in central Indiana because of her illness. I'm the oldest grandchild by four years, so care for my grandma during the day falls to me. Both my dad and his only sister have to work.

I hear crying in my grandmother's bedroom and quickly go see if I can help. My grandmother is standing naked from the waist up, with a large red scar where her left breast used to be. She is bright red all over her chest from the radiation treatment she is receiving. I am terrified, both at my grandmother's sobbing, and at seeing her nude and (as I see it then) mutilated. But I'm here, and I listen to her upset, and I try to comfort her.

Five years later, months after being pronounced "cured," she discovers the cancer has spread to her lungs. I am the overnight caregiver for the six weeks before she goes into the hospital. I listen to her cough and cough and try to breathe, and I try to calm her fears about death even though I am still only 16. I am traumatized by her disease and her prolonged and painful death a few months later.

I carry a lifelong fear of breast cancer.

"It is very small": worrisome imaging

My own story begins September 25, 2011. I am 59 years old, a mother to two adult children and the leader of a behavioral health agency that serves vulnerable children in northeast Ohio. My phone rings, and when I answer it I am told I need to return to the facility where I underwent my annual mammogram earlier that day. Upon receiving this news, an electric shock runs from my head to my toes.

I return the next morning. After another scan and twenty minutes of torturous waiting, the radiologist asks to see me. There is an "irregularity" and I will need a biopsy. I ask if it is cancer, and she gives me a noncommittal answer. I push her, and she says she believes there's a 95 percent probability that it's cancer. But it is still small and I should not delay.

She gives me the name of three surgeons before turning me over to a nurse, who spends time with me since I am obviously panicked. She describes the surgeons, and, when I push, she recommends one of them and lets me know he is very respected and that people in the department use him when they have a problem – in fact, she did herself. Despite the fact that I know him slightly from our sons both playing on the high school baseball team and feel odd about him knowing about my personal health, I call him that afternoon.

The surgeon is not available but calls me back the following day. He is kind. "It is very small," he says. "Likely, it is ductal carcinoma in situ (DCIS), and we've caught it very early." He suggests that we meet on Friday, three days later, at his office to discuss this more and to determine next steps. I tell my husband, but I ask him not to tell anyone else. I also ask him to come with me on Friday, which he does.

"It can't wait": biopsy, confusion and fear

At the appointment, I am shown the pictures of the "irregularity" and told that a biopsy is essential for accurate diagnosis and treatment recommendations. I'm offered the reassurance that "it could be nothing," but the surgeon has nevertheless already set up a biopsy time with the radiologists at the Breast Center for four days later. Importantly, he has also honored my request for medication to tranquilize me for the procedure, given my claustrophobia and the need to keep perfectly still for up to thirty minutes during the procedure.

I go to the Breast Center as directed; but despite many attempts (and many more x-rays), they are unable to biopsy the site. I am told, "It's probably very slow-growing and can be watched for six months." But I receive a call from the surgeon that afternoon strongly disagreeing with the morning radiologist's "watchful waiting" assessment. He has already consulted with the head of breast radiology, who agrees that given what they see on the previous pictures, in his words, "It can't wait." This was the first of many conflicting stories I would experience from the medical establishment during my diagnosis and treatment decision-making. Two days later, I undergo an additional, painful biopsy performed by the head of breast radiology. I am told it will take a week to receive the results.

"I have breast cancer": informing family

At this point, now mid-October, I decide that I need to tell my adult children. I first call my son, who greets the news with stunned silence and then quick caring and empathy. Spontaneously, he steps forward to actively help me navigate the medical system with its gaps and contradictions, and to support me – much as a mother rushes to the side of her injured toddler, not knowing how badly he is injured, just needing to, wanting to, being driven to help.

Mother-child, that most primitive and powerful of bonds. I remember when he had unexplained bleeding and was wheeled into surgery in a red wagon at the age of four. I remember my only slightly controlled panic and how I leaned on my own mother, who rushed to my side from Indiana to help me through the fear of the unknown status of my little boy.

And now my son, cutting the cord fairly successfully at age 29, was pulled back powerfully into my orbit, leaving his emancipating self behind in order to symbolically cradle his ill mother and to use his knowledge of the medical world and his love for me to come to my aid without being asked.

"I'll be at the doctor's appointment, Mom," he said over the phone from his office at a medical school six hours away. And he was – asking good questions and then researching what we had been told.

My daughter was also quiet at learning the news. Characteristically, her fear drove her to create more distance. Having just moved to Chicago two months earlier and trying to make her way in a new career and forge a social life, this was simply too overwhelming for her to open up to emotionally. She maintained distance throughout the entire experience, willing to hear updates but never seeking them out.

My husband of thirty years diligently "showed up" when asked. He cared deeply, but he tends to get lost in his emotions; wanting to help so much somehow makes him unable to hold the inevitable pain and ambiguity of the decision-making ahead. But he is steady, always present and unwavering in his support of my process.

Danny

When I learned about my mom's diagnosis during a phone call, which I took in my office at a college of medicine where I'm on faculty, I felt a rush of panic. To me, this news felt like a small tear in the fabric of the universe – a fundamental realignment in the order of things after which nothing is ever quite the same. How do you even respond to such news? Truly, there is no playbook when cancer is involved – a diagnosis so heavily freighted with cultural meanings and existential dread. Assurances that "it will be ok" seem to fall flat, both emotionally and empirically. Saying "I'm so sorry ..." feels more honest, but also verges on being unintentionally fatalistic. Still, our underlying impulse as humans is to create order and meaning out of chaos.

I don't recall what inadequate words I mouthed during our phone call, but I do remember taking (what I hope were inaudibly) deep breaths and saying that I would be there for her next appointment and any procedures thereafter. Knowing from my training as a medical anthropologist just how difficult it is for patients to think straight in the midst of a medical crisis, I also reassured my mom that I would comprehensively research everything we learned, documenting and cross-checking every statement from the doctors and nurses, googling every obscure medical detail, and asking colleagues at our teaching hospital for their insights. Information would be our life raft as we navigated the vast waters of fear and anxiety, and this aspect of the journey would be personally calming for me, since gathering quantitative and qualitative data on medical issues was the most normal, familiar, and outwardly useful thing I could do to help. After we had spoken, I remember walking around outside the hospital and just feeling numb.

Once I got back in my office, I recall setting up Google Alerts (essentially a tool where Google bots cull the most recent churn of web-based information on a particular topic that is then sent via email to a user) to deliver daily information about breast cancer and DCIS. Every morning, in addition to scanning the links for Alzheimer's disease that I'd set up for my academic research, I would now scour the latest literature and headlines on cancer research sent by Google's algorithms and click my way into a strange new frontier of cancer journals. To share the information I was finding with my family, I created an online Google Doc, a shared space where everyone I invited could see the research I was gleaning from all the links and journal articles. My role was clear: Despite the rip I felt in the broader order of things, I would be emotionally supportive, and I would exhaust every resource to bring clarity and comfort for the difficult decisions ahead.

Deb

Taking the reins: dissent and decision

Though the doctor initially said to me, "I can do a double mastectomy and you won't have to worry about this again," he quickly backed off when I anxiously responded with "That seems like overkill if it's as minor as you've indicated." The revised recommendation of the whole "breast team" (a week later) was a lumpectomy. The surgery was scheduled for Nov. 11. I let both children know.

Danny responded immediately: "I'll be there with Dad for your surgery, Mom. I'll stay till the next day to be sure you are ok." His stay turned into four days at my side while I was recovering, more from the shock of now being a person recovering from cancer than from the physical trauma of the surgery itself.

Danny

"Taking a plug": the day of the surgery

Driving the five-plus hours to Cleveland for the surgery was a no-brainer for me. Even though you never feel more powerless than when a loved one is being wheeled away from you into surgery, I knew it was essential to be present and help carry the emotional weight of the procedure. I will say, it was a bit surreal to be leaving my mom's fate in the hands of someone whom I'd known as a father figure at little league baseball games. While the morning of the surgery is a bit of a blur, I do have a memory of the procedure being described by someone on the healthcare team (I can't recall who) as "taking a plug" out of my mom's breast. This was one of those all-too-common moments I'd studied as a medical anthropologist when, for patients, the seemingly innocuous medical shorthand used on the wards evokes a rather unfortunate (and menacing) image for those unfamiliar with clinical idioms.

As my dad and I sat in the waiting room, the "taking a plug" dysphemism and overall tensions of the procedure weighed heavily on us both. I recall the television in the lobby filling the space with the white noise of daytime TV. I also remember watching his foot twitch back and forth rapidly and feeling the aura of his anxiety. At some point, we decided to walk around outside. Even though it was a cold, gray November day in Cleveland, being out of the medical environment helped dissipate some of the tension. We talked about sports, work – anything but the eldritch "plug-taking" that was transpiring in the surgical theater. Thankfully, when we returned, we were told the procedure had been successful and were taken back to see my mom who sat in bed groggy and with a weary, post-anesthetic smile on her face.

Deb

"You need anything, Mom?": postoperative convalescence

My initial feeling was of profound relief: "It" was out of me. I had made it through the surgery. The pain was minor. But I was tired and scared about what might lie ahead after the pathology report came back. I was grateful for the presence of both my husband, George, and Danny.

    I remember especially post-op day four, a Monday, when Dan should have been back at work but had decided to stay "just one more day." The living room. I am sitting in an easy chair, cat on my lap. A fire my son has made makes the darkness of the November day transform into dancing warmth beside me. My son on the couch working on his computer, glances at me from time to time as if to assure himself that I am still there. "You need anything, Mom?" He asks repeatedly. "No, Dan," I say. "I'm fine; and, to myself in this moment, in this womb of love, I realize I truly do have everything I need to be fine.

Danny

Elasticity of time: restful and restive

I'm fortunate to have a job that doesn't necessitate my being in the office every day; so the decision to stay with my mom post-surgery was easy, and I remained in town until she seemed to be stable and self-sufficient.

We spent some wonderful down time in the living room, with fires going throughout the day. Usually, this sort of "leisure time" was reserved for rare holidays when we were able to carve out a day or two away from work, incessant email and responsibility. In this way, the procedure and convalescence had sort of suspended all the other "stuff" of life, and we were able to "just be" as my mom healed. However, given my perhaps unhealthy inclinations as a researcher, I also used this time to tweak my Google alerts to feed me information on treatment options and preventions against cancer recurrence. I began populating the Google doc with new information.

Eventually, this document would become a repository not only of research, but also notes from doctors' visits, emails from colleagues providing input about the decision, and other helpful links (e.g., book recommendations) we'd gleaned from others. I'm not sure if anyone ever closely read the "doc," but it felt important to keep amassing information and constructing some semblance of order.

Deb

"If this were you, what would you do?": arriving at a treatment decision

Days later the final pathology report and recommendations of the team were given to me by the surgeon. Dan and George were present with me when I met with him. It was a clean biopsy with good margins. The team recommended radiation and three years of hormonal therapy (tamoxifen or an aromatase inhibitor). I was instructed by the doctor to see the radiology oncologist and, if I wished, a medical oncologist (though he was clear that he could oversee the medication regimen.)

While I respected the breast team's post-pathology recommendations, I felt a powerful need to review the facts with others, research the options, and come to my own conclusions. I believe this comes from my nature: I am a curious person who has faith in my own thinking and analytical abilities, and who tends to question almost everything! It also comes from my experience as a leader in three non-profits over a forty-three-year career. Given this experience, I am acutely aware of how positions of authority – including in a medical setting – can create a perception of being "all-knowing." I am also painfully aware that leaders seldom have knowledge that makes their decisions or recommendations unambiguously "right." Because I have been uncomfortable with people *not* questioning my ideas as a leader, I automatically question the assumptions of others in leadership roles. In this case, while I respected my doctor and the rest of his team, I had to look at my situation from all possible angles and come to my own conclusions. Danny quickly joined me in researching the recommendations as I received them. Though the entire team had recommended the same treatment protocol, I realized that, at least in my case, this might not be the right path for me.

I saw the head of breast radiology, a female doctor in her early 40s. One of her initial statements after explaining what I could expect from the treatment was, "In your case, about 50% of women would get radiation and about 50% would not." I pushed hard to understand why, but I got lost in the medical language. Finally I asked, "If this were you, what would you do?" She paused for perhaps ten seconds. "I wouldn't do radiation," she said, quickly adding, "But I would take the medication." I left saying I would get back to her social worker to let her know what I decided. I felt relief that that the radiation wasn't inevitable, but this ironically heightened my anxiety about whether or not I should do it.

My next stop was with a medical oncologist. The recommended person was not available for three weeks, so I got an appointment with another person, also a female doctor, who spent an hour with me, answering every question my son and I had come up with. She went over the relative benefits and possible side effects of both hormonal therapies. I appreciated her thoroughness and kindness, but the ambiguity of what was right for me remained heavy.

One concerning factor for me about tamoxifen, the top recommendation, was that it carries increased risk of stroke. My mother had died suddenly several years earlier from a stroke, so I made an appointment with a hematologist who specialized in analyzing risk for strokes. A week later I was told that I had no elevated risk factors; however, the fact that I had likely experienced phlebitis when on birth control pills years earlier might warrant caution with regard to developing blood clots.

As the weeks went by, my anxiety continued to rise. I sought out the oncology social worker who listened with great patience and intervened to get me a quick appointment with the radiologist and an appointment with another medical oncologist.

My question for the radiologist was clear: Exactly why wouldn't she do the radiation therapy if she were in my shoes? Again, she was patient and forthcoming. She pulled up research on her computer and showed me the most recent finding that boiled down, to a single factor, the many variables identified in previous research: How clean and how wide are the margins following the lumpectomy? In my case, she pointed out, the margins were completely clean and far in excess of what the research deemed predictive of a low likelihood of recurrence. I left feeling very reassured, with reduced anxiety and greater clarity.

The second medical oncologist, also a woman, was more clipped in her assessment. "My belief is that if you do nothing you have a three in ten chance of recurrence in the next ten years." (This was higher than the 30 percent *lifetime* risk of recurrence that I had previously been told.). She indicated that she would not recommend the aromatase inhibitor because of recent research showing that the drug could quickly lead to advanced bone loss, but it was up to me how much risk I wanted to take. "Only you can decide that." I left with a prescription ... and more uncertainty.

I returned to the first medical oncologist and laid out all I had been told and what my son had uncovered, including non-medical options for preventing recurrence. Again, she spent a lot of time with me. She emphasized the value of exercise (at least thirty-five minutes a day "and more is better"), which could cut my risk in half; and not drinking, either at all or minimally. She said little else was proven, though clear trends in nutrition pointed to the value of a plant-based diet low in soy products and few, if any, meat proteins. I left with her warmly hugging me and saying, "If I were you I honestly don't know what I would do."

My final stop in the fact-finding journey was with a medical librarian at a local cancer support center. I asked her about tamoxifen research, stating that I was very reluctant to take it but was having anxiety about "doing nothing." Without telling me what to do, she drew a simple diagram for me with 100 dashes across the page. She crossed out all but fifteen of them. Then she crossed off seven more, representing the preventive factor of exercise at the prescribed amount. Only seven dashes were left. The tamoxifen could reduce the remaining percent of recurrence only by half, or three to four. The question became clear: how much real benefit from tamoxifen versus how much risk of side effects and negative impact on quality of life. "Some women," she stated, "can't even exercise because the medication is so debilitating. Sixty percent of people who take tamoxifen are non-compliant because of side effects." And she confirmed that there is no evidence that life expectancy is greater with the administration of tamoxifen.

Dan continued consulting the medical professionals he knew and adding the research he amassed as a scholar.

The journey would continue – the research analyzed, the data collected, the contradictory recommendations and possible side effects addressed, the terror controlled in part through a carefully developed spreadsheet and shared computer document curated by my son.

Finally, at the end of January, it was time for decisions about treatment. "Danny," I said gently, "You can't make this decision with me, because if it turns out to be a bad decision I don't ever want you to feel responsible. I am interested in your thoughts and opinions, but I have to make the decision alone." Even at my most vulnerable, a primitive need to protect my child remained my top priority.

And I do make decisions. They are at odds with the medical team's advice. I turn down radiation and tamoxifen. I go it alone, with plentiful exercise and healthy diet my sole arsenal against possible recurrence. My son supports and agrees with my decision.

Danny

Fieldwork: notes from the other side of the desk

When my mom had her follow-up appointment about the pathography report, I was indeed there, taking copious (ethnography-like) field notes and trying my best to ask clarifying questions without sounding too pushy or neurotic. When you are in the patient's chair and bad news is coming at you, there's just no way to digest everything through the low-grade panic and flood of emotions. When you're a family member, it's only slightly less unnerving, but that little bit matters a lot.

Again, it felt odd to be talking to a doctor who, in my solipsistic youth, had appeared merely as a floating stock figure in the bleachers during baseball games. But here, sitting across from us in his white coat, he was patient, honest, and forthcoming in answering our fusillade of questions. I seem to recall my mom asking him what he would tell his wife or mother to do in this circumstance, and his answer – the details of which neither of us can quite remember now – seemed to carry considerable weight in the moment.

After the appointment, my mom and I continued to find information and add it to our Google doc. We also read narratives by other people diagnosed with breast cancer – some who had pursued treatment, others who had declined treatment. Back at work, I made an appointment with a colleague at the campus Breast Center. She generously took time to sit with me (even though my mom wasn't a patient at her clinic), gave me a folder of information, drew diagrams with DCIS margins and risk curves, and answered the ever-weighty question about what she would do in the same circumstance. In an email correspondence, another colleague who was an expert in functional medicine generously sent me numerous resources about diet and cancer with strategies for how women could deal with DCIS by naturally reducing estrogens and inflammation.

Admittedly, as we got deeper into the weeds of the decision to treat or not, I found myself in a rather difficult position. By disciplinary convention, medical anthropologists often take a posture critical of Western biomedicine, particularly the tendency to overmedicalize and overtreat conditions. But when a loved one has cancer, when it is so raw that "plugs" are being taken from her body, it becomes necessary to deal with the biomedical cancer diagnosis not as an abstraction to be intellectually interrogated, unpacked, and challenged, but as a viscerally real life-or-death threat. Even though my research seemed to be guiding me toward the conclusion that someone with my mom's risk profile could feel reasonably secure in a decision not to treat, I constantly wrestled with myself and my disciplinary biases. I was also aware of the physical toll that treatment – whether radiation, hormonal therapy, or mastectomy – would have on my mom, and this weighed heavily on me. The research seemed to be showing us a way out, a route of nontreatment that could be justified with evidence-based data, independent of my own biases. But I was still worried that I was seeing what I wanted to see in the vast Rorschach test of the cancer literature.

I hoped that we'd arrived at the best possible decision for my mom's wellbeing. Mostly, as things moved forward, I realized how imprecise and probabilistic modern medicine is, and how our exhaustive attempts to impose order and find a "right answer" – though perhaps not fruitless – were ultimately feeble.

Lessons learned: how love heals

Danny

In retrospect, what stands out most was that, given the giant rip in the universe I felt upon hearing the news, the ability to create streams of information was psychologically mollifying – perhaps more than it was practically useful. I felt I was able to funnel pertinent information to my mom, and this helped us put a plan in place that led to a decision we ultimately all felt comfortable with. Over time, this system has – I think – also supported my mom's long-term wellness. In the wake of the surgery and decision not to treat, she made significant lifestyle changes, lost a lot of weight, and got into excellent shape. To this day, she still tracks her daily steps and insists on walking until she breaks a sweat (I believe sweat-inducing exercise was a protective variable we had turned up in the cancer prevention literature).

The Google doc was fueled by many forces – anxiety, fear, escapism, an unhealthy Protestant work ethic, etc. – but in retrospect it was sustaining and necessary. I recently signed into the document again and saw that the "last edited" date was May 14, 2012. I'm beyond grateful that we've been able to leave the whole thing behind us and move forward.

As I think about our experience, I'm aware of my own privilege in terms of having institutional access to otherwise paywalled research, opportunities to speak informally with expert colleagues in the field, an education that had inculcated solid research habits, and a job that gave me relative freedom to dive deep into the data and be with my mom throughout her journey. I feel for people who lack these "invisible advantages" and wonder how we could set up a more humane healthcare system that would close the gaps.

Significantly, in the decade following my mom's treatment, I have committed to not taking things for granted, coming home as much as possible, trying to be there for holidays, and striving, above all, to be a present and supportive presence for both my parents. That, perhaps, is the most important lesson learned.

Deb

I remember a diagnosis of breast cancer and a sea of conflicting data and opinions, which destroyed my illusion that the medical establishment has iron-clad and coherent treatment recommendations.

I remember women physicians, nurses and social workers talking to me on- and off-the-record – how their recommendations were often contradictory both among them and from any one of them.

Over time, Dan, my partner in this medical crisis, slowly grows distant again, resuming the role of a 29-year-old adult son. We touch base on this topic at exam time for a while and then not; he periodically, and less and less frequently, sends new research articles. I miss his more constant presence, even as I know the rightness of his receding from my life in this personal way.

But in my heart lives the memory of his call to action, his coming when the need was greatest. "Post-op Day Four" is filed in my memory under "perfect love," an image that emerges when I am asked to conjure up such things in guided meditations. While I will never know if I made the right treatment decisions, I will always know beyond any doubt that the primal bond between us is deep and true and will never be severed. In a vortex of unsettling medical contradictions, this assurance of love is what is coherent and real. Perhaps it is, in fact, the most healing element of all.

KATHRYN H. SCHMITZ

I Promise You Will Feel Better: The Importance of Exercising During and After Cancer Treatment

I am an exercise oncology researcher. In my work, I prescribe exercise to people living with and beyond cancer. The conversation is predictable:

ME: I'm going to give you a pedometer. For the first week you will just note the number of steps you take every day, and then increase by about 10% or 1000 steps per day, whatever is easier for you to remember.

PATIENT: But, I can't walk. I'm fatigued.

ME: Yes, but I promise you, the walking is going to make you feel better. Just try it.

PATIENT: What part of "I'm fatigued" isn't translating here?!

ME: Okay, let's try an experiment. You try the walking. If you DON'T feel better after 10 minutes, stop.

... weeks go by ...

ME: So how did it go?

PATIENT: You're right! I feel so much better!

Know this: There is no drug on the market that will treat your cancer-related fatigue better than physical activity. This is a scientifically documented fact that you can take to the bank ... perhaps to withdraw funds to buy a pedometer and some walking shoes.

The field of exercise oncology is relatively new. Twenty years ago there had only been about four clinical trials of exercise in cancer patients. Most of those were in breast cancer, and most of them could best be characterized as pilot studies: small, flawed and in need of replication. Fast forward twenty years and we have over 1000 clinical exercise trials in the scientific literature that have documented the safety and efficacy of exercise for people living with and beyond cancer. I have been working in exercise oncology since those early days. I have personally completed over ten clinical trials, including work published in well-respected clinical medical journals such as the *Journal of the American Medical Association* and the *New England Journal of Medicine*. And I am not alone. There is now a small army of us all doing clinical exercise trials in people living with and beyond cancer.

Multiple national and international medical advocacy organizations have published evidence-based guidance recommending that exercise become standard practice during and after cancer treatment. The most recent advice from the American College of Sports Medicine is that people living with and beyond cancer do 150 minutes per week of aerobic activity and/or strength training twice weekly to prevent recurrence of breast, colon and prostate cancer. In fact, there is compelling evidence that as little as thirty minutes of aerobic exercise three times a week and/or resistance exercise two times a week is effective to treat eight common cancer health-related outcomes, including fatigue, pain, depression, anxiety, physical function, sleep, lymphedema and bone health!

Amazingly, despite the wealth of scientific and anecdotal evidence that exercise during and after treatment promotes well-being in both the short and long term, it has not yet become standard practice. The reasons have mostly to do with the way we focus on sickness more than on health and wellness – and the fact that no one has figured out how to make money from getting people living with and beyond cancer to exercise. Similar challenges exist for nutrition in the setting of cancer and, in both cases, these obstacles are perhaps mostly the result of historical and cultural norms.

Time for a story ...

Back in the 1950s, sitting president Dwight Eisenhower had a heart attack. He was treated at Bethesda Naval Hospital and his cardiologist, Dr. Paul Dudley-White, was sharply criticized for getting President Eisenhower out of bed so soon: *three weeks* after the cardiac event! Today, we get people out of bed the very next day after a heart attack. And if you ask the average person on the street if their dad who had a heart attack a month ago should be exercising to strengthen his heart, the common answer would be "Yes! Of course!"

So what happened? How did we get from the 1950s and three weeks of bed rest to today when we all know that exercise is good for the heart? Certainly there was science involved. But science was not the only factor. There were advocacy groups such as the American Heart Association and popular press books such as Jim Fixx's *The Complete Book of Running* and Kenneth Cooper's *Aerobics Program for Total Well-Being*. It's not clear exactly when it happened, but there was definitely a paradigm shift sometime in the last seventy years about exercise and heart disease.

For exercise and cancer, we are at a point when we need a similar paradigm shift. We have a beautiful scientific evidence base supporting the notion that people living with and beyond cancer should exercise regularly. And yet, if you ask the average person on the street whether their Aunt Betty who is getting chemotherapy for breast cancer should be exercising to help her get through the treatment, that average person is likely to say no. Stop for a moment and think about it. When you imagine a person with cancer, do you think of them resting? Or moving? Most people I ask say they think of a person with cancer resting. We associate cancer with rest. This was once for good reason! Cancer treatments used to be so toxic that patients received all treatments during an in-patient hospital stay. But somewhere along the line, the toxicities started to decline. It has become common for the average person to function, care for self/family and continue working during cancer treatment. If the average cancer patient can work, cook and do chores at home, why can't that person exercise? As a researcher in exercise oncology, I want to change this misconception. That's why I'm writing this chapter: to let you in on the big secret that exercise is helpful during and after cancer therapy.

Norma would agree ...

When Norma arrived to join one of my studies, multiple family members assisted her with walking. She was shaped like a question mark (curved over) and using a walker. She had heard we were doing a "supportive care" study and wanted to give it a try. Norma had advanced breast cancer and had undergone spinal surgery that had left her in a lot of pain.

To get a baseline level of activity, we measured her physical function with a few simple tests, gave her a pedometer and asked her not to change anything for a week. Then she increased steps by 1000 per day every week. By the end of the three-month intervention, she came back in to have measurements taken using only a cane; the walker was gone. She swung the cane like Charlie Chaplin to show she didn't really need it, and she was walking an average of 10,000 steps per day. She had started with extreme fatigue and pain. But she trusted us enough to try ten minutes of exercise, to see if it got better or worse. The study has been over for months now, but we still hear from Norma occasionally, just so she can tell us her daily step counts. I'm pretty sure that if Norma can do it, you can too.

Now, that's not to say that exercise is a panacea. Nor am I saying that exercise will cure your cancer. But it will change your sense of feeling out of control during and after your treatment. Gabrielle Grunewald's story illustrates this point well. "Gabe" was a collegiate runner when she was diagnosed with a rare abdominal cancer. She made the decision to keep living her life and to continue her running career, despite a serious cancer diagnosis. Gabe was a nationally ranked US track and field athlete, with a professional sponsorship from Brooks (a shoe company), and she won the 3000-meter U.S. national championship in 2014. She placed fourth for the 1500-meter race for the London U.S. Olympic trials. Gabe succumbed to her disease in 2019, at the age of 32 – well over a decade after her grim diagnosis. She had a saying over her couch that embodied her life, and the point I am trying to make: "There are two ways to live your life. One is as if nothing is a miracle. The other is as if everything is a miracle." As Gabe's story illustrates, exercising doesn't mean you won't get cancer; but it will delay the onset and minimize the spread and severity of the disease. Nor will exercise make your cancer go away. But it will put you back in the driver's seat. Besides, don't you want to be in the shape of your life for the fight of your life?

I've started a new initiative called "Moving Through Cancer": <exerciseismedicine.org/movingthroughcancer>. Here, you will find the exercise guidelines I mention above and some infographics that might help, as well as an international registry of exercise programs for people living with and beyond cancer. Head there for more. But first? Go for a walk. I promise you'll feel better.

ELIZABETH REID

Food as Medicine: How to Eat During and After Treatment for Breast Cancer

As an advanced practice dietician, my professional knowledge of nutrition and breast cancer became very personal in January 2011, when I was diagnosed with breast cancer and had a bilateral mastectomy and chemotherapy treatment. Despite a lifetime of exercise and eating well, there were factors beyond my control that affected my health, and I was not immune to cancer. I sincerely believe that following the nutrition principles that I have outlined below – combined with exercise – helped me tolerate the treatment plan my medical team prescribed and enabled me to move beyond the experience and live free from cancer. I wish the same for you and your loved ones.

After a breast cancer diagnosis, it is common to review our diet and lifestyle, searching for answers to what might have caused the cancer to occur. It's a hard question and there are usually no satisfactory answers because breast cancer is a complex diagnosis with many contributing factors that are beyond our control – age and genetics, for instance. We can try to control some factors such as physical activity, body weight and diet, and research is ongoing to help determine which types of food and dietary patterns help fight cancer. While there is no magical healthy food or ultra-healthy diet that will prevent or cure cancer, certain nutrients in food help make our bodies more inhospitable to cancer cells and help us heal from surgery, chemotherapy and other cancer treatments. Doing what you can to take care of yourself will improve your mood and energy level, and a healthy diet that includes vegetables, fruits and protein will give you the reserves of nutrients you need to keep yourself as strong as possible. These reserves will help you heal and fight infection as well as tolerate possible side effects of treatment.

Sometimes the plethora of nutrition advice on the internet and from well-meaning friends can feel overwhelming, and it may be tempting to take immediate action. It's best not to make any drastic dietary changes or buy any supplements, though, unless these suggestions have been specifically recommended by your cancer treatment care team. A registered dietitian nutritionist with knowledge regarding a healthy diet for cancer treatment would be a good option if you would like individual guidance. With or without such advice, a good place to start is planning meals that are nutritious and satisfying, and contain some of the basic nutrients that can help your immune system function at its best.

Two common drawbacks are that people think they don't like healthy foods and that they have too many changes to make while feeling stressed because of cancer therapy. Gradual small adjustments can be made to add some of the foods that have particular cancer-fighting qualities and to decrease the number of foods that don't have positive benefits – or may even be associated with an increased cancer risk.

Basic nutrition-related recommendations for people with breast cancer are as follows:

- plant-based diet
- high fiber and whole grains
- low-fat diet with emphasis on healthy monounsaturated and polyunsaturated fats
- healthy protein sources with minimal processed and cured meats
- limited processed and refined grains/flours/sugars
- high fluid intake
- healthy weight
- physical activity

Plant-Based Diet

To reduce cancer risk, the American Cancer Society (ACS) and the American Institute for Cancer Research (AICR) recommend a plant-based diet rich in fruit and vegetables (ACS 2017; AICR 2018). One large study of 91,000 women found a 15 percent reduction in breast cancer risk in women who consumed a plant-based diet (Link 1524). Similarly, a Mediterranean-style diet that emphasizes vegetables, olive oil, fish, legumes and fruit was also associated with a lower risk for breast cancer (Turati 326).

You should aim for at least three cups of vegetables and two cups of fruit daily. Vegetables and fruits can be added to both meals and snacks. For example, berries could be added to Greek yogurt or cereal for breakfast, or blended into a smoothie for an afternoon snack. Carrots and sweet potatoes can be added to soups and/or roasted and eaten with a meal. Several websites, including AICR (<https://www.aicr.org/healthyrecipes/#>), have healthy recipes to choose from. AICR also features information about a cancer-preventative diet called the "New American Plate," which is made up of 2/3 (or more) vegetables, fruits, whole grains or beans and 1/3 (or less) animal protein. Check out their programs for guidance and support as you to transition to a more plant-based diet (AICR 2019).

The reason fruits and vegetables are recommended so highly is that they contain vitamins, minerals, fiber and various cancer-fighting nutrients called phytonutrients. "Phyto" means "plant," and phytonutrients (also called phytochemicals) are produced by plants. These phytonutrients have antioxidant and chemo-preventive properties which are believed to protect cells from damage that could lead to cancer: They help protect cells from DNA damage (Chakraborty 215), they help stop the formation of cancer-causing substances (carcinogens) and they have anti-inflammatory properties (Elliot 147). Reducing inflammation is important because, left unchecked, chronic inflammation can damage DNA, which may lead to cancer over time.

Some of the most beneficial phytochemicals – and the foods that contain them – include:

- beta carotene and other carotenoids (carrots, yams, butternut and other types of squash, broccoli, cantaloupe, apricots). Many vegetables and fruits that are dark yellow, dark orange or green are rich in carotenoids.
- isothiocyanates (in cruciferous vegetables, including broccoli, cabbage, brussels sprouts, cauliflower, bok choy, kale, collards, turnips and rutabaga)

- polyphenols (tea, especially green tea, garlic, flax seed, pomegranates)
- sulforaphane (broccoli sprouts, lightly steamed broccoli, bok choy)
- anthocyanins (purple grapes, blueberries, black raspberries, cranberries, black rice)

Food is the best source of these important phytochemicals. There is no evidence that taking phytochemical supplements in pill form is as beneficial as eating a balanced diet that includes five cups or more of a variety of fruits, vegetables, beans and grains daily. Many researchers believe that these compounds work best together in food (Kapinova 36).

Organic or not?

So far, no studies demonstrate a scientifically proven link between the consumption of non-organic foods and an increased risk of breast cancer. However, female farm workers are at an increased risk of several medical conditions (Kachuri 343), and laboratory studies indicate that some of the most commonly used pesticides act like estrogen (Gray 94), which can increase risk for breast cancer. It makes sense to err on the side of caution and avoid unnecessary exposure to these potentially harmful compounds. Although washing and peeling non-organic fruits or vegetables may help to reduce pesticide residues, it will not eliminate them. Therefore, whenever possible, it's a good idea to eat organic fruits, vegetables, dairy and meats to limit your exposure to pesticide residue and hormones that may have been added. Furthermore, although more research is needed, recent evidence indicates that organic foods contain significantly higher amounts of cancer-fighting phytochemicals than conventionally grown produce (Ren 5122). And by the way, it is important to know the terms "natural" and "organic" do not mean the same thing. "Natural" is overused and has very little meaning when it comes to industry standards. "Organic" food – that is, produced without using pesticides or fertilizers made with synthetic ingredients or sewage sludge; antibiotics and growth hormones; bioengineering; or ionizing radiation – is generally more expensive than conventionally grown food, but eating non-organically grown fruits and vegetables is better than not eating fruits and vegetables at all. There are some ways to reduce costs, such as checking the prices of frozen organic fruits and vegetables, shopping at local farmers' markets or buying produce right from the farmers.

The Environmental Working Group (EWG), an environmental health advocacy organization in the U.S., analyzes pesticide studies and ranks contamination of the most popularly consumed fruits and vegetables in a shopping guide which is updated every year and published on their website (<https://www.ewg.org/foodnews/full-list.php>). The 2020 list ranks forty-seven fruits and vegetables along a continuum from the highest degree of contamination, called the "Dirty Dozen," to lowest, called the "Clean Fifteen." Utilizing this information can help you make decisions about when to purchase organic versions of foods that otherwise probably contain more pesticide residue.

The EWG's 2020 Shopper's Guide to Pesticides on Produce™:[1]
Dirty Dozen™

1. strawberries
2. spinach
3. kale
4. nectarines
5. apples
6. grapes
7. peaches
8. cherries
9. pears
10. tomatoes
11. celery
12. potatoes

---

[1] In keeping with the statement in the Introduction – that, because this book includes many perspectives, not every detail will be true for everyone – please note that these lists are different in the UK. Please reference <https://www.pan-uk.org/site/wp-content/uploads/Pesticides-in-our-food-multiple-residues-June-2019-1.pdf> Accessed August 2, 2020.

Clean Fifteen™

1. avocados
2. sweet corn*
3. pineapple
4. sweet peas (frozen)
5. onions
6. papaya*
7. eggplant
8. asparagus
9. kiwi
10. cabbage
11. cauliflower
12. cantaloupe
13. broccoli
14. mushrooms
15. honeydew melon

* A small amount of sweet corn, papaya and summer squash sold in the United States is produced from genetically modified seeds. Buy organic varieties of these crops if you want to avoid genetically modified produce (Environmental Working Group).

High Fiber and Whole Grains

Fiber found in fruits, vegetables and legumes is essential to keep the body feeling and functioning at its best – including aiding the intestines to promote regular bowel movements. Fiber can help ease both constipation and diarrhea and help control glucose levels (Anderson 188), which can lower the risk for diabetes and help promote a healthy weight. A high-fiber diet may also lower cancer risk by reducing inflammation (Farvid 335). The research on fiber and breast cancer isn't conclusive, but overall studies suggest a high-fiber diet may reduce cancer risk and/or reduce the risk of cancer progression (Farvid 335). Here's why.

Fiber can bind to toxic compounds and carcinogens so that they have less contact with the intestinal surface and are eliminated at a faster rate. Experimental studies in both humans and animals demonstrate that higher levels of dietary fiber can reduce levels of estrogen in the blood. This decrease in excessive estrogen levels in the blood may potentially reduce the risk of hormone-related cancers, such as breast cancer (Li 217). For adults up to age 50, the United States Department of Agriculture (USDA) recommends 25 grams of daily fiber for women and 38 grams for men. For adults over fifty, the recommendation is 21 grams for women and 30 grams for men each day. Many adults in the United States don't meet these recommendations, consuming only about 10–15 grams daily. You can increase fiber by eating fruits and vegetables with the peel on if possible, trying more beans and legumes and eating whole grains.

For bread, check the label to make sure "whole grain" is listed as the first ingredient. Breads and cereals that claim to be "multigrain" may or may not be whole grain, and it can be hard to tell without checking the ingredient list. Choose breads and crackers with three or more grams of fiber per serving, cereals with six or more grams of fiber per serving and pasta with four or more grams of fiber per serving. You can also check to see if a whole-grain food has at least 1–2 grams of fiber for every 10 grams of carbohydrate. Note: If you need to increase your fiber intake, make gradual increases in fiber-rich foods and consume extra water to help the intestines adapt.

As with phytonutrients, evidence suggests that eating foods that contain fiber is more likely to reduce the risk of breast cancer than taking supplements like Metamucil® or Benefiber® (Holscher 172). Whole foods provide both soluble and insoluble fiber (both of which are good for us), plus vitamins, minerals and other beneficial nutrients not found in fiber supplements. Some good sources of soluble fiber are kidney and black beans, lentils, brussels sprouts, avocados and melons. Sources of insoluble fiber include whole wheat flour, wheat bran, chia seeds, cauliflower and figs. One study showed that women who ate legumes such as beans and lentils at least twice a week had a lower risk of developing breast cancer than women who ate them less than once a month (Sangaramoorthy 2131).

Low-Fat Diet with emphasis on healthy monounsaturated and polyunsaturated fats

The role of dietary fat in breast cancer is the subject of ongoing research. Some studies suggest that high-fat diets, as well as diets high in saturated fat, increase the risk of developing breast cancer (Schulz 942). The potential elevated risk of breast cancer may be because high-fat diets may increase estrogen levels. Furthermore, diets high in fat – especially saturated fat – are associated with heart disease (Wang 423), so it makes sense to limit general fat intake to 30 percent (or less) and reduce saturated fat intake to 8 percent (or less).

There is evidence that following a low-fat diet may lengthen survival for postmenopausal women diagnosed with breast cancer. Results from the Women's Health Initiative Trial suggest that postmenopausal women who reduced the amount of fat in their diet seem to lower their risk of dying from breast cancer by 21 percent (Chlebowski 2919). There is growing evidence that the omega-3 fatty acids alpha linoleic acid (ALA), eicosapentaenoic acid (EPA) and docosahexaenoic acid (DHA) may reduce the risk of breast cancer growth and metastasis (Fabian 2015), and can enhance the immune system. Good sources of ALA are flaxseed, canola oil, chia seeds and walnuts. DHA and EPA are plentiful in fatty fish such as salmon, herring and mackerel. A Mediterranean-style diet that emphasizes healthy monounsaturated and omega-3 fatty acids may be a good model to decrease breast cancer risk and progression. Aim for a low to moderate fat-intake, focusing on the type and quality of fat. Limit animal fats and avoid hydrogenated fats, and increase intake of omega-3 fatty acids. Note: Remember that all fats are equally high in calories, so be careful of weight gain. General recommendations for fat consumption include the following:

- Limit the intake of highly saturated fat such as beef, lamb, organ meats, cheeses, cream, butter and ice cream.
- Decrease hydrogenated fats containing trans fatty acids, such as commercially prepared baked goods, crackers and margarine.

- Focus on consuming moderate amounts of monounsaturated fats such as extra-virgin olive oil, avocados, nuts such as almonds and pistachios and seeds such as pumpkin and flax as healthy fat sources.
- Increase your intake of fish to three times per week. This will increase omega-3-polyunsaturated fat intake. Research has suggested that these fatty acids may inhibit the growth of breast tumors.

Healthy Protein Sources with minimal processed and cured meats

Protein is part of a healthy diet. Include some protein in every meal, and include plant-based protein at least once daily. Protein helps build and repair tissues, maintains muscle mass, and enhances important metabolic functions like repairing cells and making new ones. Aim for healthy protein sources with little, if any, processed and cured meats. Higher intakes of red meat are associated with an increased risk of breast cancer. A large seven-and-a-half-year prospective study of women's health and diet data and breast cancer risk reported that those women with the highest red meat intake were 23 percent more likely to develop invasive breast cancer (Lo 2019). (Women who consumed white meat had a lower incidence of breast cancer.) The association was stronger for breast cancer in postmenopausal women. A meta-analysis of studies performed prior to January 2018 found a 9 percent increased risk of breast cancer in people who consume a high percentage of cured and processed meats, compared to those who ate the least amount of processed meats. While cutting down processed meat intake may reduce breast cancer risk, experts caution that the studies do not prove that higher consumption of processed meat directly causes breast cancer. Choose a variety of protein foods, including seafood and lean meats, poultry, eggs, legumes, beans and peas, nuts and seeds. Smaller amounts of protein are found in vegetables and whole grains.

Note: The relationship between soy intake and breast cancer has been controversial. The American Institute for Cancer Research reports that soy is safe in moderate amounts and contains isoflavones, a phytonutrient with cancer-fighting properties. Whole-soy foods (rather than powders) are safe and may be beneficial up to three servings daily (Collins 2019).

Limit Processed and Refined Grains/Flours/Sugars

An observational study published in the *British Medical Journal* analyzed five years of dietary questionnaires from 105,000 middle-aged men and women (average age 43 years) in France, looking at the consumption of processed foods. The researchers also examined the participants' medical records and tried to isolate the specific risks that food processing played, taking into account some commonly known risk factors, including age, gender, educational level, family cancer history and physical activity level. They found for every 10 percent dietary increase in packaged snacks, sweetened beverages, sugary cereals and other highly processed foods, cancer risk increased by 12 percent. The incidence of breast cancer was associated with greater consumption of mass produced, highly processed foods, including instant soups, frozen or ready-to-eat meals, commercially made desserts and products processed with preservatives (other than salt) such as nitrates. Many of these items contain hydrogenated oils, modified starches, colorants, emulsifiers, texturizers, sweeteners and other additives. Minimally processed foods such as fresh, frozen and canned fruits and vegetables, rice, pasta, eggs, meat, fish and milk were associated with a lower risk of cancer, including breast cancer. The study doesn't prove that ultra-processed foods cause cancer, but that there is an association between the consumption of highly processed foods and increased cancer risk (Fiolet 2018).

An additional concern is that a diet rich in processed foods is likely to be high in calories and contribute to weight gain, which is a known risk factor for many cancers – including breast cancer. Highly processed foods are likely replacing other foods that are rich in phytonutrients, fiber and other healthy ingredients. High-sugar foods are also usually low in nutrient density and fiber. These foods may increase serum insulin and insulin-like growth factor, which may stimulate cancer cell growth.

What about alcohol?

Research consistently shows that drinking alcoholic beverages on a regular basis increases the risk of breast cancer. Alcohol can increase the levels of estrogen and other hormones in the body that are associated with an increased risk of estrogen-receptor-positive breast cancer. It may also damage the DNA in cells. Women who have three alcoholic drinks each week have a higher risk of breast cancer than women who don't drink at all, and experts estimate that the risk of breast cancer increases for each additional drink that is regularly consumed (Ellison 740). All types of alcohol count. One drink equals twelve ounces of beer, five ounces of wine or one-and-a-half ounces of hard liquor.

High Fluid Intake

Staying well-hydrated is essential for our well-being and helps our bodies function optimally. It is especially important during cancer therapy, when treatments may affect the balance of fluid in our bodies, because adequate hydration helps reduce the fatigue that often accompanies cancer treatment. Maintaining the proper balance of fluid in our bodies plays a vital role in the following:

- controlling heart rate, blood pressure and circulation
- maintaining body temperature
- digesting and absorbing food, and preventing constipation
- transporting nutrients throughout the body to help nourish and heal
- transporting and eliminating wastes and toxins from the body
- protecting organs, tissues and joints

We can't rely on thirst to measure hydration, and it's easier to prevent under-hydration or dehydration than to catch up when we're behind in fluid intake. Aim to drink sixty to eighty ounces of water and non-caffeinated beverages daily. It's important to drink before, during and after treatment, and several strategies may help you accomplish this. It may be easier to drink more in the morning than toward the end of the day when you may feel more tired. It usually helps to begin the day with a glass or two of water. Some people find it easier to fill a large glass to start with, and may even use a glass pint or quart mason jar to drink from. You may find it easier to keep track of your intake by filling some bottles or containers with water at the start of the day and aim to finish them by the end of the day. It doesn't matter if it's cold, room temperature or hot with a squeeze of flavor. In addition to water, you can also try sport drinks, milks, and decaffeinated tea and coffee. Foods that are liquid at room temperature such as soup, popsicles, gelatin, fruits and vegetables count too. Some fruits (like watermelon and grapes) are especially high in water content. Note: A good indicator of hydration is the color of your urine, not related to excreting chemotherapy or other medications. Urine should be a pale yellow or straw color.

Some signs of underhydration are:

- headache
- fatigue or feeling weak
- irritability
- dry lips, tongue and mouth
- dizziness
- constipation
- dark-colored urine (not related to excreting chemotherapy or other medicines)
- rapid weight loss

If you experience any of these symptoms and can't keep them under control by taking in more fluid, contact your healthcare team for advice. Dehydration can be serious. If you are ill with vomiting or diarrhea during cancer treatment, you are at higher risk for becoming dehydrated and should ask your healthcare team for advice on how best to manage safely.

Healthy Weight

Maintaining a healthy weight can lower the risk of getting breast cancer as well as reduce the risk of recurrence in women who have breast cancer, especially after menopause. If you are overweight, there is good evidence that getting to a healthy weight and maintaining it will reduce the risk of breast cancer recurrence or of developing other health problems, including types of cancer. Research studies suggest that excess body fat causes higher levels of estrogen, which, again, increases the risk of breast cancer and breast cancer recurrence. If you do need to lose weight, partner with your healthcare team for guidance and support. If you are starting breast cancer treatment, you may want to focus on eating well, exercising moderately and taking care of yourself throughout the treatment phase – and address weight loss afterward.

Physical Activity

Regular exercise is an important part of optimizing health. Research shows that regular moderate exercise such as walking three to five hours per week can reduce the risk of getting breast cancer and also reduce the risk of breast cancer recurrence. There is also good evidence that exercise can help breast cancer survivors live longer and have a more active life. Exercise builds muscle and burns fat and can, when used in conjunction with a healthy diet, help you attain and maintain a healthy weight.

It is safe to exercise during cancer treatment as long as the healthcare team has no objections and as long as you follow any needed precautions or modifications. Exercise can improve common side effects from cancer treatment such as fatigue, nausea and lymphedema which some women experience following mastectomy. It can also help improve circulation to the whole body, including the legs, which reduces the risk of blood clots. Exercise stimulates the digestive tract and can help promote elimination, thereby preventing constipation. Regular exercise will help you fall asleep faster and sleep more deeply to provide healing rest for your body.

Some treatments for breast cancer cause bone loss. Women are more likely to experience bone loss after age 50. Weight-bearing exercise such as walking, dancing and running can counteract these effects and help promote strong bones. Exercise also builds muscles and helps improve strength, stamina and overall quality of life.

Finally, exercise promotes a feeling of well-being, as it triggers the release of endorphins that contribute to feelings of joy and relaxation and can help control the anxiety and depression that may accompany a cancer diagnosis. Regular moderate exercise can be like meditation, helping you focus on good health and maintain a calm state of mind. (See also Professor Schmitz's essay on the benefits of exercise elsewhere in this book.)

Some trustworthy online resources for nutrition information during cancer treatment include the following:

Breast cancer.org <https://www.breastcancer.org/tips/nutrition>

American Institute for Cancer Research: What to eat to lower cancer risk

<https://www.aicr.org/reduce-your-cancer-risk/diet/>

Diet, Nutrition and Breast Cancer pdf:

<https://www.aicr.org/continuous-update-project/reports/breast-cancer-report-2017.pdf>

How to find a nutrition expert:

<https"//www.eatright.org/find-an-expert> search by cancer/oncology nutrition expertise

Bibliography

ACS 2017. "ACS Guidelines for Nutrition and Physical Activity." cancer.org online (2017), <https://www.cancer.org/healthy/eat-healthy-get-active/acs-guidelines-nutrition-physical-activity-cancer-prevention/guidelines.html>. Accessed November 30, 2019.

AICR 2018. "World Cancer Research Fund/American Institute for Cancer Research: Continuous Update Project Expert Report (2018): Diet, Nutrition, Physical Activity and Breast Cancer." <dietandcancerreport.org>. Accessed November 30, 2019.

AICR 2019. "AICR New American Plate." <https://www.aicr.org/cancer-prevention/healthy-eating/new-american-plate>. Accessed November 30, 2019.

Anderson, J. W., P. Baird, R. H. Davis Jr., et al. "Health Benefits of Dietary Fiber." *Nutrition Reviews* 67.4 (April 2009): 188–205.

Chakraborty, S., M. Roy, and R. K. Bhattacharya. "Prevention and Repair of DNA Damage by Selected Phytochemicals as Measured by Single Cell Gel Electrophoresis." *Journal of Environmental Pathology, Toxicology and Oncology* 23.3 (2004): 215–26.

Chlebowski, Rowan T., Aaron K. Aragaki, Garnet L. Anderson, et al. "Low-Fat Dietary Pattern and Breast Cancer Mortality in the Women's Health Initiative Randomized Controlled Trial." *Journal of Clinical Oncology* 35.25 (September 1, 2017): 2919–26.

Collins, Karen. "Soy and Cancer: Myths and Misconceptions." AICR online (February 19, 2019), <https://www.aicr.org/resources/blog/soy-and-cancer-myths-and-misconceptions>. Accessed November 30, 2019.

Elliot, Ruan. "Mechanisms of Genomic and Non-genomic Actions of Carotenoids." *Biochimica et Biophysica Acta (BBA) – Molecular Basis of Disease* 1740.2 (May 30, 2005): 147–54.

Ellison, R. Curtis, Yuqing Zhang, Christine E. McLennan, et al. "Exploring the Relation of Alcohol Consumption to Risk of Breast Cancer." *American Journal of Epidemiology* 154. 8 (October 15, 2001): 740–7.

Environmental Working Group. <https://www.ewg.org/foodnews/>. Accessed November 14, 2020.

Fabian, Carol J., Bruce F. Kimler, and Stephen D. Hursting. "Omega-3 Fatty Acids for Breast Cancer Prevention and Survivorship." *Breast Cancer Research* 17.1 (2015): 62.

Farvid, Maryam S., Eunyoung Cho, A. Heather Eliassen, et al. "Lifetime Grain Consumption and Breast Cancer Risk." *Breast Cancer Research and Treatment* 159.2 (September 2016): 335–45.

Fiolet, Thibault, Bernard Srour, Laury Sellem, et al. "Consumption of Ultra-Processed Foods and Cancer Risk: Results from NutriNet-Santé Prospective Cohort." *British Medical Journal* (February 14, 2018): 1–11.

Gray, Janet M., Sharima Rasanayagam, Connie Engel, et al. "State of the Evidence 2017: An Update on the Connection between Breast Cancer and the Environment." *Environmental Health* 16.360 (2017): 1–61.

Holscher, Hannah D. "Dietary Fiber and Prebiotics and the Gastrointestinal Microbiota." *Gut Microbes* 8.2 (2017): 172–84.

Kachuri, Linda M., Anne Harris, Jill S. MacLeod, et al. "Cancer Risks in a Population-Based Study of 70,570 Agricultural Workers: Results from the Canadian Census Health and Environment Cohort (CanCHEC)". *BMC Cancer* 17.343 (May 19, 2017): 1–15.

Kapinova, A., P. Kubatka, O. Golubnitschaja, et al. "Dietary Phytochemicals in Breast Cancer Research: Anticancer Effects and Potential Utility for Effective Chemoprevention." *Environmental Health and Preventive Medicine* 23.36 (2018): 1–18.

Li, Q., T. R. Holford, Y. Zhang, et al. "Dietary Fiber Intake and Risk of Breast Cancer by Menopausal and Estrogen Receptor Status." *European Journal of Nutrition* 52 (2013): 217–23.

Link, L. B., A. J. Canchola, L. Bernstein, et al. "Dietary Patterns and Breast Cancer Risk in the California Teachers Study Cohort." *American Journal of Clinical Nutrition* 98.6 (2013): 1524–32.

Lo, J. J., Y. M. Park, R. Sinha, et al. "Association between Meat Consumption and Risk of Breast Cancer: Findings from the Sister Study." *International Journal of Cancer* (August 6, 2019). doi: 10.1002/ijc.32547. [Epub ahead of print]

Ren, Feiyue, Kim Reilly, Joseph P. Kerry, et al. "Higher Antioxidant Activity, Total Flavonols, and Specific Quercetin Glucosides in Two Different Onion (Allium cepa L.) Varieties Grown under Organic Production: Results from a 6-Year Field Study". *Journal of Agricultural and Food Chemistry* 65.25 (2017): 5122–32.

Sangaramoorthy, Meera, Jocelyn Koo, and Esther M. John. "Intake of Bean Fiber, Beans, and Grains and Reduced Risk of Hormone Receptor-Negative Breast Cancer: The San Francisco Bay Area Breast Cancer Study." *Cancer Medicine* 7.5 (May 2018): 2131–44.

Schulz, M., K. Hoffmann, C. Weikert, et al. "Identification of a Dietary Pattern Characterized by High-Fat Food Choices Associated with Increased Risk of Breast Cancer: The European Prospective Investigation into Cancer and Nutrition (EPIC)-Potsdam Study." *British Journal of Nutrition* 100.5 (November 2008): 942–6.

Turati, F., G. Cairoli, F. Bravi, et al. "Mediterranean Diet and Breast Cancer Risk." *Nutrients* 10.3 (March 8, 2018): 326.

Wang, Dong D., and Frank B. Hu. "Dietary Fat and Risk of Cardiovascular Disease: Recent Controversies and Advances." *Annual Review of Nutrition* 37.1 (2017): 423–46.

AMY HOLIDAY

A Future on Ice

We were two people waiting in a waiting room. I had breast cancer, he was my fiancé.

It was an October morning. Early enough in the fall that it was neither hot nor cold, but crisp enough that you regretted leaving home without a light jacket and hat. As I sat, I wondered how it would feel to be bald in the winter. It felt too abstract, sad, so I snacked on breath mints instead. He flipped mindlessly through a promotional magazine celebrating the hospital's newest robotic nurses. I was nervous. Time dripped by slowly as it does in a waiting room.

Around us, the rhythm of a doctor's office pulsed. Couples walking in holding hands, checking in, sitting down, settling in. A receptionist sat high behind a tall counter.

There were framed prints of watercolor flowers, perfectly aligned rows of green chairs, a conspicuously placed medical-grade hand sanitizer. The magazines on the table were *Working Mother* and *Popular Mechanics*. The lighting was fluorescent. The air was purified. Jazz played on a speaker poorly hidden behind a potted indoor plant. The room was trying to feel calm and upscale.

The room was full of people, waiting just like us. I tried to find myself in them but couldn't.

They looked content, at ease and okay. They seemed roughly middle-aged, with crisp looking clothes and expensive bags. Their waiting room small talk and waiting room laughter seemed hopeful, bordering on happy. They recognized the nurses when their names were called; they smiled as they went on back. The women looked professional and healthy, alert and prepared. The men tired, but supportive.

Everything seemed routine and familiar, to everyone but us.

We were at the NYU Fertility Clinic. It was our first time in this waiting room. I felt like a reluctant intruder, lurking around a scene in which I didn't belong. I was cautious. I felt young and underdressed. And for the first time, Sick.

Two weeks before, I had been diagnosed with stage 2, invasive ductal carcinoma. Like so many cancers, it came out of nowhere – a pain, a lump, a biopsy. The cancer had a Ki-67 rate (a protein in cells that increases when they're preparing to divide into new cells) of sixty, meaning a high number of cells in my left breast were dividing and growing into new, deadly cells. It was aggressive cancer. I was 28, on the verge of everything.

The immediate space between cancer diagnosis and treatment is a demilitarized zone. It is a pause between two terrors. It is learning a new identity, calibrating to a new future. It's appointments and tests, as doctors work to develop a treatment plan and understand the boundaries of your disease. It's the space where a provocation evolves into a war.

The weapons most commonly deployed against cancer – chemotherapy and radiation – have toxic effects on the body. In the short term, they kill cancerous cells. But they are ruthless and do not discriminate. In the longer term, they can render patients sterile. So it is in this zone between diagnosis and treatment that some patients attempt fertility preservation. That is, before fighting for their own lives, they fight for the privilege to potentially create new life in a hypothetical future.

Fertility preservation is elective. It is, relative to cancer treatment, a privilege. As more and more young cancer patients enjoy the prospect of living disease-free, many doctors now recommend fertility preservation before beginning certain types of treatment. For a woman, fertility preservation is a process of overstimulating the ovaries, harvesting the eggs, and freezing them for implantation at a future time.

It is a scientific manufacturing of potential conception.

The window to decide to undergo fertility preservation is often narrow, forcing a fast – and expensive – decision in this liminal zone of pause. The urgency of starting cancer treatment and the cycles of a woman's body mean she must act quickly, usually while she is emotionally overwhelmed and unable to think quite clearly.

I had two days to decide whether I would attempt fertility preservation. I had one shot. We talked about it and decided to try, juggling the money we had allocated for a wedding to make the process possible. We decided to postpone our wedding in part to freeze my eggs.

We never spoke these words out loud, but there was an assumed agreement: Cancer could kill me, but this was the future we wanted to fight for.

I was determined to live through cancer. And I was determined to become a mother.

That is how we found ourselves between two worlds. One hour, I was among women – bald, thin, dying – and the next, at a fertility clinic with happy couples on the precipice of starting bigger, child-ful lives. I felt different from them and much smaller.

Because cancer is often invisible before treatment starts, you look regular until one day you look like a cancer patient. So in this place – before treatment started, as I attempted to ensure my fertile future – I looked like everyone else.

They called me back, and we stood and walked together, past the plant and the hand sanitizer, and into the doctor's office.

****

We were 28 and 29. The babies were coming. Our friends, their worlds – and soon, our shared worlds – filled with birth announcements, birth days and everything that follows. We were watching, and pregnancy was feeling imminent. And logical.

When the world around you is procreating, and you are merely living, it can feel just like that: like you haven't started the race yet, you're waiting. You're making meaning, of course, embracing the *independence*. But when something feels imminent, that's when you begin to live. Everything happening now, before the *thing*, is the *before*.

The first would be named Francis, after his family. She would have his sense of adventure and precision for problem solving. I would take her running. With the dog. We'd be the family that took their infants camping; we'd make it work.

We'd have to move out of the city at some point. We were laying the foundation.

****

The goal of ovarian stimulation is for a woman's body to produce eight to fifteen feasible eggs, which are harvested surgically after seven to twelve days of treatment. The eggs can be fertilized, frozen, and stored for future implantation. In the case of a cancer patient, the frozen eggs are an insurance policy before chemotherapy and radiation kill them off.

The process is a cocktail of drugs, monitoring, and lab work.

It generally involves three types of drugs, all self-administered at home. First, a medication to stimulate the development of multiple eggs. Second, a medication to suppress ovulation. And third, a trigger injection to cause the eggs to mature. Dosages and cadence of the drugs vary each day, so women make daily clinic visits for monitoring.

If the ovaries are overstimulated, it can cause serious threat to the woman's body; if the ovaries are understimulated, there is a risk that the harvest is unsuccessful. So during monitoring visits, doctors decide to adjust drug dosages up or down to manufacture progress. They are looking for the development of multiple, maturing egg follicles – perfectly sized, perfectly ripe. When they are fully developed, the patient administers a trigger injection; exactly thirty-six hours later, the eggs are surgically harvested.

Each afternoon during the ovary stimulation phase, the nurses call with a verdict: The drugs are working or we need to adjust.

Depending on their counsel, a patient will adjust her drug dosage for evening injections and hope that the following day's results are positive.

It's physically and emotionally exhausting. The injections override natural process and body regulations.

It is a repetitive, precarious, needle-ful routine.

****

I gave myself the first injection alone in a hotel room in Dallas. The room was generic: two large, plump, perfectly made beds, tan-colored everything, a window overlooking other buildings overlooking other buildings. The carpet was patterned dizzyingly with shapes turning into other shapes. It was cold outside. It felt hot inside my room.

A Future on Ice

It was a work trip. I could have stayed at home. But I ignored the doctor's recommendation and went anyway, because I didn't want to feel defeated by cancer before treatment had started.

I didn't know what to wear. The informational videos that I had watched about this injection – my shaking, needle-wielding hand pushing repeat repeatedly – were full of happy couples. Always dressed in neutral colors with neutral backgrounds. The people in the videos were healthy, just a little infertile. I was envious of the concreteness of their problem.

My phone was positioned on the pillows. His face took up the whole screen, the video pixels coming in and out. He was trying to figure out what to say to be supportive. His reassuring voice was fighting against the Wi-Fi in the room, words muffled and missing. At some point I turned it off because I needed to do this alone.

My body, my choice. Or something.

Everything seemed sweaty.

I tried sitting on a chair, standing by a mirror, kneeling against the bed. I tried to find a posture that was secure, that I knew I couldn't recoil from. I had never injected myself before. I tried to get comfortable.

Everything felt significant. The cost of this injection was nearly $1,000.

My belly button was an anchor. A target. I grabbed a roll of fat and looked at it. It was regular-looking, a little tired. I counted to ten and on nine, at 7:15 p.m., I pierced the needle into the skin just under my navel.

Proud of myself for finding some levity as the needle emptied, I thought that I should have worn maternity pants.

The syringe emptied, the needle clicked, and it slipped out of me. I waited for the site to bleed, but nothing happened. As I held the needle, a single clear drop dripped from the needle head onto the carpet. Pants off, shirt up, stomach still glistening from the antiseptic wipe. I wondered what that was, that drop: a tiny part of the start of motherhood. And I wondered where I was now; my feet suddenly felt cemented to a runway that was moving. Everything that was hypothetical suddenly felt real.

I was done, and it was dinner time, so I put the needle into a box and walked alone, down the hall and into the world that didn't know what I had just started.

****

Every day for eleven days, I was obedient to the rigid routines of fertility preservation.

I grew tired and emotional. Each day felt harder, a little heavier. My body and my mind were bloated.

The fertility treatment process can be summarized by pricks, probes, timelines, and stirrups. You spend a lot of time exposing your body – both physically, but also emotionally – to the toll of daily blood work, morning transvaginal ultrasounds, nightly injections, the fear of misstepping, the doubt that your body will comply. You must give in for the process to work. You must give up to give in.

In the mornings I woke up at 5:30 a.m. and took the subway to the Upper East Side. It was that sacred time, when the city is still sleeping and your sense of purpose in being awake – walking alone, on wide empty sidewalks – feels exaggerated. I walked from the train station, but as soon as I crossed the threshold into the elevator, I became an automaton.

Check in. Confirm date of birth. Settle into the room of watercolor flowers, green chairs, and hand sanitizer. The jazz music was always playing.

When your name is called, you walk back to wait in the blood draw lab, flanked by other women. The nurses tie a tourniquet around your arm, make small talk, and draw your blood. Then you progress to an exam room, wiggle into a gown, onto the bed and into the stirrups. The doctor dims the lights and sticks a slick ultrasound probe into your vaginal canal.

I would watch the doctor watch the ultrasound screen. There were objects and outlines on the screen that I could not decipher. Since being diagnosed with cancer, I was getting used to discerning doctor's expressions as they processed images of my body. I could predict good news, or bad news, based on what their faces said.

My ovaries, displayed there on the screen, looked like the spongy mass inside bones. There were holes and gaps, dark spots and bright circles. It looked like a jumble to me. The doctor's face looked pleased.

Things were progressing, she said as she slipped the probe out of my body.

Your body is doing great, she said as she walked out of the room.

I got out of my gown and walked out of the exam room. I passed many other women walking in and walking out, our routines nearly identical except for the one significant difference.

Each morning, after my monitoring appointments, I went to the cancer center. The cross-town bus transported me from a place of women of health to women in treatment, from styled hair to baldness, from power suits to wheelchairs. I was getting ready for cancer treatment to begin; the tumor was being scanned, the breast cancer being analyzed, the chemotherapy drugs being decided.

The other women went on with their days and their careers.

I wanted life to speed up – to spit me out of this pause zone, to let me click back into something that felt regular. But at the same time, I wanted everything to stop. I was terrified of what would happen to me next.

****

I gave myself the trigger shot at exactly 10:10 p.m. on Thursday. It was Halloween. Everyone around us, on the street, with their families, seemed light and happy. We did this last one together. He held my hand, I sucked on a candy and slipped the needle in.

****

Once again, we were two people waiting in a waiting room. I had breast cancer, he was my fiancé.

It was Saturday morning, the day of the retrieval. It was colder now. I was wearing a hat and a sweatshirt. As I got dressed, I wondered how women decided what to wear on days of such significance – when you have your baby, when you lose your hair.

A few other couples sat beside us, some holding hands, some reading magazines. I felt at ease and realized that in some ways, I had become them. I felt older than I had eleven days ago, a little more weathered, my stomach like a swollen pin cushion.

They called him and me back at the same time, but in opposite directions. He was to go down the hall into a Specimen Deposit Room, and I was to walk into the operating room.

When I woke up, I cried. It was the hormones and the pain, and the relief of being done. My body felt swollen and I felt pain in places that had never been activated before.

Everything was successful. They harvested twenty-eight eggs. In the haze of anesthesia, I remember the doctor telling me I should be proud.

****

I am done with chemotherapy now. I am done with the mastectomy that destroyed my breast and the reconstructive surgery that attempted to rebuild it. I am cancer-free.

Harder things seem easier now. And easier things can be debilitatingly hard.

Because my cancer feeds on estrogen, I am on hormone therapy. Pills and injections have catapulted my body into menopause and keep it there, suspended in a period of barrenness and dryness. After five years, my doctors will evaluate whether it is safe for me pause this drug regimen and have an embryo implanted. If not, they will say to wait another five years. They'll suggest, as they do now, surrogacy and adoption. Or a life without kids.

All of these paths seem abstract now. Far away and hypothetical. I am not upset about them as much as I am intimidated by the distance between now and then. Right now, I am focused on now.

I find myself, like survivors of any sort, in a strange territory of recovery and discovery. I am happy and I am devastated, trying to find a little plot of land between the two poles to rebuild the foundation of my life and start again.

Breast cancer strips away womanhood in so many ways. I am a 28-year-old woman in some ways, but in so many ways, I am not. I am something else and I am figuring out what that is.

I pass the fertility clinic now and wonder how they are doing. I imagine the rent I'm paying for their comfort. And I wonder about the freezer and the canister that holds a future.

ELVA J. WINTER

Intimacy and Sexuality in the Context of Breast Cancer

"My new 'girls' don't look quite right and don't feel quite right; and coloring nipples on them when I want to look good for some dude is a bother, but I guess I'll get used to it."

"I'm against skin tattoos. When the radiology techs told me they were putting three pinpoint tattoos in my breast area to mark radiation targets, I got angry – even though they're pinpoint."

"My breasts now are always perky – a little out of context for a seventy-year-old. But contrast them with the natural pendulous ones I had before ... I'd say the change is about 50:50."

"The chemo results weren't so bad as I thought they'd be."

"I don't mind loss of breast sensation because I never liked my husband touching my breasts."

"I miss breast sensation."

"The skin under my arms feels like corrugated cardboard."

"I still have nipple sensation because the surgeon sewed part of my intact nipple onto skin over my implant."

"Even though I don't want to have another child, the thought of not being able to create life and give birth because I had a hysterectomy as part of treatment threw me for a loop."

"The experience gave me the courage to try online dating in hopes I'd discover positive sexual relating I'd never had. My experiment worked ... sexually, but not relationally."

As these comments from some of my therapy clients who have had breast cancer indicate, responses to the disease and its treatments vary widely. Many people demonstrate positive adjustment to their breast cancer experience, and I suspect just as many even thrive, given the human capacity to grow. One woman told me, "My sense of being a woman doesn't come from having breasts – it comes from my intellect and heart. In relationship I'm the same woman I've always been." She said, "Cancer took away my two breasts, not me." Another woman, diagnosed and treated while she and her husband were in the process of divorcing for reasons not related to cancer, received support from her husband. He said he would stay with her through her treatment, surgery and breast reconstruction – and he did.

But grief over losses in sensation and self-image, along with relationship challenges, are common concerns among most people who are diagnosed and treated. Surgery for breast cancer removal and reconstruction means bodies are cut into, body parts are cut off and out, skin is bruised and nerves may be injured or deadened. Scars and altered range of motion in the arms and back can result. Radiation treatment can cause skin inflammation and chest skin burns. Chemotherapy can cause nausea, vomiting, changes in appetite and weight, profound fatigue and hair loss to the degree of baldness. How a body looks and feels is of central importance to people's sexual sense of self; and even the fear of these side effects can impact sexual interest, desire and expression. Grief is inevitable when people begin to consider themselves as no longer healthy and no longer the sexual persons they had been. Grief takes time to resolve. People need the freedom to grieve.

Women often struggle with their identity as a woman, particularly if their breasts have been a significant part of love-making or of motherhood – but also even if breast importance occurred in seemingly more simple ways such as dress, appearance and feeling attractive. When a woman begins anti-estrogen therapy (if her tumor is hormone-positive) or has her uterus and ovaries removed (if a genetic disposition to uterine and ovarian cancer has been discovered through genetic testing and she elects prophylactic hysterectomy), she experiences what is commonly called "induced menopause" because of lack of estrogen. Changes in her body temperature cause hot flashes and night sweats, and changes in vaginal tissue cause burning, dryness and irritation, which contribute to painful sexual intercourse. Bladder leakage and infections can become more likely. These changes may affect a 35-year-old woman differently from an 80-year-old woman, but they do affect the sexual sense of self of both.

Men often grapple with embarrassment because they've been diagnosed with what is typically considered "a woman's disease." Side effects of surgery, radiation and chemotherapy in men are similar to those in women. In addition, men who are accustomed to going bare-chested may be bothered by a scarred chest and/or the lack of nipples – and questions about same. Hormone therapy, when indicated, can cause weight gain, hot flashes, mood swings, loss of sexual desire and erectile dysfunction.

Having breast cancer challenges a couple's relationship too: variances in mood (especially anxiety and depression) in either partner; communication between partners; the ability to be mutually supportive; the need to maintain or modify established family and social roles; changes that arise from one individual's or the couple's evaluation of the meaning of their lives and, potentially, a determination to actualize latent desires (Zimmerman 102–8). While it may seem burdensome for persons experiencing breast cancer to pay attention to their significant sexual relationships and to communicate openly and regularly with partners, doing so is a positive approach to stave off or minimize discord between them.

For all these reasons, even though breast cancer is the most common cancer women experience, is a rare occurrence in men, is treatable, has a low mortality rate and is considered a chronic disease, enduring it can be traumatic. Upon breast cancer diagnosis and with each new intervention and side effect, a person confronts a new sense of self and degree of wellness. And because breast cancer treatment and recovery can require months or perhaps years, it is not unusual for people to seek counseling for sexual issues a year or more after treatment ends. Among their first struggle with sexuality is the difference in their appearance and how to be comfortable when interacting physically. Sexual therapists can help people regain (or gain for the first time) a positive sexual sense of self. My efforts include broadening people's understanding of sexuality in general, and supporting them as they explore how they want to express themselves.

Initially, what most people experiencing breast cancer need in therapy is permission to be compassionate with themselves. Therapists of any discipline can offer permission for self-compassion. They also can give permission for clients to incorporate sexual desires and practices. Therapists can do both to the degree they're comfortable hearing clients' sexual concerns and desires, and are knowledgeable about human sexuality. What distinguishes sexual therapists is that they've generally been educated in dimensions of sexuality that include historical and cultural antecedents and emerging practices. This additional training enables sexual therapists to suspend their own values and judgment as they listen to clients' sexual concerns. Consequently, clients usually become comfortable talking openly about sexuality – which is a crucial first step toward healing.

Sexual therapists often utilize a model of intervention called PLISSIT: Permission, Limited Information, Specific Suggestion and Intensive Therapy (Annon). I find that using PLISSIT encourages me to keep asking myself the question "What does this client need at this particular time?" as therapy evolves.

Diana's Story

Diana had a caring relationship with her girlfriend, Emma, who was gentle and attentive. Diana couldn't understand, then, why, a year after her recovery from breast cancer treatment and seeming recovery, she startled when Emma physically drew her close. Diana's entire body stiffened. She desired sexual activity but found herself detaching as their interaction moved beyond kissing. She was inexplicably angry with Emma for wanting sexual intimacy, yet she recognized that she was the one whose ability to connect was compromised. Diana's startle effect, detachment and displaced anger were evidence that she had experienced breast cancer as trauma; hers were posttraumatic stress responses.

Six months of weekly talk therapy that included education about trauma and its after-effects enabled Diana to see a connection between the present crisis and a previous girlfriend's behavior. Having never resolved that situation, she had carried forward anger, reflexive recoil and detachment as a means of coping. After giving herself permission to feel self-compassion for having these natural responses, and after learning more about crisis and its resolution, Diana was able to return to positive sexual relating with Emma. In this way, Diana benefitted especially from two aspects of the PLISSIT model – "Permission" to talk in depth about experiencing breast cancer as trauma and "Limited Information" that validated her experience.

Gretchen's Story

Gretchen, aged 48, sought treatment with me early because she was particularly shocked upon her diagnosis. She had been eating healthfully as vegetarian and exercising assiduously to avoid dying from heart disease in her early fifties as her mother had done. Whereas she had felt prepared to deal with developing heart disease at some later point in life, she felt blindsided and totally at a loss to deal with what would follow her breast cancer diagnosis.

Gretchen felt guilty. She feared she was being punished with breast cancer because she was trying to ward off the fate of developing heart disease. She also thought that having breast cancer was appropriate pay-back for having rejected her childhood learning that "having sex" before marriage was wrong, and "enjoying sex" was even more wrong. Preparing for treatment side effects before radiation therapy had kept her guilt at bay for short periods of time. She secured appropriate skin lotion, selected non-irritating clothing and made list after list of ways she would treat herself on therapy days. "Forewarned is forearmed," she said. "But I didn't forewarn myself about this guilt."

What she needed at that time in therapy was help to resolve those feelings. Cognitive Behavioral Therapy (CBT), in which people learn to examine their thoughts for accuracy and then modify them to be more realistic, was helpful. Just as important was examining how her parents had come to believe what they believed – and had taught her to believe – about sexuality. This process enabled her to identify and affirm what she had learned through experience to be valid – something different from her parents' point of view.

After several months of sexual therapy that focused on her beliefs and attitudes, she decided to end counseling. Weekly sessions had been adding to her physiological tiredness from chemotherapy, radiation treatment and mastectomy with reconstructive surgery. She had gained self-compassion, and her struggle with guilt had resolved; and she was able to look at fatigue as her body's call to rest. We welcomed this sign of self-awareness and self-care.

Gretchen had not prepared for resuming sexual sharing with her partner, however, and she returned to therapy about three months later. Now, she was ready to address a more sexually explicit issue. She revealed that her previous sexual relating patterns had consistently been breast-focused – for both her partner and herself. As an adult, she had never been able to receive vaginal penetration because of vaginismus, an involuntary contraction of muscles around the opening of the vagina that creates pain on attempted penetration. She had attributed the condition to having been vaginally "probed" against her will as a teenager by a fellow teen during a party game. She had settled into receiving pleasure and orgasm through her breasts and at times simultaneously through her clitoris. Her partner had been satisfied with their sexual sharing in that way.

But now she had no nipples, just a flat tattoo, so the source of her primary arousal was gone. She had no deep breast sensation, only the feel of light touching which was not enough to enable physical and emotional arousal. To both her and her partner, her breast prostheses felt like water-filled balloons – too cold and uncomfortable to lead to the penile stimulation he enjoyed or to an orgasm for her, as direct clitoral stimulation without breast arousal was insufficient to bring about climax.

"What can I do?" she asked. "I don't want to give up having sex. And I don't want to just go through some meaningless motions so my partner gets off."

Gretchen didn't have to do either. She opened her thinking to consider that addressing her vaginismus might result in a new arousal pattern and sexual fulfillment. She agreed that her situation might warrant the more Intensive Therapy aspect of the PLISSIT model. Before we began intensive therapy, though, she wanted to "try it" on her own. "Just give me some suggestions," she said. I obliged and gave her **S**pecific **S**uggestions, as per PLISSIT.

I suggested she study the topic of vaginismus – something she had never done – by gathering information from internet sources. I also suggested that she and her partner experiment with touching each other's full naked bodies in every place imaginable, including her genital area. They were to touch with hands and mouths as well as feathers and other objects agreeable to them, but only for brief periods of minutes, giving no one part of the body any more time than any other. The goals were to identify areas of positive sensation, encourage relaxation and possibly to reduce, physically and mentally, her sensations of fear.

Gretchen tried my suggestions for about two months, then returned saying, "I think we're getting closer to success, but I get frustrated. I'd hoped my vagina would spring to life and open a little, but it's still angry." At this point, I suggested that we focus on intensive therapy because she wanted to become newly receptive to sexual experience. A plus was that both she and her partner had talked about her new learning, and he was as invested as she was. Her sense of humor added positivity, too.

Intensive therapy with Gretchen included involving her obstetrician to prescribe pelvic floor physical therapy. As she progressed through weeks of physical therapy, she became aware of and comfortable with sensations other than pain in her genitalia. When it became possible for her to slip her little finger into her vagina without pain, we discussed how vaginal moisturizing suppositories could be helpful, possibly along with bioidentical hormones (also in suppository form). The hope that they might decrease discomfort and pain gave her impetus to proceed with vaginal dilator treatment.

As Gretchen moved through the treatment with dilators, she and I discussed the effect on her vagina as well as the past sexual assault she'd called "probing." Eventually she became able to welcome the presence of her partner's finger – and later his penis – in her vagina. The force of his thrusting movements remained a challenge for her, but she expected their humor would help with that concern. They laughed often, alone or together, during intercourse, and discovered that laughing disrupted the pain she sometimes experienced. Gretchen also wanted to identify some ways to incorporate past breast pleasure into their love-making. Learning to watch erotic movies with her partner and reading erotic passages about women's breasts became a way to prompt memories of their past breast enjoyment and provide pleasure in the present.

Redefining Sex

Consider the state of a person experiencing an unexpected breast cancer diagnosis and the cumulative physical and psychological effects of treatment over time. "Sexy" is probably the *last* thing she or he feels – or expects to feel. Reconsidering what constitutes "sexy," though, can broaden sexual horizons and deepen interpersonal intimacy. "Sexy" includes making eye contact; smiling genuinely; being curious, interested and interesting; listening closely; embodying self-confidence; valuing and taking care of oneself (it shows); being kind. And that's just the beginning! Sexy is in the eyes of the beholder. Fortunate is the person who understands this about herself or himself. And fortunate is the partner who enjoys these more nuanced forms of sexuality.

Textbooks often describe sexual desire as a condition that happens automatically, as something a person spontaneously feels emotionally and/or physically, something that gives rise to genital and full-body arousal. This description is incomplete, however, without crediting the brain for setting the process in motion. Our mind-brain provides motivation to engage sexually. Sexual desire typically stems from a person's being fully present with what is happening – either with a partner or merely in her own mind. Desire, then, is the impetus for "more," however people conceptualize that "more": acts such as hugging, kissing, genital stimulation, penetration, etc., that bring about mutual (in the best of all possible worlds) pleasuring.

A person's sexual self is an amalgam of many different influences: facts about sexuality (incomplete, usually); folklore (much); cultural, family, and religious teachings (many and varied); sexual experiences (negative and positive); plus physical responses, emotions and attitudes that result from all these factors. Although born with sexual expression potential, we become a fully sexual person throughout the course of our lifetime, and thus, at any moment/day/year we are newly experiencing and expressing ourselves sexually. Understanding that the brain is critical in bringing about sexual interest, it is easy to appreciate that mental desire and fulfillment are key to a lifetime of discovering joy in continuously becoming sexual. Clear thinking, reasoning and decision-making about sexuality and one's own sexual nature are critical too. These elements operate the same way in sexual expression after breast cancer experience as before. Breast cancer time can be an opportunity for growth and even discovery of new ways of sexual expression, as is any season of a person's life.

Ways of Sexual Pleasuring

There are many ways of sexual pleasuring. Recently I heard a comedian say that most people have a repertoire of six sexual acts. Six, to me, does not constitute "a lot." The comedian also said that by the time number four of the six is reached, the sexual sharing is usually over because the partners have reached their goal of orgasm or have given up trying to reach it. Comedy is based on truth. The truth inherent in this comedy routine is disheartening, but it need not be so.

Part of the truth is that as humans we become victims of the routines we establish to allow us to move as comfortably as possible through life. This is true even for sexual habits. Routines are not inherently negative. They give us satisfaction and allow us to put our energy into interests and activities that keep curiosity and wonder alive within us. But sexual interaction often (dare I say "usually"?) becomes routine because we learn that certain actions bring about the sexual satisfaction we seek. We stop exploring other possibilities once we've discovered what works.

Innate curiosity and wonder become the best allies of sexual partners faced with the challenge to change because of breast cancer. When they use the opportunity to learn additional ways to pleasure each other and themselves, additional ways of expressing care (and for many, love), they become more fulfilled as sexually sharing humans. To be "fulfilled" is more than to be "satisfied." To me, satisfaction indicates supporting and reinforcing a present human condition, whereas fulfillment connotes the actualization of human possibility – many opportunities for what "might be" if we only set our minds to pursue natural curiosity. "Fulfillment" bespeaks a use and manifestation of creative force, something far beyond performance of routine, some deeper human experience.

Sexual fulfillment is available to anyone who is willing to move out of an established routine of sexual interaction. With all people seeking sexual counsel I provide educational material, clarify information and help them overcome obstacles to their permitting themselves pleasurable activity. Since many people need only that approach to move toward sexual fulfillment, I present here some aspects of what I consider fundamental learning.

Consider this about human sexuality: The skin on our body covers about twenty square feet, making it our largest organ. Skin is massively responsive to touch, and touching is a primary component of sexual sharing. As babies, most of us learn to experience full-body touch as pleasurable. Skin responds to sensations from stroking, pressure, light tickling, air movement, moisture, temperature and more; we call these sensations sensual. Stimulation of our senses of sight, hearing, taste and smell can be sensual too when they evoke pleasurable feelings related to sexuality. Not surprisingly, then, a typical first intervention for couples seeking sex therapy of any kind is "sensate focus," a prescribed series of touching exercises to help people expand ways of giving and receiving full-body (as compared with genitally focused) pleasure. The main goal of sensate focus is to improve sexual intimacy and overall relationship satisfaction (Weiner and Avery-Clark).

The pleasure to be experienced through our skin can be especially exhilarating when we actively engage our brain. Pleasure to the senses is processed in the brain. Again, the brain ... creates imaginative contexts in which quality sexual interactions can develop; the brain ... readies us to be interested and willing to engage in sexual activity; the brain ... processes whole-body sensuality as meaningful. It is difficult to really "get" that brain preparation is essential for sexual fulfillment when mainstream media all around us suggest that "it" (sex) just happens ... and happens spontaneously. Attention to all of our senses brings about more pleasurable – and perhaps more meaningful – sexual relating than will happen by trying to fit our experiences into a media model of immediate and athletic body penetration that leads to orgasmic release worthy of fireworks. Because genital stimulation feels so powerfully pleasurable we sometimes forget about engaging in equally pleasurable acts that can precede – and prepare us for – genital pleasure.

For instance, incorporating sexual toys can heighten pleasure, especially as physiological sexual response cycles change in the contexts of illness and aging. Integrating elements that provide a sensual atmosphere to expand touch – like fantasy, visual or written erotica, music, aromatic oils, tastes of varied range and texture and hand-held implements like feathers or scarves – await invitation. Full bare-being body contact – that is, bare-human to bare-human physical presence and humans emotionally and fully being-with-each-other – is arguably the most powerful turn-on. The brain comprehends genitally induced orgasm as one aspect of sexual experience, not the only goal. Even so, if a person has previously experienced genital orgasm, the brain can make it possible to experience orgasm via stimulation of other areas of the body – earlobes or inner arms, for instance – when genital orgasm becomes impossible through, say, paralysis or nerve damage.

Years ago, giving and receiving pleasure above the neck was called "necking." Pleasuring below the neck, but without penetration, was called "petting." Later, those experiences were known as "making out." Now, "vibing" is a term that teens and young adults use to describe their synchronicity and interest in each other – interest that may or may not include making out. None of these activities is worth discarding once genital pleasuring is discovered. Young people just opening to their sexuality find great pleasure in vibing and making out. Oldsters once took pleasure there and can do so again. So can persons of any age who have experienced breast cancer.

Indeed, discoveries of the young can lead those who are older, including those of breast cancer experience, toward new pleasuring activity. "Soloing," which is focused on getting to know one's own sexual self and sexual expression, is a contemporary term that sounds to youth more accurate than terms like self-pleasuring (sounds indulgent) and masturbation (sounds like bad behavior). Soloing can help people consolidate a gender sense of self, connect erotically and lovingly, and improve their overall health. Persons of any age, ones of breast cancer experience included, could opt to test that theory and so expand pleasuring skills.

The experience of breast cancer does not inevitably alter cognitive ability and it does not kill creative potential. One still has a body with sensory capacity. One is still a sexual person. One still has soul (a topic for another time). A breast cancer experience may alter expression of a person's sexuality but need not annihilate future sexual experience nor its quality. So ... instead of claiming that humans have a repertoire of (only six!) sexual acts, a more accurate statement about sexual pleasuring is that there are as many permutations and variations of sexual pleasure as our minds can create and feel at home with, alone or partnered.

There are many books (including academic sexuality textbooks) about how to create meaningful sexual experiences after cancer. I suggest to clients they search the internet for the topic "sexuality after cancer" and read the tables of contents of books that speak to their specific questions and individual needs. Reading historical material about breasts, breast cancer, and sexuality in different cultures can enlarge a person's view of who we have been as sexual people. A helpful consequence of reading about sexuality in general as well as sexuality after breast cancer is that it gives one something other than her or his personal cancer experience to talk about with others, and a means to educate others by sharing new knowledge – which adds to a positive sense of self. Ultimately, exposure to new ideas can help a person reclaim her sexual potential and alter the way she expresses herself sexually.

Books that have been helpful to clients include the following:

A History of the Breast, by Marilyn Yalom, 1998.

And in Health: A Guide for Couples Facing Cancer Together, by Dan Shapiro, 2013.

Breasts: A Natural and Unnatural History, by Florence Williams, 2013.

Radical: The Science, Culture, and History of Breast Cancer in America, by Kate Pickert, 2019.

The History of Sexuality, Vol.1: An Introduction, by Michael Foucault, 1990.

The History of Sexuality, Vol. 2: The Use of Pleasure, by Michael Foucault and Robert Hurley, 1990.

The History of Sexuality, Vol.3: The Care of the Self, by Michael Foucault and Robert Hurley, 1988.

The History of Sexuality Sourcebook, by Matthew Kuefler, 2007.

Additionally, many videos and internet websites – as well as sexual counselors and therapists – can be valuable resources.

Conclusion

Through the expression of oneself sexually, a person can give and receive pleasure, care, comfort, compassion and joy. Sexual sharing provides opportunities to create, to grow and to know wonder in ways that can make us more fully human. The experience of breast cancer and breast cancer treatment need not limit people's ability to express themselves sexually. Not as long as they stay alive to possibilities.

Bibliography

Annon, J. S. *Behavioral Treatment of Sexual Problems: Brief Therapy*. Oxford: Harper & Row, 1976.

Weiner, Linda, and Constance Avery-Clark. *Sensate Focus in Sex Therapy*. New York: Routledge, 2017.

Zimmerman, Tania. "Intimate Relationships Affected by Breast Cancer: Interventions for Couples." *Breast Care* 10:2 (April 2015): 102–8.

PART III

Shaping Cancer, (Re)Shaping Self

DEBORAH BOWMAN

On Being Constant and Changed: Breast Cancer in Six Acts

Act 1: Frankenstein's Breast and the Vanishing Woman

It was a Sunday evening when my reflection shocked me. I was undressing for my ritual pre-working week bath. My right breast was distorted: Frankenstein's breast. The nipple was inverting, the breast was misshapen and lumpy with skin that appeared puckered and wizened. I looked in disbelief. I had showered after exercising that morning and all had been normal. What had happened? How could a body alter and mutate into a monstrous appearance within hours? I lay in the bath staring at my alien right breast.

> It will be fine.
> I am going to die.
> Most lumps are innocuous.
> This isn't 'a lump' – my breast has collapsed.
> Do not Google.
> Where is the computer?
> Do not Google.
> Oh my God. This is obviously cancer and a nasty one at that.
>
> *Repeat to fade .....*

A sleepless night yielded to a tense morning. I work in a medical school and mentioned, casually, to my colleague that I was going to need to see my doctor because I'd noticed some changes in my breast. I watched as her clinical composure struggled with fear and pity for me.

> Deborah, you must go.
> Today.
> Go today.
> Promise?
> Ring me.
> Promise you'll go and ring me?

I picked up the phone and rang the surgery. I say the words aloud to a stranger down the line.

> I think I need an appointment. My breast has, well –
> It is weird, kind of –
> Well, it's changed, suddenly.
> Yes, yes, a lump, but more than that too.
> My nipple, is, well, vanishing –
> And, the skin looks, well –
> Oh, okay. Yes, I can come this afternoon.
> If you think it's necessary?
> You've been kind, thank you.
> Where do I come?
> You see, I don't really come to the doctor often or ever, really.

It was my first experience of the altering and altered self. I knew, with every rational part of me, that I needed to see a doctor. I wanted to do anything but see a doctor. I was disoriented by a sense of guilt, almost shame. The considered woman who had worked in medical settings for her entire career was clearly and calmly explaining her surprising symptoms, whilst the same woman was trembling inside.

> I think we need to refer you. It looks like an infection, but just in case.
> Yes, I thought maybe an infection. Perhaps if it settles with the antibiotics, I can pass on the referral?

On Being Constant and Changed: Breast Cancer in Six Acts

> No, I think just to be sure, you should go.
> Oh, right. Yes, of course. When might the antibiotics have an effect if it is an infection?
> It can vary, but I'll prescribe a week's course and get that letter to the oncologists. Where would you like to be seen?
> I, erm, well, I don't know really. I guess not at my own hospital. I think that would be difficult for me …

I have often written about autonomy. The word means "self-rule." I believe that individuals should be able to choose what happens to them in their care and that ethical practice attends to the differences amongst people. Nonetheless, autonomy isn't unproblematic. The notion of people as separate, rational and self-determining may overlook the connectedness and relationships that shape not only our own choices, but that also inform what it is to be part of a flourishing community. Autonomy depends on trust and understanding for it to be meaningful – a credible choice cannot be made without an appreciation of one's situation and the key variables at play. I have wondered too about the notion of prospective autonomy: the extent to which anyone can really know what it is he or she would want in unexperienced, hypothetical circumstances. Nonetheless, autonomy is, for me, central to clinical ethics.

At this first GP appointment, I faced my first choice and expression of autonomy – which hospital did I wish to attend? Yet, every fiber of my being resented this apparent choice. There was, I knew, little to choose here: If I did not attend the specialist cancer hospital and begin the pathway of mammograms, biopsies, scans and blood tests, my life was at risk. Autonomy seemed fragile and choice illusory in that moment. It was an exemplary consultation and I appeared contained, constant and recognizably myself; yet I was changing and vanishing as a result of crossing into the land of the sick. It would reveal autonomy to be more complex, more contested, more nuanced than I could ever have imagined.

Act 2: She Appeared Bored and I Was Altered

> Professor Bowman? It is good to meet you. I am Mr. B, a breast surgeon here, and this is M, one of our clinical nurse specialists.
>
> Hello, it is good to meet you both.
> *[I don't want to be here. A clinical nurse specialist in the room is a terrible sign, isn't it? What does her expression mean?]*
>
> I am afraid the results show that you do have cancer in the right breast and also your lymph nodes. I am sorry.
>
> That's okay, I was expecting it really. I, well, when the antibiotics had no effect and the lump under my arm got bigger. Well, you know – anyway, I guess we need to talk about what's next?
>
> *[I don't want to hear what's next. Hold it together. Just let me go home. I need to ask if I am dying. Am I dying? I need to know. I really don't want to know. Am I sicker than others in the waiting room? Stage 3 isn't great. Better than stage 4. I want to run away.]*
>
> Actually, before we talk about what's next, can I ask a question? *[You can do this. You have to do this. You need to know for the kids.]*
>
> Sure, what is it?
>
> Am – well, I need to tell my kids, you see. I need to be open and honest with them. So, well, I need to know if – I have to understand whether – if, if I am – dying?
>
> *[Tell me the truth. Don't tell me I am dying. Be honest with me. Don't make me tell my children I am dying. Tell me. Don't tell me. Why is he pausing so long?]*
>
> Well, I understand why you'd ask and no. No, I don't think you are dying.

This gentle, kind and clear breast surgeon explained that because of the size of the tumor and the spread to my lymph nodes, I would have chemotherapy before surgery. An appointment was scheduled with the medical oncologist to prepare for chemotherapy. The notion of choice, whilst there in theory, was for me a remote and theoretical construct at that appointment.

In these early appointments, I learned a great deal about autonomy. First, the experience of being ill changes us in ways that potentially both enhance and detract from our identity, sense of self and, perhaps, autonomy. I was more reflective, enquiring and focused than ever before. A forensic wish to understand, to consider, to question and to analyze the information and possibilities presented to me drove me. I was hypersensitive to the weight and meaning of words, gestures and facial expressions. I was also emotional: scared, overwhelmed, shocked and protective of those I love whom I longed to shield from the impact of my diagnosis.

I realized that to attend properly to autonomy is to attend to all the different "ways of being and knowing" that co-exist in a clinical consultation. It is about much more than the provision of information and the facilitation of choice, although those are sound enactments of respecting autonomy. To have real meaning, autonomy requires that a clinician accommodate and shift among competing forces: forensic rationality, insatiable questions and emotional responses. It is possible to make choices and difficult decisions with someone who recognizes that what might be unexpressed – fear, shame, sadness, anger and doubt – was also in the consultation room along with the apparently composed, professional woman talking calmly about surgical options and chemotherapy.

Time matters to facilitating autonomous choices - from the purely practical matter of how much can be shared in a single meeting to a more abstract but powerful sense of the extent to which information can be borne at a specific point. I am someone who believed I needed to know everything: all of it, at once. Leaving aside the impossibility of such an insatiable appetite for knowledge and an unrealistic wish for certainty, I discovered that when illness strikes, the sharing of information in a paced, careful, caring and gentle way allows space for it to settle and to sift. Had

I been allowed, I would have made significant and irrevocable choices on that day my diagnosis was confirmed. Uncertainty – my oldest foe – was to be vanquished by knowing as much as possible and simply "doing something." Yet, my wise, experienced and caring clinical team instead slowed me down, sharing what I need to know at that point and answering my questions, but also cautioning against hurrying and gently letting me adapt to the new normal whilst walking alongside me without judgment.

I will never again underestimate the value of written information and supportive resources. However, no matter to what extent the patient may consider herself intelligent and informed and irrespective of the exemplary communication skills of the clinician, there is simply nothing that compares to having materials that can be explored at home and at a time that works for the individual. Being in touch with others who have navigated this testing terrain is uniquely therapeutic when a person is learning to make choices in circumstances no one would choose. I confess that initially I took the booklets and details of support organizations with reluctance. But in the end, they were invaluable.

The treatment pathway began, and the changing nature of self was brought home to me regularly. At my first meeting with the oncologist to discuss chemotherapy, there were two other people in the room: another clinical nurse specialist and a health care assistant. Their role was non-speaking. I could feel the nurse's warmth, compassion and attention shining a light of confidence on me even as I felt frightened and overwhelmed. The healthcare assistant, however, appeared bored and uninterested. As I nodded and questioned the oncologist, I became increasingly aware of the woman at the edge of my sightline whose demeanor was unengaged. I watched her eyes begin to close as she inadvertently jerked, struggling to stay awake before submitting to the pull of sleep under the autumn sun that was streaming through the window.

Constant Deborah: It isn't ideal for her to fall asleep in a clinical consultation, but perhaps she has worked a double shift, perhaps she is ill herself, perhaps she was up all night caring for a relative. Healthcare professionals are people too with vulnerabilities. Don't judge or presume – we're all carrying more burdens and pains than others know. Meet people with compassion and openness. I wonder if I can offer feedback about what I have seen without criticism or complaint.

> *Changed Deborah:* How could she? It is a devastating and life-changing moment for me. I'm grappling with a life-threatening diagnosis and the details of a horrible treatment path, and she sleeps. All she has to do is stay awake. But she can't even do that – what kind of a person is she? She shouldn't be in healthcare if she can't do the basics. I should complain. She needs not to do this to people at their most vulnerable.
>
> *Contradictory Deborah:* I am furious. I shouldn't be furious. There are probably good reasons she has fallen asleep. Yes, but she can't do that – it is upsetting, disrespectful and insensitive. There'll be reasons, and it is easy to judge from a distance. Maybe, but the patient comes first. I don't want to complain. I want to complain. I just don't want it to happen to anyone else. I resent that it has happened to me.

My response to this sleeping woman revealed the constant, the changed and the contradictory in my identity.

I became increasingly aware that I was simultaneously myself and yet fundamentally different, and this was changing what I *thought* I knew about clinical ethics. Since I walked into the hospital and at every subsequent consultation, I wanted both to know and not to know, to understand and to deny, to reject and to accept, to question and to trust. Of course, sometimes, one preference was stronger than the other. I cannot conceive of not wanting to know my diagnosis or of undergoing surgery without an appreciation of what is involved and why. Yet, more often than not, there was a curious doubling, whereby competing and conflicting impulses co-existed.

Act 3: Performing Autonomy and Doubling Deborah

As my treatment progressed, there were many points when I had to revisit concepts that I took for granted as a Professor of Medical Ethics. It was, I am embarrassed to admit, a shock to experience the impact a standard consent form could have on a patient who had previously considered herself to be informed, rational and enquiring. When consent was being sought both for chemotherapy and for surgery, I was taken aback by the rising impulse to stop reading as I went through the possible side effects and potentially serious and fatal complications. I noticed that when I returned home, I hid my copy of these consent forms even as I knew it was absurd to do so.

At the beginning of my treatment, I asked to be copied into correspondence from the specialists to my GP. Professionally, I've even challenged doctors who'd argued that there's a risk of causing harm by copying patients into letters. But that apparent ethical clarity was challenged when the letters began to arrive. I am used to reading medical records and letters in my professional life. Nonetheless, the effect of seeing my own experience captured in clinical terms with its brutal specificity, detached evaluation and the unavoidable facts laid bare, was disruptive and painful. I quickly learned to recognize the envelopes and to expect a lurch of my stomach. I would pick up the letters from the doormat as if handling a grenade before bracing myself to read the contents. I should stress that I wanted to receive these letters and I am grateful that copying in patients to correspondence has become common in clinical practice. I believe in openness and I am committed to sharing information. My response was borne of the doubling that had occurred.

My academic understanding of, and commitment to, disclosure, choice and information remained, but illness rendered me simultaneously scared, vulnerable and overwhelmed by the impact of what I sought. I learned I could both crave and be undone by a consent process that was exemplary. I understood that I both yearned for, and wanted to run from, the information that was being offered in a gentle and patient-centered way.

I have reflected on what it is to be a clinician in such a context. Perhaps professionals too are susceptible to doubling. Doctors may believe in the value of information-sharing whilst wishing they did not have to impart painful news or life-changing knowledge. They may want always to be honest and realistic but also yearn to offer hope. A professional will draw on his or her scientific training and a rational evidence-base whilst remembering the patients who surprised them. To be pulled in different directions – whether as a patient or as a doctor – by competing and opposing forces is perhaps not merely just common but inevitable. Yet, I do not recall it being discussed in clinical communication "training" to which I have contributed. That seems like an omission.

> I'm doing well, thank you. A few side-effects – you know, a bit sick, tired in that first week of the cycle, but coping on the whole.
>
> That's good to hear. Pop up on the couch and we'll take a look. The last ultrasound showed great things, didn't it? I can see from the report – the tumor's getting much smaller and the lymph nodes look normal.
>
> Yes, it was just the sort of result that you need when you're in the chemo tunnel.
>
> Okay, here we go. The gel will be a bit cold.
>
> *Silence. A stretching silence. The air in the small room becomes heavy.*
>
> Hmm, excuse me, I'm just going to check the report from last time again.
>
> Sure ...
>
> *The silence closes in. A tear falls from the patient's right eye as she watches and waits.*
>
> Okay, so I think it was probably always the case that there is a bit of the tumor we can't easily see on all ultrasounds. It means the shrinking isn't quite what we thought.
>
> Right.
>
> I reckon it was probably always there. It isn't likely to be new. Are you off to clinic now?
>
> Yes.
>
> I'll get this report down to them, so you can talk it through when you see the consultant.
>
> Okay. Thank you.
>
> *The tears flow freely as the woman leaves.*

That cold morning of the ultrasound scan, about halfway through eight cycles of chemotherapy, undid me and the version of autonomy that I had been performing to date. I was devastated by the scan and its findings. I was exhausted, resentful and terrified. I wanted out of treatment. I needed treatment. I wanted to know what these unexpected findings meant. I couldn't bear to hear what these unexpected findings might mean. I wanted to talk about risk and prognosis. I yearned for someone to tell me that my prognosis was better than I feared. How my oncologist responded to the tearful, undone version of me revealed that, fundamentally, autonomy is relational. It is predicated on interaction and exchange. It does not and cannot exist without the kindness, patience, sensitivity, wisdom, honesty, commitment and expertise of professional staff. I was, for the first time, perhaps, able to be vulnerable enough to express fears. I trusted that he would answer my questions truthfully, but not without sensitivity and attention to the emotional import of his responses. I knew that, even in my distress, I was experiencing the most precious form of connectedness which gave autonomy meaning.

Act 4: The Ambivalence of Certainty

As chemotherapy ended, I had another stage of treatment to consider: surgery. Axillary lymph node clearance and a right-sided mastectomy were planned. I had always intuitively felt that I would prefer to have a bilateral or double mastectomy. That was a surprise to me in many ways. I knew from reading the literature (as an academic, that is, after all, what I am trained to do) that, in the absence of genetic mutations, there was no evidence that women who had double mastectomies reduced their risk of recurrence or metastatic disease. I considered myself a rational, evidence-based person who made choices according to what the data showed. And yet, when it came to my own care, my own body and my own choices, I could not shake the belief that a bilateral mastectomy was preferable, that is, the removal of both breasts even though, as far as anyone knew, there was no disease in the left breast.

In ethics, a distinction is commonly drawn between needs and wants, with greater moral weight afforded to "needs" which must be met, and lesser weight given to "wants" which are a negotiation among doctor, patient and health system. It is a neat distinction in theory, but in practice – in my life – those clean categories were confusing and unhelpful. Was my wish for a bilateral mastectomy – a decision that was neither evidence-based nor clinically indicated – a need or a want? And why was I making such a decision at all? Did I not work in a health sciences university and hospital? Was scientific evidence not the best basis on which to make medical choices? I had thought so since I was a teenager, so why was I doing something else now? I had underestimated the psychological and emotional. The knowledge of self, which meant I realized that I would find it harder to live with being "lopsided" after a single mastectomy than to be flat. The insight to recognize that to have a breast to continue to examine for changes would be more stressful, for me, than living without the breast at all. The confidence to know that my appearance was less important to me than other considerations and that I could and would adapt to my new appearance. These and other factors played out with a certainty that surprised me, but nonetheless made my decision to have both breasts removed clear.

Alongside my thoughts about mastectomy were questions about reconstruction. I wasn't sure about having any type of reconstruction, whether in the form of implants or grafting tissue from another part of my body. I was in a minority in not seeking reconstruction, but it simply didn't make sense to me. It was a decision made, to some extent, in the abstract though. Much as I looked at photos of women who had undergone bilateral mastectomies and declined reconstruction, and read their stories of adapting to being flat-chested, I could not know how I would respond when I looked in the mirror for the first time and saw a large scar where my breasts used to be. It was a contingent autonomy. I made a decision that was predicated on the best knowledge I had of myself at the moment, whilst recognizing that I could never be certain.

What's more, even though I was certain about my choice both to have a bilateral mastectomy and to decline reconstruction, ambivalence remained. I had not previously understood that it was possible both to be clear that a choice was the right one but also to question and even dislike that choice. Ambivalence was not an indicator that I was making the wrong decision or that I would come to regret my surgery. It was recognition that I was having to make a decision that I would prefer not to have to make at all. It was acknowledgment that it was possible both to be grateful for life-saving surgery and to hate that it was happening. Although I still feel ambivalence about the operation, that does not mean it was a "wrong" decision or a poor expression of my autonomy. It means I am human, and it reflects the real burden of cancer and its treatment. It gives meaning to the complexity of the experiences I have had. Autonomy is multilayered, complex and sometimes contradictory. It is rarely neat, linear and consistent when the choices are unwelcome, upsetting and difficult.

On the morning of the operation, I handed over my consent form to the surgeon. I did so with a necessary sadness and considerable apprehension. I was met with acceptance and kindness, no more so than in the anesthetic room before the operation. One of the recurrent challenges for me since I began having investigations and throughout treatment, especially during chemotherapy, was my fear of needles. I was a source of amusement for the patient nurses in the chemotherapy unit who would take bets on how much local anesthetic cream I would apply before anyone attempted to access my portacath. Every time there was a procedure to be performed, my first question was always about the needles. To give autonomy meaning is often to attend to priorities, concerns and questions that are absent from the consent form or the medical textbook. So it was that morning in the preparation room just outside the operating theatre.

> Hello, how are you doing this morning?
>
> I'm probably a bit of a flight risk.
>
> Oh dear. Well, we'd best make sure you get the best sleep of your life sooner rather than later then.
>
> I'm embarrassed to admit this, but well – I am – you see – it might be in my notes –
>
> What might?
>
> I – I'm really scared –
>
> It's normal to be scared before surgery and having an anaesthetic. It's a big deal.

> No, well – yes, I am a bit worried about that, but mostly I am dreading you putting a line into my hand. I hate needles you see. Really hate them.
>
> Ah. I see. Lots of people do. How about I use the mask instead?
>
> The mask?
>
> Yes, you just need to breathe deeply and before you know it, you'll be asleep. Then we'll put the cannulas in your hand.
>
> You'd do that? Isn't that meant for children?
>
> Of course. And it's for anyone who would find it makes things a bit easier for them. Do you have any other questions or stuff on your mind before we get going?
>
> No, I don't think so, but thank you, thank you so much.

I woke to find my chest tightly bandaged, a cannula in my hand and a new perspective on what it is to give meaning to someone's autonomy: from the major decisions about which body parts to remove to the apparently minor, but deeply significant choices about needles. I learned that I could hate and embrace a decision. To acknowledge the potential, maybe even the necessity, for these simultaneous and yet contadictory responses is to acknowledge the essential humanity of healthcare. It is to recognize that facts, knowledge, skills, experiences and emotions collide in illness and the clinical consultation. It is to give permission to us all – doctor and patient alike – to meet and to interact in a context that is complex, uncertain, challenging, but ultimately, potentially transformative.

Act 5: Hope and the Clinical Trial

During chemotherapy, my oncologist explained that he would be including a note about potential trials for which I might be eligible once I had completed active treatment. Knowing me well, he emphasized that this was included as an *aide-memoire* for the team and research nurse, not a proposal that I should spend hours researching on my own. (There is little as frustrating for a clinician as a Professor of Ethics with PubMed access and an anxious disposition.).

Shortly before I began radiotherapy, I discussed the trial again, but this time in more specific terms. I was introduced to the research nurse who, along with my oncologist, described the trial for which I might be suitable. The pace, sensitivity, responsiveness and clarity with which they discussed the trial, its aims and its methodology demonstrated not only skill, but the characteristic ethical commitment and patient-focus that I had come to learn imbues their practice.

I went home from that initial discussion about the specific trial carrying large bundle of paper: patient leaflets, background information, the trial protocol and a weighty consent form. I read them all diligently. I was discomfited by my reaction to what I read. I had expected, on digesting the information and reflecting on the consultation, to be focused on the uncertainty inherent in equipoise, the risks of volunteering for research, the burden of continuing to visit the hospital regularly and the potential to contribute to scientific and clinical knowledge. These were the fundamental discussion questions when I had taught and written about research ethics as an academic. Yet it was a deep-seated urge to "try anything possible" to prevent recurrence and/or secondary disease that dominated and shaped how I interacted with the information I had received.

I took myself in hand and asked expert colleagues and friends to review the data that had been published from earlier trials of the drug. They generously gave their time and shared their dispassionate analyses and informed thoughts with me. I deliberately read the material several times, making myself focus on the information about risks as well as potential benefits. I spoke to trusted confidants about the trial and encouraged them to challenge my impulse to sign up. I reminded myself that I could be randomized to the control arm of the trial. These were important disciplines, yet I remained determined to participate in the trial in a way that surprised me.

I have thought a lot about that determination and impulse to participate in a clinical trial and the implications for research ethics. Although I have often framed discussion of research ethics with reference to vulnerability,

I had underestimated – indeed been ignorant of – the urge to pursue hope in the face of serious illness. Irrespective of training, professional background and efforts to be rational, there was, for me, an overriding wish to "do everything possible." Much as I deliberately slowed myself down and challenged that impulse, it dominated. I found easy narratives to support my decision *ex post facto*. I told myself that altruism and the prospect of contributing to knowledge resonated with my values. The results from earlier trials of the drug had shown promise, and impartial colleagues agreed (although as good scientists and researchers, they pointed out that those results were from a group of patients who were in different circumstances). I would continue to be a regular visitor to the hospital, which would allow for surveillance. All of those narratives are true, but they were not the driving force for my decision, which was an irrational, almost primitive, search for hope and control.

> I can't make Wednesday morning as I have to go to the hospital for my regular review.
>
> Poor you. You must get really fed up of being there all the time.
>
> Hmm, it isn't my first choice of destination, but I'm lucky, you know, to be able to be part of a clinical trial at all.
>
> I know, but I suppose, well –
>
> What?
>
> Well, I guess I am kinda surprised. You seem to have so many problems on the trial – the infections, the risks, the transfusions, the endless appointments. I thought you might have wanted to avoid hospitals and all that stuff after everything you've gone through.
>
> Oh, so did I. I thought that too. A year ago. And then, well- then I got sick and everything changed. I changed.

As the trial has progressed, I have encountered problems along the way. The drug is potent and has considerable side-effects. My neutrophil count regularly drops to dangerous levels, rendering me at risk of infection – which is particularly tough for someone who works in a hospital environment. On other occasions, I have been anemic and exhausted because of the impact of the drug. And yet, when I wait to hear whether my blood results are sufficient to enable me to continue with the next cycle of the drug, I yearn to minimize the impact of these side-effects. I find myself overwhelmingly hoping that I can remain on the trial above all else. When there has been talk of whether someone can continue as a participant if her immune system struggles, I want to shout that I must be allowed to continue, even as I know it may not be in my best interests to do so. There are limitations to my autonomy and choice: I cannot demand or even request to continue to receive the trial drug if it is causing me too much harm, however much I might be willing to bear that harm. I have to learn to quell the visceral wish to remain in the trial at all costs. I have to recognize that my autonomous choice to be a research participant is born of something primitive and irrational and that it has limits. For now, I continue in the trial, but I have to accept that may not be possible for the duration of the study because whilst I might continue to consent, my neutrophils and hemoglobin may prevent it.

How then might researchers approach potential participants about enrolling in trials and studies? Perhaps the first step is, alongside the emphasis on time, space and information, to acknowledge the complex drivers and influences that shape an individual's thinking about trials. I do not presume to generalize from my experience – I have met many patients in my professional life who appeared to take a more interrogative and rational approach to enrolling in research along, of course, with those who decide it is not something in which they wish to participate. However, I do suggest that the individualism of anyone who is approached as eligible for a trial or research study cannot be captured in leaflets, forms, protocols and papers. Whilst research is often concerned with populations, cohorts and groups, it always involves working with, and responding to, individuals and their own needs, values, priorities, hopes and concerns. And those individual and specific dimensions of choice and decision-making may be unarticulated, surprising, contradictory, confusing, changing and hidden. What might be needed is someone who both knows the individual and is independent of the individual, a recruitment process that is both consistent and adaptive – that is attentive to signals and cues and that acknowledges that the prospect of a trial may represent much more to the participant than can ever be expressed or understood.

Act 6: Constant and Altered

Autonomy is elusive and complex .... it ebbs and flows. It is often characterized as the expression of an essential self. Yet, illness changes us; who we are is both constant and altered. I have thought often of the Samuel Beckett quotation from *Happy Days*, Act II:

> "To have been what I always am – and so changed from what I was".

As a breast cancer patient, I've learned that when we talk about "self-rule," we're describing a shifting and sometimes confusing idea of who we are. People give autonomy meaning. The ethical challenge is often to find that meaning. It takes time, patience, skill and attention. I now think about autonomy as a complex, shifting negotiation between people.

My life will never be as it was before cancer. I will never be who I was before cancer. Yet the narrative threads of my life and the person I am remain. Autonomy does not mean being certain about difficult choices. It will not protect against doubt, fear and anxiety or act as an ethical shield against an uncertain future. Contradiction and complexity persist, even as one makes considered and informed decisions. Autonomy is made possible by people rather than consent forms. It is predicated on dialogue and discussion and that, in turn, depends on connectedness, trust, attention and compassion. Autonomy is always a work in progress, as is life with cancer. There are scenes and acts to come which are unknown and cannot be captured in this story. I am grateful to all those who have walked, and will continue to walk, alongside me in my simultaneously constant and altered state. Together we recognize that our autonomy, identity and wellbeing are inextricably linked and interdependent. That realization is profoundly moral in character, and it is central to what it means to care for ourselves and for others.

JOHANNA SHAPIRO

Women's Breast Cancer Poetry: Voice, Identity, Contingency and Death

Introduction

Breast cancer has been described as a biographical disruption that catches women between longing for what was (life before cancer) and fear of what will be (assaults on the body, pain, uncertainty and even death) (Martino and Freda 622). Cancer alters the relationship between the woman's body, the woman's sense of self and the surrounding world (Smit, Coetzee, Roomaney et al., 231; Herndl 221). How women process and interpret the experience of breast cancer – with its uniquely gendered, nurturing and sexualized associations – becomes a revealing exercise in finding one's voice amidst the pressures to narrate experience in certain societally and medically approved ways. In particular, I became interested in the disjuncture between the messages implicit and explicit in the medical model, and the points of view and understanding of women actually undergoing the experience of breast cancer.

In an attempt to better understand how women with breast cancer express their experiences with doctors, medicine and healthcare in writing, I reviewed poetry (and some prose) dating back to the 1980s and extending into the first two decades of the twenty-first century. To my surprise, I found many more poems written in the 1990s and early 2000s than in the following decade. Although I am not sure why, it is possible that contemporary women are more likely to turn to blogs and YouTube videos for self-expression rather than to poetry. Thus, the majority of this analysis is based on poems produced in the latter years of the twentieth century and the very early part of the twenty-first century. It may also be relevant to know that I read great poets and "ordinary people" poets – women who, not necessarily with any formal training, applied pen to paper or fingers to keyboard to express their thoughts, hopes and fears. As such, this survey is representative of many voices, while not inclusive of all. Because this work is not a literary analysis but rather a "data mining" exercise considering poetry as data (Shapiro 172), I treated all these works equally, paying less attention to craft and wordsmithing and more attention to the insights, stories and perspectives each woman discovered.

The Medical Model and the Poetry of Women with Breast Cancer. A large literature exists about the medical model and the medicalization of the body. For the purposes of this chapter, several aspects of this model have special salience. First is the emphasis on professional priorities and attitudes that can create a context of clinical coldness in the overall healthcare system, including hospitals, physicians and other health professionals involved in care of the patient. The hallmarks of this faux professionalism are a stress on efficiency and productivity (the smooth running of the system), transmission of information with the purpose of reaching medically approved decisions and thus a timely path forward, and instrumental intervention in the form of medications and surgeries (Kellerman A12). In this paradigm, compassion and empathy are implicit but not always manifest. Second is a determined focus on cheerfulness and optimism (McGrath, Jordens, Montgomery et al. 665–7; Setchell, Abrams, McAdam et al. 1891), which can support flagging spirits but, with inappropriate application, can also suppress the patient's authentic voice. Third, with its emphasis on the recovery of existence "as it was" prior to the intervention of disease, the medical model assumes the desirability of prostheses and reconstructive surgery in an effort to "fix" the apparent deficit caused by breast surgery/mastectomy (Davis and Gonzalez 33–62; Remen 16). Finally, the medical model tends to celebrate survivorship (Ristovski-Slijepcevic and Bell 167; Ehlers 88), consonant with societal movements such as Pink Ribbon (DeShazer, *Mammographies* 9), rather than admit the real possibility of recurrence, metastasis and death.

The healthcare system is a powerful one; therefore, its medical model is hard to resist. Indeed, who would want to stand against a model that works toward restitution and "normalcy," a concept which, although shrouded in the science of statistics, has come to mean "the legitimate way of being in the world and the only version of a good life" (Michalko and Titchkosky 5)? Many women who undergo breast cancer, however, bump into the limitations and shortcomings of this model. Historically silent under the weight of social and medical pressures toward conformity and compliance, women in the 1980s began to find their voices in many permutations of the written word, including poetry.

Writing poetry about breast cancer initially seemed odd, even transgressive. When an early multi-authored collection of poetry about breast cancer appeared in 1988 (Lifschitz 1988), even the author of the foreword was somewhat nonplussed by its content. Echoing Sontag's assessment eleven years earlier in *Illness as Metaphor* that "cancer is a rare and still scandalous subject for poetry" (20), P. H. Thompson described the topic as "a curious and rather narrowly defined theme ... [that] strikes a note at the least very peculiar. Who in particular would find appealing a book so bizarre in its limits [...]?" (Lifschitz xix). In a similar vein that reflects widespread mistrust at the time about addressing such an "abject" topic in poetry, Hilda Raz, in her poem "Day-Old Bargain," records a male voice imploring the poet not to write about breast cancer: "When you give your breast/to cancer, for God's sake don't/write about it" (*Divine* 23). Since the last decades of the twentieth century, we have discovered that literary depictions of breast cancer can provide healing, resistance and commemoration (DeShazer, *Fractured* 7). Women have certainly reclaimed their voices, in both prose and poetry; and that reclaiming raises further questions about their experiences and interpretations of breast cancer.

Cancer is by definition unruly, expansive, unpredictable and unregulated. Can poetry, often although not always a rigorous undertaking, somehow exert formal control over cancer? How can a poet match her art to the challenge of cancer? (Twiddy 12). In the end, these poets, spanning thirty years of verse about breast cancer, generally seem to conclude that although poetry may not be able to prevent death, and does not always even provide consolation, it does offer witnessing and the satisfaction of truth-telling. As Audre Lorde and Lucille Clifton bravely urged, poetry is an expression of the determination to share one's story. Poetry of course can be political (Faulkner 89), especially in the sense that it offers hitherto unperceived ways of discernment as well as radical visions of new possibilities and new worlds, even when these understandings and worlds make others uncomfortable. Poetry relies on the particular and the personal for its power, but it has implications beyond itself.

Restitution Stories and Experiences of Women with Breast Cancer in the Healthcare System. In general, in the period reviewed (1980s to early 2000s), medicine and its practitioners still embodied a modernist view (Coll-Planas and Visa 885–6): The body is brought under control by medical knowledge, which can avoid or postpone death. The desired state of the body is predictability, order and cleanliness – as close to perfection as possible. In narrative terms, medicine relied then (and still relies today, in large part) on what the medical sociologist Arthur Frank called a restitution story, in which the patient is returned to her previous life, and her body is returned to its previous state of familiarity, predictability and control (75–96). In this model, the surgeon has the task of saving the life of a passive victim; the doctor's heroism is valorized, and women's expressions of suffering are silenced (Bahar 1027). For obvious reasons, the restitution story has great appeal. A 2016 study of women bloggers with breast cancer confirmed that the majority told restitution narratives that legitimized health professionals, made extensive use of medical vocabulary, trusted medical knowledge and expressed gratitude to health professionals (Coll-Planas and Visa 888–9).

Quest Stories. However, the restitution story is not possible for many (perhaps most) cancer patients – even those who recover – for reasons discussed in more depth later in this paper. Another common story Frank identifies is the quest story, based on the work of the mythologist Joseph Campbell, in which a hero goes on a journey, suffers trials and tribulations and emerges transformed as a wise and noble leader (Campbell 63–94). Jackie Stacey's book *Teratologies* illustrates the ubiquity of this model, offering an astute analysis of cancer narratives at the time (1970s): The patient receives a diagnosis that shocks and bewilders, is thrown into despair, reassesses her values and the meaning of her life and ultimately rises up from the encounter a new and better person (12). This narrative also appears in many poems, albeit with certain variations. Other writers, however, have acknowledged the inadequacy of the quest narrative. For example, Ruth Picardie, a British journalist who documented her experience with breast cancer, asserted that breast cancer was not "an opportunity to live better, but an opportunity to resist the sentimentalization of suffering" (13).

Chaos Stories. Because of the inherent out-of-control nature of breast cancer – wildly proliferating cells, uncertainty due to the possibility of metastasis or relapse, and the contingency of mortality – it may be more accurate to say that breast cancer's narrative conforms best to yet another Frankian construction, a chaos story (Bahar 1031–32). In the chaos account, there is little understanding, no resolution, and great suffering (Frank 97–114). As we will see, many women writing about breast cancer express this sort of crying out, giving voice to an anguish that at times appears to have no other outlet. The women poets I reviewed tended to oscillate among the following Frankian narratives: longing for restitution while recognizing its impossibility; immersion in the suffering, anger and helplessness of a chaos narrative; and seeking transformation through a quest story (Frank 113–36). Unlike the Campbell model, these poets' depictions of transformation and transcendence avoid the sentimentality and uncomplicated, happy endings usually characteristic of quest narratives. In other words, their quests, although sometimes taking the classic heroic form, are often primarily focused on self-definition and identity formation, and are cast in the context of solidarity with other women with breast cancer past and present. (This sense of solidarity seems particularly strong in the poetry of African-American and Jewish women, many of whom come from families and communities decimated by breast cancer.) These poems acknowledge, even actively pursue, posttraumatic growth (Tedeschi and Calhoun 58–60; Calhoun and Tedeschi 138–75), while acknowledging suffering and rage, and insisting that identity is one's own to define.

Women with Breast Cancer in Healthcare Settings

Losing and Reclaiming Voice. The traditional medical model can impose a kind of colonization, or takeover, of the body that reduces the woman to an object of scientific attention (DeShazer, *Fractured* 13) and privileges the authoritarian single voice of the physician (Bahar 1027) with a consequent loss of the patient's perspective. This "narrative surrender" (Coll-Planas and Visa 885) may be especially true for female patients, as women's bodies and the diseases of women's bodies traditionally are perceived as particularly unruly, unpredictable and in need of control (Faith 1–10; Holliday and Hassard 1–18). In this model, the patient's role is to be obedient to the physician's authority and expertise, passively fulfilling medical instruction. The implicit trade-off, as noted, is a promised restitution or a fulfilling journey.

Linda Pastan, writing "Clinic" in the 1980s, notes the medicalization of the body and the consequent loss of narrative control:

> [...]we stand in line
> for X-ray and EKG,
> dressing and undressing,
> clutching the charts
> which slowly accumulate –
> the only autobiography
> we have left.
>
> When did we stop
> being part of our bodies
> and start simply to inhabit them [...] (60)

"Abstract/Concrete (about Louise)" is a piece of found poetry that concludes:

> Being a cancer patient is like being an object in a factory,
> Like going through an assembly line.
> Each person at each station does something to me,
> Disassembled [...]
> Assembled [...]
> Pieces put back together to make the new me,
> And then, when it's all done,
> I'm just going to be spit out. (Reilly, Lee, Lauz et al., 204–5)

After contemplating an image of her skeleton in "Bone Scan," Amy Ling realizes that the technology of medicine has erased her identity: "how can that be you? / Where are your Asian eyes / yellow-tinged skin, / flat nose,

/ straight black hair / – all the things that make you you [...]" (112–3). It seems there is little in the hospital experience to provide succor or support, or to acknowledge the uniqueness and individuality of each patient.

Reclaiming Voice. Scholars generally pay tribute to Audre Lorde as one of the progenitor "mothers" of writing about breast cancer as an explicit form of resistance against this medical colonization of the body. In her iconic *Cancer Journals* (diary format) and later in the poetry of her collection *The Marvelous Arithmetics of Distance* (written after her breast cancer had metastasized to her liver), Lorde put forth clear criteria for meaningful writing. Perhaps most important to her was resisting the silence that had surrounded breast cancer in the 1970s and early 1980s. She led the resistance, even though talking back – especially among minority women – is often seen as evidence of a troublemaker (Ashing-Giwa, Padilla, Kraemer et al. 418).

Lorde was one of the first to advocate for women to give expression to the particularities of their breast cancer experiences. Conceptualizing her own encounters with breast cancer, Lorde herself was firmly rooted in gendered, racial, environmental and feminist perspectives; but she did not require that other women uniformly share this approach. Rather, she stressed that all women speak their particular truths, and many followed her counsel. For example, in her poem "Isaac Stern's Performance," Hilda Raz instructs the reader, "I'm telling you cancer" (*Divine* 7); in other words, she is telling *her* cancer story. Judith Hall, in "Rimbaud's Cancer," issues a call to speak out, be angry: "Complain! Stamp a tiny foot against God" (36–7). Still, despite Lorde's uncompromising leadership, the twenty-first century poet Felicia Johnson observes, "Breast cancer had bound us with paralyzing fear [...] / All I could hear were the silent voices of those affected" (2010). In "Silent No More," Helen Keys implores, "We can no longer remain silent / [...] Listen to the many voices of breast cancer" (60–2).

Though reclaiming voice from silence is crucial, there are pitfalls in figuring out how to tell one's story. Consider, for example, what is an authentic voice vs. a co-opted voice? Does narrating a standard plot – a restitution story, for example, or a quest story – necessarily make it inauthentic? How much of the "expected" or "normative" story has the teller internalized? To what extent is she telling stories others wish to hear vs. stories that she longs to hear for herself? What is the purpose of the story? Authenticity? Truth-telling? Consolation? Who gets to decide? These sorts of questions come to mind as we read poetry about breast cancer, noting that, in authors who have written at length about their cancer, different elements – of restitution, longing, fear, anger, acceptance – emerge in different poems (and sometimes within the same poem).

One possible thread of these women's stories is an examination of how they represent their perceptions of their relationships with the overall healthcare system, physicians and ancillary health professionals committed to their care. Despite intentions of goodwill on both sides, these relationships are fraught from their inception for reasons that are not so much personal as structural and systemic. Interestingly, many poets never or rarely write about these topics, perhaps not wanting to waste precious time on people and places they see as peripheral to and often uninterested in their daily struggles. In reading their poetry, we must attend to absences as well as presence, noting all those places where we might expect a physician or other health professional to make an appearance, but instead find only aloneness.

Clinics and Hospitals. The healthcare environment described in these poems is usually cold and indifferent, starting with the impersonality of the intake experience. In "Impersonation," Julia Darling attempts to subvert the mandatory medical paperwork by reinventing herself in an act of resistance:

> I take time with
> your NINETEEN PAGE FORM
> in re-invented handwriting
> I write a false name [...]
> she [the woman she invents] will have no
> category or shoe size.

But she can't circumvent the system; she knows the receptionist will

> [...] rip it [the form] to confetti
> and hand me another
> *start again properly*
> *Mrs. Darling* she'll snap
> *forms aren't funny.* (11–2)

Next comes the mindless waiting for the doctor. Darling's poem, "A Waiting Room in August," portrays the polite, cooperative waiting to which most patients conform, which signals their acquiescence to the rules and expectations of the healthcare system: "This morning we polished // our shoes, so that they should wait / smartly. Our wigs lie patiently / on our dignified heads / Our mouths are ironed." Then she erupts in fury, rebelling against the dehumanization of this system: "Haven't we waited long enough? / Haven't we waited beautifully?" (14–5). Conformity to the rules of the system does not yield the expected reward for the doctor to appear, and beyond that, for cancer to conclude.

The hospital experience itself is equally dehumanizing, a place of spiritual barrenness that invites metaphors of deconstruction, disassembly and objectification, paralleling what is happening to the poets' bodies. The poem "In the Hospital," by Patricia Goedicke, notes the harshness, even cruelty of this supposedly healing environment: "When they came at me with sharp knives [...] / When they asked me embarrassing questions [...] / When they laid harsh hands on me [...]" (2). In "Cancer Winter," Marilyn Hacker describes the hospital as "bright and false as treason" (*Winter* 80), while Darling refers to her hospital as "half-built wastelands" (13). Darling's poem "High Maintenance" speaks with mingled defiance and desperation: "And if I sing, / and wear ear plugs, / I never hear the word / demolition" (9), reminding us that the institutions that care for the ill are places of disintegration and decay. As Helene Davis writes in "Here and There,"

> [...] Here, they cart away parts of your body piece
> by piece and your hair and your eyelashes fall out [...]
> [...] No one will take them away and
> say prayers over them to make magic so that you will
> become whole again. Here, no one forgives you [...] (61)

Using similar language in "Separation," Miriam R. Krasno describes the hospital as an environment in which the body is "ripped apart [...] / [...] strangers take parts of you away" (17).

In the end, the hospital is often a place to flee – into either the liminality of survival or the certainty of death. In Darling's words, "and the impossible hospital lay down its chimneys [sic] / its sluices, tired doctors, and waiting room chairs. / And I came here / It was easy to leave" (56). Of course, although I did not actually find any laudatory descriptions of hospitals in the poetry I reviewed, this does not mean such examples do not exist. As in the discussion of physicians below, there may be many factors to explain this relative absence of positive representation.

Women with Breast Cancer and Their Doctors. Although one would expect physicians to be empathic, compassionate and concerned, when doctors (often surgeons) do appear in these poems, they usually appear as rather distant, occasionally arrogant figures in their self-confidence and certainty. It is, of course, important to remember that the poems I examined are only patients' representations of their physicians, in contrast to actual physician behavior. Many breast cancer patients feel positive about their surgeons (Dean 1748), although this is less true for women of color (Sheppard, Hurtado de Mendoza, Talley et al. 143). However, since we have no record of these encounters, all we know is that these overwhelmingly negative portrayals of their doctors is what these poets wished to preserve. It may be that critical portrayals make for better poetry. Perhaps these poets remembered their negative encounters more vividly than the more pleasant ones. Further, many of the poets were academics and/or feminists with an ingrained skepticism of establishment institutions, including medicine. Their discontent could have stemmed as well from a time when most surgeons were male, interacting with their female patients in a historical context that was itself often sexist and racist. Regardless, from their poetic accounts, it seems these women at times endured hurtful, insensitive behaviors from their physicians. Sometimes they confronted them; more often, they kept silent in the exam room. But they documented their mistreatment in verse.

Barriers of Communication. As represented in the poetry reviewed, the language physicians choose with their patients is harsh and unfeeling. For example, Clare Best's consultant in "Vital Statistics" mercilessly informs her that, based on family history, she has an 85 percent chance of developing breast cancer. Best retaliates by comparing this number to other statistics (some apparently factual, some patently not) to show the absurdity and meaninglessness of such analyses. (Of note, she eventually decides on a prophylactic mastectomy.) (30). In "Swallowtails," V. Jane Schneeloch describes how the language of medicine begins to colonize her: "The doctor points/to small white flecks/on the dark film. /*See?* he says, some *abnormality*. / Another doctor says, *Cancer,* / and I must put that word in a sentence beginning with my name" (58). Similarly, in Darling's poem "Too Heavy," the medicalized language weighs her down, crushes her spirit, and deprives her of her voice:

> Dear Doctor,
> I am writing to complain about these words
> you have given me, that I carry in my bag
> *lymphatic, nodal, progressive, metastatic*
> [...] I'm bent
> with the weight of them [...]
>
> [...] they tick like bombs and overpower my own
> sweet tasting words. (16)

Instead of sympathizing with Darling's sense of being overrun by the language of cancer, the doctor mocks her silence: *"Where are your words, Mrs. Patient?/ What have you done with your words?"* (16).

In "This Breast Surgeon," Alysa Cummings records her surgeon's obtuse stream of consciousness in reviewing her imaging: "Oh, I don't like this. I don't like this one bit," he mutters to himself, although she is sitting right next to him in the exam room. As the surgeon continues, she tries to regain a sense of control by comparing him to Picasso, perhaps ironically, perhaps hopefully: "He is good at drawing breasts. / He is good at cutting breasts. / He knows breasts" (2002). In Linda Pastan's "Routine Mammogram," the radiologist explains in a sexist and condescending metaphor, "We are looking for a worm / in the apple-" (46). Although we might hope that such misogynistic behavior has vanished, a 2017 poem by Janay Cosner ("I Knew, I Didn't Know") describes how two men – the surgeon and the patient's doctor-husband – talk over her head to each other: "I am a wilting wallflower in the room / as they discuss appointments- / a PET scan, blood tests, x-rays" (4). In these poems, the depersonalization and misdirection of physicians' language only serves to further wound an already vulnerable, hurting patient.

Physicians as Usurpers. Other poems express the sense of being overrun by the physician's view of their situation, with the result that the women feel exiled from their own lives. "Living in the New Extension" shows

Darling employing the metaphor of "doctor gardeners" who have taken over her home: "Then, what was once my home was given over / to a team of doctor gardeners, to phantom nurses" (26). They have literally colonized her house (a metaphor for her life). In this usage, the doctors are not benign cultivators but purveyors of pesticides who at the end of the day leave the narrator alone with her ruined life. In a poem that uses another garden metaphor, "That Was the Fruit of My Orchard," Goedicke laments that her breast, this precious fruit, was plucked from the field of her body, and trampled by harsh, clumsy doctors (21–2).

Masks of Cheerfulness. In "Ink and Green Wash: In the Oncologist's Waiting Room," Hall comments unfavorably about doctors who "offer laughter constantly," their unrelieved cheerfulness grating on her as she waits once again for her oncologist to arrive (31–2). This observation echoes Samantha King's reference to the "tyranny of cheerfulness" (101–5) that plagues much of the breast cancer movement. Fleur Adcock, in "The Soho Hospital for Women," also notes sardonically this fake ritual of cheerfulness: the doctor

> turns his practiced smile on me:
> "How are you this morning?" "Fine,
> very well, thank you." I smile too.
> And possibly all that murmurs within me
> is the slow dissolving of stitches. (1745)

The wonderful insertion of the adverb "possibly" conveys her protest and frustration. Darling appreciates that the physician's falseness requires similar fakery in the patient, as portrayed in her poem "Macaroon": "I must never be pale. I smile fiercely. Run. / There are words I must not say: pain or Macmillan [sic]. // [...]Let me show you / how heartily I can eat a macaroon" (36).

The Breast Cancer Marketplace. The ancillary members of the healthcare team who appear in poetry are mostly women, who we might expect to offer more personalized, compassionate care. The majority of poems reviewed, however, are more likely to render them as representatives of Cancer Inc. (DeShazer, *Fractured* 87) and the Breast Cancer Marketplace (Ehrenreich 43–53) – more interested in "selling" the restitution story than in understanding the individual needs and desires of their patients. For the most part, in poetry they seem willing accomplices of the doctors and the healthcare system that employs them. In poems that do not shy away from anger, the poets reserve special wrath for these individuals and the products they promote to restore a certain stereotypic femininity. For example, in "Breast Care Nurse" Best describes the blithe cheerfulness of her nurse: "She whistles in flat shoes, primary colours, / wide smile," and she nonchalantly advises her patient, "Remember to take some softies when you leave – / nobody'll guess. Then call and make a date / for silicone ones, any size you fancy [...]" (38). The poet resists this automatic assumption that a patient will want to masquerade her new appearance from others, as well as the supposed "benefit" of having the opportunity to select her breast size. In "'Girl' Friends" Cosner writes:

> The topic today areola nipple tattooing-
> [...] The "breast" specialist talks about women
> recapturing our former selves.
> She has other services available -
> [...] to make our beauty everlasting.
>
> You can look even better than you did.
> Some of us frown, others' eyes tear up. (62)

This author, who in other poems mourns the loss of her sexy, alluring appearance in very stereotypical terms (the forfeiture of her blond hair, bikini, tan and flat stomach) (65), feels defiant as she asserts that women are more than their beautiful bodies. She adopts the language of Lorde and other feminist writers as she concludes, "we are .... warriors" (63).

Communitarian Dimensions of Breast Cancer

In *Welcome to Cancerland*, Barbara Ehrenreich notes the "ultrafeminine" cancer narratives in mainstream breast cancer culture that are characterized by gratitude and positivity, with little or no anger or reference to the larger issues of race, class, access to care and environmental contamination implicated in breast cancer (Lorde, *Cancer Journals* 65–6; DeShazer, *Fractured* 12). Indeed, because society by and large accepts the medicalization of cancer, it tends to see the disease primarily as an individual problem, and relies on personal blame or heroics to resolve it. Women whom others perceive as "not caring about their health" do not take preventive and screening measures to protect themselves from cancer, do not seek treatment early enough and consequently may die. Heroic women and their heroic doctors fight valiantly against the disease and triumph over it.

In claiming their voices, many of the poets I reviewed also emphasize a triumphalist individual autonomy, privileging the search for personal self-growth and transcendence over more socially situated communitarian approaches (Bahar 29–31; Klawitter 74; Hunsaker Hawkins 193). Focusing on the systemic and structural aspects of breast cancer is only occasionally in evidence, and is more likely in writings of African-American and Jewish women, who often have suffered generational and communal losses to breast cancer. Perhaps in consequence, they appear more motivated to look beyond their individual experience toward what they perceive as the greater evils of environmental pollutants, racism, anti-Semitism and militarism.

Race and Ethnicity. Unsurprisingly, given their history of exploitation and mistreatment in the healthcare system (Williams, Mohammed, and Shields 2138–49; Heiney, Hilfinger, Felder et al. 217–24), African-American women are most adamant in their suspicion of the medicalization of the body and their physicians. In "No News is BAD NEWS," an anonymous woman writes,

> They sit you in the room
> They wait for hours
> and hours and hours
> before they tell you anything.
> No hurry now – I've told myself
> and I done decided it's BAD NEWS. (Kooken, Haase, and Russell 907)

The patient sees the endless waiting as a lack of caring, a lack of communication, and she reclaims control, deciding on her own what the outcome will be. Similarly, in "The Pink Ribbon Shield," another

African-American woman writes, "You have to watch / when you go to the doctor. / Sometimes, they be in a hurry / [...] But they come in the room / [...] never looking at me" (Kooken, Haase and Russell 909). Finally, in "ERAC" (care spelled backwards), the anonymous poet describes

> Two doctors examining me
> talking to each other,
> as if I am not there.
> I guess I should be glad
> at least they talk among themselves.
> It is the only way to get
> information about myself. (Kooken, Haase and Russell 911)

In the same poem, she wonders whether her doctors are "scared to touch me / [...] because I am ... African-American?" (911).

As already noted, Lorde consistently interprets her breast cancer within her experience as a black woman in a racist, sexist culture. Like Lorde, many of Lucille Clifton's poems routinely place her own breast cancer in a similar context. In "1994," she warns women to avoid denial and speak their own stories: "You know how dangerous it is // to be born with breasts / you know how dangerous it is / to wear dark skin" (493). In "Watershed," Tracey K. Smith, an African-American poet, tackles environmental contamination from a DuPont factory as a possible contributor to her own and others' breast cancers. She understands this as just one more sign of oppression and inequity:

> Dupont: did not make this information public
> declined to disclose this finding
> [...] They knew this stuff was harmful
> And they put it in the water anyway [...]
> *I suspect that the Earth may be a place of education* [...]" (2017)

In "We Carry: I Carry Personal Stories," Felicia Johnson writes about the cost of breast cancer's legacy across generations: "I am a generational breast cancer overcomer [...] / We carry breast cancer disease attacking our women [...] / We carried our tears [...] / We carried the shared experiences ..." (2010).

Marilyn Hacker, who was Jewish, repeatedly situates her personal suffering within larger, collective suffering. She demonstrates awareness of other women living and dying with cancer and acknowledges "how lives are braided / how those women's deaths and lives, lived and died, were / interleaved [...]" (*Winter* 75–6). When she can't sleep because of her terror about recurrence of her cancer and imminent death, she tells herself her circumstances are not as bad as Auschwitz. Like most post-Holocaust Jews, she commits to life, all the while noting her own unimportance in the scheme of things: "I'm still alive, an unimportant exiled Jew" (81).

Environment. Alicia Ostriker locates her cancer within the larger context of the Gulf War, thereby gaining perspective on her private suffering, and declares in favor of activism rather than despair: "[...] although we can perhaps do little to heal either the world or ourselves, we can do *something*. Something is not the same as nothing" ("Scenes" 197). In "The Mastectomy Poems: The Bridge of Fantasy," pursuing the theme of profit-driven environmental contamination she notes that a carcinogenic world has created the cancer cells that have planted their "Judas kiss / Inside the Jerusalem of the breast" (1996). Jo Shapcott peppers her thoughts about breast cancer with allusions to the Iraq war and climate change: "[...] those other / places where all the frontiers end with a question" (4). Susan King also addresses possible environmental factors in her disease (30–1) and situates marches advocating for breast cancer research and funding within a long tradition of political activism (95–7). What all these writers have in common is a refusal to define breast cancer only as an individual affliction, rather acknowledging it as complicated by larger societal and structural concerns – only one instance of suffering in a world filled with injustice and sorrow.

Loss and the Quest for a New Identity: Appearance vs. Transformation

Mastectomy as a Threat to Identity. Breasts are socially constructed in the sense that, at least in modern Western culture, they have come to be synonymous with feminine desirability. But obviously breasts also have subjective, very personal meaning for the women to whom they belong; and this meaning often involves their identity as maternal, erotic and sexually desirable beings. Thus, a cancer that threatens the breast may also threaten identity, both in the eyes of others and in one's own eyes.

In "A Wait," Caroline Webb-Wiltshire grieves the disappearance of a breast that a man once held and kissed, that a child suckled (2016). Other writers regretfully celebrate the form, functions and delights of the breast. In "Breast Count," Irish poet Marie Cadden remembers her breasts "brimful of squashy / choice for the mouth, / lush pasture for the eyes, / undulating landscape / on a balanced horizon" (22). Others, like Che'Vonceil Echols, fear that without a breast they will no longer be lovable or desirable:

> My perfectly lovely round brown breasts
> Aren't so perfect, lovely, or round anymore
> And I can't help but wonder
> Will he still love me tomorrow? (8)

After her mastectomy, Echols reflects in "Who Am I?": "My Name Is Self-Hatred / Yeah, Call Me That! / 'Cause Nobody Love A Woman With No Breast" (80–1). The contrast between the plumpness of the breast and the flatness of the mastectomy scar is a constant reminder of the sense of diminishment in her own eyes and in the eyes of society. In her poem "Mastectomy," Kay Schodek focuses on the ugliness of mastectomy: "My terrain's dry / and flat as baked clay" (40). Ostriker describes her scar as "… a skinny stripe / That won't come off with soap / A scarlet letter lacking in meaning" (*Little Space* 203); she's been branded not for the temerity of adultery, but for having a fallible body.

Women often find the resultant absence of symmetry particularly distressing, reverberating symbolically as an existential threat to wholeness, balance, equilibrium and what society has told them is the "normal" condition. In "After Surgery," Alice J. Davis views herself with disappointment: "I am lopsided / flatter than a boy" (41). Cummings reflects sadly on a blue dress, a reminder of her "before" when she had "both sides matching" (2002). When Goedicke looks in the mirror, she wonders, "Who is that lopsided stranger?" (33), and King confesses that she doesn't "have the guts to greet the world each day/as an amputee [...] / [...] Think of the connotations of 'unbalanced'" (59–60).

While appearance does matter, many poets are ready to "forsak[e] symmetry for survival" (Shaughnessy 17). Best, for instance, is unambiguous about what she has gained. In "Consolations," she begins with a list of trivial benefits – hearts closer when she hugs her lover, no bras to ruin in the wash, no bouncing boobs when running, but ends poignantly by pointing out she has traded her breasts for life: "Press your ear to this ribcage, / hear me live" (54). After the passage of time, in "Seduction," she writes that her breasts have been "excised, remembered, grieved / and almost, now, forgotten" (56).

Prostheses and Reconstruction. Rosemarie Garland-Thomson identified the role of appearance in the medicalization of women's bodies: Socially constructed ideologies of normalcy and beauty see the female body as something primarily to be gazed at (1557–8, 1567). Cancer makes the already less-than (because not-male) female body "leaky" in Shildrick's terms – unpredictable, unstable, contaminated (10–4). The role of the surgeon is to restore the patient from the margins where disease has relegated her back to life at the normative center through vanquishing the unruly cancer but also through recreating the body that existed previously (i.e., with two breasts).

There is no question that many women long for their pre-cancer breasts, in part because they symbolize pre-cancer lives. In "Untitled (About Carol)," the authors channel her voice: "My life was smooth before. / But there's this rough patch. / Having cancer. / But now it's getting smooth again" (with reconstruction) (Reilly, Lee, Lauz et al. 196). Susan Krebs Deerfield writes about the importance of reconstruction for her: "Being whole is worth any cost" ("My Breast Cancer Journey"). After initial stanzas that show estrangement from her body, mourning the loss of her hair, and wondering if she will ever feel like a woman again, she writes, "My body has changed but I'm now so alive / my future no longer looks bleak, / I see myself now as the woman I am, / I'm no longer, in my mind, 'the freak'" (2013). With reconstruction of her breast, she appears to feel restored to her pre-cancer state.

In the restitution narrative, the idea that reconstruction or prosthesis could be rejected seems irrational and unthinkable, because it restores (an approximation of) external appearance. This narrative is one that is comfortable for many breast surgeons because it conforms to their training to "fix things." Interestingly, as various poets sort through their sense of loss and mutilation, their disappointment at the emphasis on appearance, their frequent rejection of prostheses and reconstruction and their eventual (although sometimes ambivalent) embracing of their status as "one-breasted women," in their poetry itself they do not share any of this journey with their doctors. Of course, we don't know *why* there is no poetic evidence of such conversations. Did they not occur? Were they not deemed important enough to be transformed into poetry? It is possible that, because of the dominance of the restitution narrative and the medical model, women accepting their one-breastedness might have worried about negative judgment from their physicians. Regardless, I did not discover poetic evidence that such conversations occurred.

Early feminist poets uniformly questioned the push toward prostheses, and Lorde unequivocally saw prosthetics as a step that disempowered women, an expectation that forced them to deny the truth of their current situation. Later writers often similarly resisted what they deemed a misplaced emphasis on appearance rather than subjective sensuality or chosen self-image. Other more contemporary poets echo the dismay and anger Eve Kosofsky Sedgwick expresses in her essay "White Glasses." Participating in a hospital support group, Sedgwick is shocked when a social worker reassures the participants that "with proper toning exercise, makeup, wigs, and a well-fitting prosthesis, we could feel just as feminine as we ever had and no one (i.e., no man) need ever know that anything had happened" (69). These poets comprehend that restoring appearance is not, in fact, the same as regaining their pre-cancer body. Best mourns the loss of her nipples in "The Nipple Place," (44) and in "Flatlands" describes her chest as "regions of polar snow-/uninhabited, no sensation" (45). In "Circles," Carol Dine reflects, "Tomorrow, I will remove a bandage / unveiling /the plastic surgeon's rendering – / my tattooed nipple / that cannot be suckled or aroused" (253). Further depersonalizing the reconstructed breast, Raz emphasizes the commercial nature of her prosthesis:

> My new breast is two months old,
> […] stays cold under my skin
> when the old breast is warm;
> catalogue price, $276. My serial number,

> #B-1754, means some sisters under the skin
> [...] my new breast is sterile,
> will never have cancer. (*Divine* 24)

The Single-Breasted Amazon. Lorde's vision of the Amazon warrior gave post-mastectomy women an alternative to the restitution story. It is important to note that Lorde offered this image not as a warlike metaphor, but as a proud adaptation to life-threatening circumstances. Deena Metzger's poem "I Am No Longer Afraid" is another early celebration of the one-breasted body: "I am no longer ashamed to make love: / [...] I have the body of a warrior who does not kill or wound" (71). In her accompanying iconic bare-breasted photograph, she proudly displays the tattoo across her chest that symbolizes life and renewal.

The image of the Amazon occurs frequently in other women's poems, sometimes in celebration, as in Pastan's unambiguous identification with one-breasted Amazon women in "Routine Mammogram" (46–7). Ostriker's poem "Wintering" includes a similarly straightforward call to Amazon status: "A woman should be able to say / *I've become an Amazon, / Warrior woman minus a breast, / The better to shoot arrow / after fierce arrow*" (*Little Space* 209). Best writes, "We are warrior women, marked by a lack of breast – / [...] We live by our wits, we live on the move" ("Amazons" 48). In her poem "Asymmetry," King affirms the value of her new form and defiantly asserts, "I am a living sculpture; I am / in-the-flesh performance art." She admonishes the reader, "Resist the impulse to center the remaining breast, / to cut it off. Live with the discomfort. / You will learn to find me beautiful" (48–9).

Some acknowledge the image while adding an ambivalent twist. Clifton welcomes Amazonian iconography: "What is the splendor of one breast / on one woman?" – but it is not an uncomplicated embrace. She warns that if she, or any other woman with breast cancer, "... begins to cry // if you do, you will cry forever" (491–2). Shaughnessy describes herself as a reluctant Amazon with a "quiver full of fears," observing that she did not choose this designation, though now "the deed is done" (19). Cosner yearns time and again for the restoration of her old self – beautiful, sexy, flirty. Still, "Now, bald, hollowed by a surgeon's knife / [...] I tunnel into my ruined self / and transition to a scarred warrior" (82).

Post-Traumatic Growth and Challenges to "Normalcy" in an Altered Body. Some poets' confrontation with their radically changed form at times suggests debased abjection (Kristeva 1–3; DeShazer, *Fractured* 43). As we have seen, this not-uncommon sentiment is promoted by medicalized understandings of breast cancer that women can internalize and experience subjectively. However, at some point many of these poets question their initial reaction and ultimately embrace their difference as transgressive. Some challenge how much the breast really matters. Joanne Selzer asks in "Breasts," "What's a breast? Illusion" (55), reflecting voices in the lesbian and transgender communities that push back against the assumed primacy of the breast. In "White Glasses," for example, Sedgwick describes her lack of attachment to and identification with her breasts, and disputes the idea that they are central to either her sexuality or her identity (69–71). In "The Lost Breasts," Pat Riviere-Seel confesses that she didn't even especially like her breasts (37). Less can be more, these poets assert.

Poets who resist the dominant definitions of femininity and what it means to be "normal" in this manner reject the idea of being less-than because they are, in one poet's humorous phrase, "… on the lighter side / that would be the front" (Hartung 15). Ostriker, in "Wintering," takes to heart a friend's words: *You know what? You're the same person / After the mastectomy as before.* An idea / That had never occurred to me (*Little Space* 210). In "Normal," when she returns to teaching, colleagues tell her she looks normal, making this judgment of course based on her external appearance. She replies defiantly, "I am normal" (211), recognizing the paradox that, were these same people to see her naked body, they would pityingly assess her as "not normal." Instead, she claims her one-breasted self as a valid way of being in the world, and in doing so upends conventional definitions of "normal." Echoing Ostriker, Lois Tschetter Hjelmstad states in "Affirmation" that while mastectomy is indeed a disfigurement, it "Need not include / My soul" (81).

Such reinterpretations and revisioning may contain an element of posttraumatic growth (Brennan 1–18; Sears, Stanton and Danoff-Berg 487; Tedeschi and Calhoun 58–60). Rejecting what they perceive as an empty pursuit of appearance, these women embrace transformation instead (Wear 81). In her poem "Reconstruction" (pp. 51-2 in this book), poet Lisa Katz asks, "Couldn't we / admire the ruined, the torn, the perfect / error [...]?"; and in "The Form," she declares "[...] I will accept / the transformation, for worse or better: / the wife into bird, the mother into stone. / Not least of all I want the story meaningful." Similarly using images from nature, Shaughnessy describes herself as "yew-burnt, / yew-red, / new" (18), including the metaphor of a trial by fire from which she emerges not unscathed, but transformed. After losing her breast, Ostriker commits to "love myself courageously" ("Scenes" 188), as she is. A sense of possibility seems inherent in Best's "The Surgeon's Album." After her doctor shows her photos of full and partial reconstruction and implants, she muses, "[...] But how would I look/ flat? No extras. Straightforward scars" (31) and then decides against reconstruction. In a later poem, "Recovery Room," Best knows that in fact she will have to reconstruct herself piece by piece (35).

Others echo this sense of potentiality. Riviere-Seel writes in "The Lost Breasts" that, with her breasts gone, she now has "a place to begin in, space that could become anything // freshly plowed earth [...] / waiting for new life" (37). Similarly, Tschetter Hjelmstad sees clearly in "Last Day" that "Life will go on, of course[...] / but I will not / be the same" (32). In "Ward Thirty-Six," Darling does "[...] the crossword, find[ing] new words / for 'wreckage' and then 'rebirth'" (49). Her life is ruined, but there is a possibility that, Phoenix-like, she will rise again. In "I've Been through Something" the anonymous author acknowledges, "The scars are the wounds from the battle. / I've been through something. / The scars are the birthmarks – renewed life" (Kooken, Haase, and Russell 913). In "Self-Portrait without Breasts," Best decides that, although she's been "manscaped, hills removed [...]," she chooses to believe her lover when she tells her she is "even more beautiful now" because she has become an explorer, a seeker – because now she has developed "an ear for truth" (42).

Baldness Is Also a Threat to Identity. Loss of a breast is devastating, but loss of hair is also traumatic because of its close association with female identity. Many authors describe baldness as a form of spectacle and nakedness, a symbol of vulnerability in a society that judges by appearance. In "The Nakedness," Christine Stoddard compares herself unfavorably to an egg or space alien (2015), and in "Cancer Cat Sonnet," Cummings compares herself to a cat losing fur (2002). When her hair falls out, Echols worries, "Does that mean I am no longer glorious? No longer favored? / No longer beautiful? / No longer desirous? / No longer wanting?" Her poem is an ode to her hair, but she also says with tough resignation, "I've learned how to live without it" (2–8).

At other times, these poets embrace their baldness as an opportunity for new perspective. Although in other writing Cosner compares herself bitterly to a "piece of popcorn waiting to be popped / a soft-boiled egg, / a Genoa jellyfish, / a billiard ball jumping off dark corners" (39), in "Christmas Cancer" she sports a hat that reads "My Oncologist Does My Hair" (20). Cummings is advised to get a wig and "Get on with it," but she is "bewitched by [her] bald head" (2002), and in "Hairless," Shapcott watches a bald woman "[...] about to raise her arms to the sky; / [...] as she prepared to sing, to roar" (8). Baldness too is an opportunity for identity transformation. Whether hairless or breastless, women resist the imperative for restitution, even as they long for new images, new ways of understanding what their bodies have become – embracing rather rejecting, seeking not appearance but a way toward compatibility with who they now are.

Facing (Contingent) Life and Death

Early feminist writers realize that silence is a malignant veil dropped not only over breast cancer, but also over death itself. In her classic poem "A Woman Dead in Her Forties," Adrienne Rich admits that *"we never spoke at your deathbed of your death/* but from here on / I want more crazy mourning, more howl, more keening / We stayed mute and disloyal / because we were afraid" (53–8). In fact, research finds that women with breast cancer think about, write about and create art about existential questions of death, meaning and purpose (Reilly, Lee, Lauz et al. 202). Sometimes these writers' views of death differ considerably from the narratives of physicians and larger society that emphasize invulnerability, predictability, certainty (DeShazer, *Mammographies* 175) and survivorship. It is well known that oncologists have difficulty broaching end-of-life discussions with their patients (Fine, Reid, Shengelia et al. 595–603; The, Hak, Koeter et al. 1376–81). Further, the medical model often fails to address the reality that, because of the instability of survival, "survival itself can constitute a crisis" (Caruth 3–12). The women in this review wrote extensively about their possible or impending death. What is striking is that these musings, at least as described in poetry, never occur in connection with physicians or health professionals, but instead remain highly personal interrogations.

Living a Contingent Life. In her book *Fractured Borders*, DeShazer points out that the fundamental problem for women with breast cancer is uncertainty as to whether the disease will recur (3). This awareness challenges a linear, coherent narrative in which the patient either dies or is cured, and highlights the ongoing disruption for many women whose lives are not necessarily better but different and uncertain. The contingent nature of their existence going forward is prominent. Adapting to her changed body, Marian S. Irwin writes in "Post-Mastectomy-Week One," "The hard new path / I follow [...] / I am my own unknown [...] / I weep the loss / and wait / whatever certainty remains" (32). Slone-Crumbie goes to Hawaii but can't escape thoughts of recurrence ("The Fear"). Tschetter Hjelmstad writes that "Perhaps maturity is / Knowing there are no answers / And finding the courage / To live without them." (108). She has, at least in this moment, learned to live without certainty, truth, perfect faith or even answers.

Contingency and uncertainty are the inevitable and often unresolvable outcomes of even temporary life. In "Waiting Room," Darling powerfully juxtaposes waiting for ordinary things with a miracle that will mark the end of cancer: "I'm waiting for / the drugs to work, / this rain to stop, for results, / the tea to brew / paint to dry, // my hair to grow, morning, / the weekend, a miracle" (23). In "Don't Worry," another poem by Darling, this staid Englishwoman counsels other breast cancer patients to "Behave badly. Lie on the floor. / Throw a tantrum if you're bored. / Be late, / Be sordid. Eat six pies." After all, she reminds the reader, "[...] Beneath your feet / worms aren't worrying" (25). Death awaits, so why worry what the living think?

Survivorship as a Quest Narrative. If contingent life is a challenge, it is also a second chance. Some poets enthusiastically embrace survivorship as an exemplar of the quest narrative, seeing breast cancer as an experience that has made them better, wiser people. Tschetter Hjelmstad sees breast cancer as a gift because it is a reminder of mortality, a way of learning about oneself and connecting with strength, courage, joy and the preciousness of life (40). In "Cancer's Impact," Slone-Crumbie uses an acrostic to enumerate all the positive impacts of cancer: It has adjusted her attitude, renewed her focus and created a purpose-driven life (2015). King analogizes her experience with breast cancer to an alchemical process, a painful but valuable transformation:

> When heated directly by fire,
> the fire of trial, the heat of disease,
> infernos of grief and penury,
> the clay we're made of,
> will it crack and shatter,
> or will it thicken against the blaze
> a shield, refractory, infusible?
> [...] Can we
> hold under the terror,
> the torment of transforming
> under the forge
> until we are
> bearers of light [...] (24)

These poems are consonant with a larger sampling of women's attitudes toward breast cancer in general. A 2019 meta-analysis of qualitative breast cancer research concluded that most studies found that women typically viewed changes brought about by breast cancer as positive and an opportunity for positive self-growth. Moreover, experiencing breast cancer often results in a strong commitment to other women dealing with the disease (Smit, Coetzee, Roomaney et al. 241–2).

Challenging the Primacy of Survivorship. Some writers push back against the elevation of survivorship that is conveyed in the quest narrative (DeShazer, *Mammographies* 1). Ehrenreich confronts the "mindless triumphalism" of survivors that denigrates the dread and the dying: "Did we who live 'fight' harder than those who have died? Can we claim to be 'braver,' better people than the dead?" (43–53). Sandra Steingraber, who experienced bladder cancer and whose mother died of breast cancer, dedicated her collection of poems *Post-Diagnosis* to "nonsurvivors." (7). In her poem "In Response to a Promotional Ad Claiming that the Number of People Who Have Survived Cancer Could Now Fill the City of Los Angeles," she makes the point, "And the nonsurvivors fill the Pacific Ocean, / the Grand Canyon, / and the whole of Antarctica. / They fill our silences / And they fill our mouths / when we try to speak" (11–2). Reflecting a similar desire to honor the dead, Hacker notes in her "Journal Entries" that when a nurse brings in photographs of former patients "This routine to induce optimism only made me think of the photos she didn't have and would never show" ("Living" 211). Elsewhere, Hacker reflects on the dead and how they died:

> If I'm one of the victims, who survives?
> If I'm – reach for it – a survivor, who
> are the victims? The heroic dead,
> the ones who died in despair, the ones who died
> in terror, the exhausted ones who died
> tired?
>
> [...] I sit, tethered to a present tense
> whose intimations of mortality
> may ultimately make no difference
> to anyone, except of course to me,
> and finally, to nobody at all [...] (*Winter* 91, 93)

The only answer? Be in the present: "My future, though, is coming toward me fast / [...] All I can know is the expanding moment, / present, infinitesimal, infinite." (Hacker, *Winter* 91–5). Ostriker too struggles against her own survivor guilt, first ridiculing the clichés about survival before finally confronting the difficult truth: "Or do I smile in order not to collapse in guilty grief at the thought of the dead?" ("Scenes" 175).

Death Itself. Acknowledging the contingency and uncertainty of survival as well as the simplicity of survivor triumphalism, requires that these poets authentically face the possibility of their own deaths. Some approach death with dread, loss of control and sorrow. After a grim metaphor of a road blocked by entropy, ending in a ruined castle, surrounded by bald and blighted trees, Hacker begs, "I don't know how to die yet. Let me live." (*Winter* 86). In "Getting Well," Raz receives a present of four hairs from the head of another breast cancer patient that have been pressed into a book. She is unsure of the message: "[...] Work / can keep us alive to the world? / Writing down some truth will help?" (*Living* 134–5). The interrogatory structure suggests she doubts the efficacy of either work or writing to ward off death. Cosner, taking a reflective pause, realizes she could vanish in an instant: "Poof! / I evaporate in a cloud / of pink dust, / return to ashes" (71). Ironically, breast cancer pink still surrounds her, only now it is a symbol of her death. Eavesdropping on the ordinary sounds coming from the people she loves in an adjoining room, Kelina Leeks wonders "If this is what it will sound like/when I am gone" (31).

For still others, sadness is tinged with acceptance. In "Remission," Pastan reflects, "It seems you must grow / into your own death slowly, / as if it were a pair of new shoes / waiting on the closet floor." (57). Aimee Grunsberger gives a rare passing nod to her physicians in "If the Doctors Are Right," in which she attempts to prepare for death: "I've got to make some order / stop wasting what little is left." She decides watching the lunar eclipse "seems worth a look," while mourning that everything will go on "without me" (54). Yet, like others, she also celebrates that she is at that moment still alive.

As Silver contemplates her own death in "Limitless," she confesses that, while she wants to stay, when she must leave, she wants her last words to be "I loved it all" (2002). A similar sense of gratitude for life's bounty is expressed in King's "As Death Approaches," where she writes, with some amazement,

> I can't believe I'm laughing!
> I'd have sworn
> I'd be shaking or sniveling
> [...] That's why I'm laughing,
> I've had so much love
> [...] So this laughter
> I had to work up to
> through so many tears

> it just keeps coming
> like a fountain, a spray.
> Let it light on you
> refreshment, benediction,
> as I'm driven away. (127–8)

Lorde knew that awareness of one's own mortality could be a means of helping both herself and other women (Barnes 775). "The whole terrible meaning of mortality as both weapon and power" must be examined, she says (Lorde, *Cancer Journals* 51). In her later work, *The Marvelous Arithmetics of Distance*, Lorde often appears ready to face her death: "*I am not afraid to say / unembellished / I am dying / but I do not want to do it / looking the other way // Today is not the day / It could be / but it is not*" (7–59). "Restoration: A Memorial 9/18/91" analogizes death to "[...] a burnt star / perched on the rim of my teacup" (Lorde, *Marvelous* 40). Here, death becomes almost friendly, familiar and even cozy. Ultimately, though, her mastectomy scar reminds Lorde of her looming death:

> I still patrol that line
> [...] along the scar
> the surest way of knowing
> death is a fractured border
> through the center of my days. (*Marvelous* 52–3)

Even reconciled to her passing, she mourns "How hard it is to sleep / in the middle of life" (*Marvelous* 60).

Final Thoughts

The medical model, which objectifies women's bodies by emphasizing the technology of care, still holds sway in the treatment of breast cancer patients. For thirty years, in their poetry, women with breast cancer both long for the promises of the restitution story and resist its controlling dominance (the silencing of their voices, the certainty of its doctors, the assembly-line organization of its systems) as well as its falseness (the substitution of appearance for reality, its denial of suffering and death). In telling their own stories, these poets often begin with a cry of chaos. Although they understandably yearn for a story of restitution, they frequently come to adopt positions very different from the narrative favored in the medical model. Often, from desire or necessity, they commit to a journey, in part a classic quest story, resulting in a more aware, more meaningful life, but absent the cheerful sentimentality that characterizes the Panglossian conclusion that everything, even cancer, is all for the best. While celebrating contingent survival, many reject the primacy of survivorship and pay tribute to all those who do not survive their disease. Still others open themselves to the possibility of personal transformations that encompass a different way of being women in the world – one-breasted Amazons who know that their vulnerability is what gives them strength.

Most of these writers know that they can never put their life back as it was before. They mourn the loss, they struggle with the contingency of the future and the possibility of death, but they also embrace their moment and their new selves, sometimes in dread, sometimes with acceptance, always with courage.

Acknowledgments: I gratefully acknowledge the foundational work of Dr. Mary DeShazer, which informed many of the ideas in this chapter. I would also like to thank Anh-Minh Nguyen BS, UC Irvine, for help with the literature review.

Bibliography

Adcock, Fleur. "The Soho Hospital for Women." In *The Norton Anthology of Poetry*. New York: W. W. Norton & Company, 1996.

Ashing-Giwa, Kimlin Tam, Geraldine Padilla, Judith Tejero, Janet Kraemer, Anne Coscarelli, Sheila Clayton, Imani Williams, and Dawn Hills. "Understanding the Breast Cancer Experience of Women: A Qualitative Study of African American, Asian American, Latina and Caucasian Cancer Survivors." *Psycho-Oncology* 13.6 (June 2004): 408–28.

Bahar, Saba. "If I'm One of the Victims, Who Survives?": Marilyn Hacker's Breast Cancer Texts." *Journal of Women in Culture and Society* 28.4 (June 2003): 1025–52.
Barnes, Sharon L. "Marvelous Arithmetics: Prosthesis, Speech, and Death in the Late Work of Audre Lorde." *Women's Studies* 37.7 (September 9, 2008): 769–89.
Best, Clare. *Excisions*. Hove: Waterloo Press, 2011.
Brennan, James. "Adjustment to Cancer – Coping or Personal Transition?" *Psycho-Oncology* 10.1 (January 2001): 1–18.
Cadden, Marie. "Breast Count." In *Bosom Pals: Eight Poets Share Their Experiences with Breast Cancer*. Ed. Marie Cadden. Inverin: Doire Press, 2017.
Calhoun, Lawrence G. and Richard G. Tedeschi, editors. *Handbook of Posttraumatic Growth : Research and Practice*. 1st ed. New York: Routledge, 2006.
Campbell, Joseph. *The Hero's Journey : Joseph Campbell on His Life and Work*. 3rd ed. New York: New World Library, 2014.
Caruth, Cathy. *Trauma : Explorations in Memory*. 1st ed. Baltimore: Johns Hopkins University Press, 1995.
Clifton, Lucille. *The Collected Poems of Lucille Clifton 1965–2010*. Eds. Kevin Young and Michael S. Glaser. Rochester: Lannan Boa, 2012.
Coll-Planas, Gerard, and Mariona Visa. "The Wounded Blogger: Analysis of Narratives by Women with Breast Cancer." *Sociology of Health & Illness* 38.6 (February 19, 2016): 884–98.
Cosner, Janay. *Dancing with Breast Cancer: A Memoir in Poems*. Naples: Reborn Phoenix Press, 2017.
Cummings, Alysa. Cummings, Alysa. *Oncolink* (2002), <https://www.oncolink.org/support/survivorship/creative-inspiration/oncolink-reading-room/poetry/5082>. Accessed January 27, 2020.
Darling, Julia. *Sudden Collapses in Public Places*. Great Britain: Arc Publications, 2003.
Davis, Alice J. "After Surgery." In *Her Soul Beneath the Bone: Women's Poetry on Breast Cancer*. Ed. Leatrice H. Lifshitz. Chicago: University of Illinois Press, 1988.
Davis, Helene. *Chemo-Poet and Other Poems*. Cambridge: Alice James Books, 2002.
Davis, Joseph E. and Ana M. Gonzalez. *To Fix or To Heal*. Manhattan: NYU Press, 2016.
Dean, Lorraine T., Shadiya Moss, Anne Marie McCarthy, and Katrina Armstrong. "Healthcare System Distrust, Physician Trust, and Patient Discordance with Adjuvant Breast Cancer Treatment Recommendations." *Cancer Epidemiology and Prevention Biomarkers* 26.12 (2017): 1745–52.

Deerfield, Susan Krebbs. "My Cancer Journey." Breast Cancer DIY (2013). <https://www.breastcancerdiy.com/readpoetry.htm>. Accessed January 27, 2020.

DeShazer, Mary K. *Fractured Borders : Reading Women's Cancer Literature*. 1st ed. Ann Arbor: University of Michigan Press, 2005.

———. *Mammographies : The Cultural Discourses of Breast Cancer Narratives*. Ann Arbor: The University of Michigan Press, 2013.

Dine, Carol. "Circles." In *Living on the Margins: Women Writers on Breast Cancer*. Ed. Hilda Raz. New York: Persea Books, 1999.

Echols, Che'Vonceil. *Songs for My Hair*. Self-published, 2017.

Ehlers, Nadine. "Risking 'Safety': Breast Cancer, Prognosis, and the Strategic Enterprise of Life." *Journal of Medical Humanities* 37.1 (June 18, 2014): 81–94.

Ehrenreich, Barbara. "Welcome to Cancerland." *Harper's Magazine* (November 2001): 43–53.

Faith, Karlene. *Unruly Women : The Politics of Confinement and Resistance*. Vancouver: Press Gang Publishers, 2011.

Faulkner, Sandra L. "Poetry Is Politics: An Autoethnographic Poetry Manifesto." *International Review of Qualitative Research* 10.1 (May 2017): 89–96.

Fine, Elizabeth, Carrington Reid, Rouzi Shingelia, and Ronald D. Adelman. "Directly Observed Patient–Physician Discussions in Palliative and End-of-Life Care: A Systematic Review of the Literature." *Journal of Palliative Medicine* 13.5 (May 1, 2010): 595–603.

Frank, Arthur W. *The Wounded Storyteller: Body, Illness, and Ethics*. Chicago: The University of Chicago Press, 1995.

Garland-Thomson, Rosemarie. "Feminist Disability Studies." *Signs: Journal of Women in Culture and Society* 30.2 (January 2005): 1557–87.

Goedicke, Patricia. "In the Hospital." In *Her Soul Beneath the Bone : Women's Poetry on Breast Cancer*. Ed. Leatrice H. Lifschitz. Chicago: University of Illinois Press, 1988.

Grunsberger, Aimee. "If the Doctors Are Right." *Uncharted Lines: Poems from the Journal of the American Medical Association*. Ed. Charlene Breedlove. New York: Boaz, 1998.

Hacker, Marilyn. *Winter Numbers: Poems*. New York: W.W. Norton & Co., 1994.

———. "Journal Entries." In *Living on the Margins: Women Writers on Breast Cancer*. Ed. Hilda Raz. New York: Persea Books, 1999.

Hall, Judith. "Ink and Green Wash: In the Oncologist's Waiting Room." *Anatomy, Errata: [Poems]*. Columbus: Ohio State University Press, 1998.

Hartung, Susan. "Mastectomies." *Cell 2 Soul: The Journal of Humane Medicine and Medical Humor* 1.4 (2005): 15.

Hawkins, Anne Hunsaker. *Reconstructing Illness: Studies in Pathography.* Purdue: Purdue University Press, 1999.
Heiney, Sue P., DeAnne K. Hilfinger Messias, Tisha M. Felder, Kenneth W. Phelps, and Jada C. Quinn. "African American Women's Recollected Experiences of Adherence to Breast Cancer Treatment." *Oncology Nursing Forum* 44.2 (2017): 217–24.
Herndl, Diane Price. "Our Breasts, Our Selves: Identity, Continuity, and Ethics in Cancer Autobiographies." *Signs: Journal of Women in Culture and Society* 35.1 (2006): 221–45.
Hjelmstad, Lois Tschetter. *Fine Black Lines: Reflections on Facing Cancer, Fear, and Loneliness.* Englewood: Mulberry Hill Press, 2003.
Holliday, Ruth and John Hassard. *Contested Bodies.* New York: Routledge, 2001.
Irwin, Marion S. "Post-Mastectomy Week 1." In *Her Soul Beneath the Bone: Women's Poetry on Breast Cancer.* Ed. Leatrice H. Lifschitz. Chicago: University of Illinois Press, 1988.
Johnson, Felicia. "We Carry: I Carry Personal Stories." Susan G. Komen (2010), <https://ww5.komen.org/Blog/Poem-of-a-Family-Deeply-Affected-by-Metastatic-Breast-Cancer/>. Accessed January 27, 2020.
Kellerman, Paul S. "Old Friends: Maintaining the Physician-Patient Connection in the 21st Century." *American Journal of Kidney Diseases* 71.3 (2018): A12–A13.
Keys, Helen. "Silent No More." In *Cherry Cheesecake: Poems Filled with Love and Hope for Women with Breast Cancer.* Ed. Carolyn F. Nemec. Long Island: Local Gems Press, 2014.
King, Samantha. *Pink Ribbons, Inc.: Breast Cancer and the Politics of Philanthropy.* Minneapolis: University of Minnesota Press, 2006.
King, Susan Deborah. *One-Breasted Woman: Poems.* Duluth: Holy Cow! Press, 2007.
Klawitter, Maren. "Racing for the Cure, Walking Women and Toxic Curing: Mapping Cultures of Action with the Bay Area Terrain of Breast Cancer." In *Ideologies of Breast Cancer: Feminist Perspectives.* Ed. Laura K. Potts. London: MacMillan, 2000.
Kooken, Wendy Carter, Joan E. Haase, and Kathleen M. Russell. "'I've Been Through Something.'" *Western Journal of Nursing Research* 29.7 (November 2007): 896–919.
Krasno, Miriam R. "Separation." In *Her Soul Beneath the Bone: Women's Poetry on Breast Cancer.* Ed. Leatrice H. Lifschitz Chicago: University of Illinois Press, 1988.
Kristeva, Julia. *Powers of Horror: An Essay on Abjection.* New York: Columbia University Press, 1982.

Leeks, Kalina. "In the Other Room." In *Cancer Poetry Project 2: More Poems by Cancer Patients and Those Who Love Them*. Ed. Karin B. Miller. Minneapolis: Tasora Books, 2013.

Lifshitz, Leatrice H. *Her Soul Beneath the Bone : Women's Poetry on Breast Cancer*. Urbana: University of Illinois Press, 1988.

Ling, Amy. "Bone Scan." In *Living on the Margins: Women Writers on Breast Cancer*. Ed. Hilda Raz. New York: Persea Books, 1999.

Lorde, Audre. *The Marvelous Arithmetics of Distance : Poems, 1987–1992*. New York: W.W. Norton & Company, 1993.

———. *The Cancer Journals*. 2nd ed. San Francisco: Aunt Lute Books, 1997.

Martino, Maria Luisa, and Maria Francesca Freda. "Meaning-Making Process Related to Temporality during Breast Cancer Traumatic Experience: The Clinical Use of Narrative to Promote a New Continuity of Life." *Europe's Journal of Psychology* 12.4 (November 18, 2016): 622–34.

McGrath, C., C. F. C. Jordens, K. Montgomery, and I. H. Kerridge. "'Right' Way to 'Do' Illness? Thinking Critically about Positive Thinking." *Internal Medicine Journal* 36.10 (September 4, 2006): 665–9.

Metzger, Deena. "I Am No Longer Afraid." In *Her Soul Beneath the Bone: Women's Poetry on Breast Cancer*. Ed. Leatrice H. Lifschitz. Chicago: University of Illinois Press, 1988.

Michalko, Rod, and Tanya Titchkosky, eds. *Rethinking Normalcy: A Disability Studies Reader*. Canadian Scholars' Press, 2009.

Ostriker, Alicia. *The Little Space: Poems Selected and New, 1968–1998*. Pittsburgh: University of Pittsburgh Press, 1998.

———. "Scenes from a Mastectomy." In *Living on the Margins: Women Writers on Breast Cancer*. Ed. Hilda Raz. New York: Persea Books, 1999.

———. "The Mastectomy Poems: The Bridge of Fantasy." *Oncolink* (1996), <https://www.oncolink.org/support/survivorship/creative-inspiration/oncolink-reading-room/poetry/5082>. Accessed January 27, 2020.

Pastan, Linda. *Fraction of Darkness*. 1st ed. New York: W. W. Norton and Company, Inc., 1985.

Picardie, Ruth, et al. *Before I Say Goodbye*. 3rd ed. London: Penguin, 1998.

Raz, Hilda. *Divine Honors*. Middletown: Wesleyan University Press, 1997.

———. "Getting Well." In *Living on the Margins: Women Writers on Breast Cancer*. Ed. Hilda Raz. New York: Persea Books, 1999.

Remen, Rachel N. *In the Service of Life*. Meridians-Columbia, 1998.

Reilly, Rosemary C., Virginia Lee, Kate Lauz, and Andreanne Robitaille. "Using Found Poetry to Illuminate the Existential and Posttraumatic Growth of Women with Breast Cancer Engaging in Art Therapy." *Qualitative Research in Psychology* 15.2–3 (February 15, 2018): 196–217.

Rich, Adrienne. "A Woman Dead in Her Forties." *The Dream of a Common Language: Poems 1974–1977*. New York; London: W.W. Norton, 1978.
Ristovski-Slijepcevic, Svetlana and Kirsten Bell. "Rethinking Assumptions about Cancer Survivorship." *Canadian Oncology Nursing Journal* 24.3 (August 5, 2014): 166–8.
Riviere-Seel, Pat. "The Lost Breasts." *Cancer Poetry Project 2: More Poems by Cancer Patients and Those Who Love Them*. Ed. Karin B. Miller. Minneapolis: Tasora Books, 2013.
Schneeloch, Jane V. "Swallowtails." In *Cancer Poetry Project 2: More Poems by Cancer Patients and Those Who Love Them*. Ed. Karin B. Miller. Minneapolis: Tasora Books, 2013.
Schodek, Kay. "Mastectomy." In *Her Soul Beneath the Bone: Women's Poetry on Breast Cancer*. Ed. Leatrice H. Lifschitz Chicago: University of Illinois Press, 1988.
Sears, Sharon R., Annette L. Stanton, and Sharon Danoff-Burg. "The Yellow Brick Road and the Emerald City: Benefit Finding, Positive Reappraisal Coping and Posttraumatic Growth in Women with Early-Stage Breast Cancer." *Health Psychology* 22.5 (2003): 487.
Sedgwick, Eve Kosofsky. "White Glasses." In *Living on the Margins: Women Writers on Breast Cancer*. Ed. Hilda Raz. New York: Persea Books, 1999.
Selzer, Joanne. "Breasts." In *Her Soul Beneath the Bone: Women's Poetry on Breast Cancer*. Ed. Leatrice H. Lifschitz. Urbana: University of Illinois Press, 1988.
Setchell, Jenny, Thomas Abrams, Laura C. McAdam, and Barbara E. Gibson. "Cheer* in Health Care Practice: What It Excludes and Why It Matters." *Qualitative Health Research* 29.13 (April 8, 2019): 1890–1903.
Shapiro, Johanna. "Can Poetry Be Data? Potential Relationships between Poetry and Research." *Families, Systems, & Health* 22.2 (2004): 171–7.
Shapcott, Jo. *Of Mutability*. London: Faber & Faber, 2010.
Shaughnessy, Lorna. *Bosom Pals: Eight Poets Share Their Experiences with Breast Cancer*. Ed. Marie Cadden. Inverin: Doire Press, 2017.
Sheppard, Vanessa B., Alejandra Hurtado de Mendoza, Costellia H. Talley, et al. "Reducing Racial Disparities in Breast Cancer Survivors' Ratings of Quality Cancer Care: The Enduring Impact of Trust." *The Journal for Healthcare Quality* 38.3 (2016): 143–63.
Shildrick, Margrit. *Leaky Bodies and Boundaries: Feminism, Postmodernism and (Bio)Ethics*. 1st ed. New York: Routledge, 1997.
Silver, Anne. "Limitless." *Oncolink* (2002), <https://www.oncolink.org/support/survivorship/creative-inspiration/oncolink-reading-room/poetry/5082>. Accessed January 28, 2020.

Slone-Crumbie, Donna C. Breast Cancer DIY (2015), <https://www.breastcancerdiy.com/readpoetry.htm>. Accessed January 28, 2020.
Smit, Anri, Beonwyne Jo'Sean Coetzee, Rizwanna Roomaney, et al. "Women's Stories of Living with Breast Cancer: A Systematic Review and Meta-Synthesis of Qualitative Evidence." *Social Science & Medicine* 222 (January 14, 2019): 231–45.
Smith, Tracy K. "Watershed." *Poets.Org*, Academy of American Poets (June 17, 2017), <https://poets.org/poem/watershed>. Accessed January 28, 2020.
Sontag, Susan. *Illness as Metaphor*. New York: Farrar, Straus and Giroux, 1977.
Stacey, Jackie. *Teratologies: A Cultural Study of Cancer*. New York: Routledge, 1997.
Steingraber, Sandra. *Post-Diagnosis*. Ithaca: Firebrand Books, 2005.
Stoddard, Christine. "The Nakedness." Breast Cancer DIY (2015), <https://www.breastcancerdiy.com/readpoetry.htm>. Accessed January 27, 2020.
Tedeschi, Richard G. and Lawrence Calhoun. "Posttraumatic Growth: A New Perspective on Psychotraumatology." *Psychiatric Times* 21.4 (April 1, 2004): 58–60.
The, Anne-Mei, Tony Hak, Gerard Koeter, and Gerrit van der Wal. "Collusion in Doctor-Patient Communication about Imminent Death: An Ethnographic Study." *British Medical Journal* 321.7273 (December 2, 2000): 1376–81.
Twiddy, Iain. *Cancer Poetry*. Hampshire, England: Palgrave MacMillan, 2015.
Wear, Delese. "Your Breasts/Sliced Off." *Women & Health* 20.4 (December 1993): 81–100.
Webb-Wiltshire, Carolyn. "A Wait." Breast Cancer DIY (2016), <https://www.breastcancerdiy.com/readpoetry.htm>. Accessed January 27, 2020.
Williams, David R., Selina A. Mohammed, and Alexandra E. Shields. "Understanding and Effectively Addressing Breast Cancer in African American Women: Unpacking the Social Context." *Cancer* 122.14 (February 29, 2016): 2138–49.

JENNIFER HAYDEN

Under the Birdcage

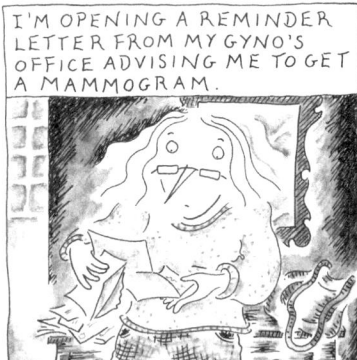
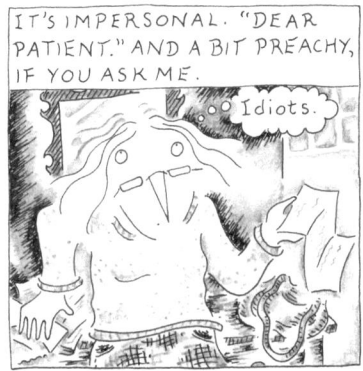
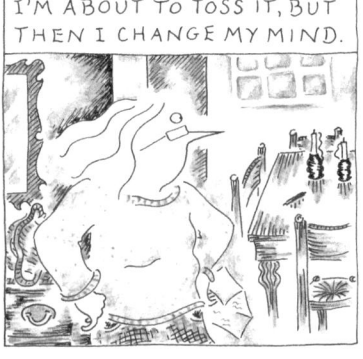
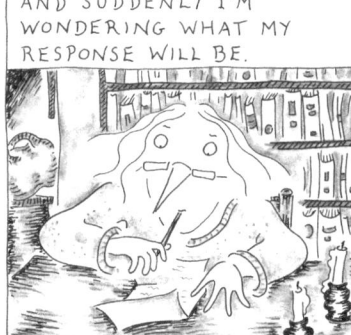
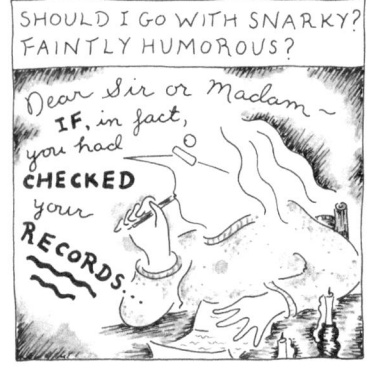

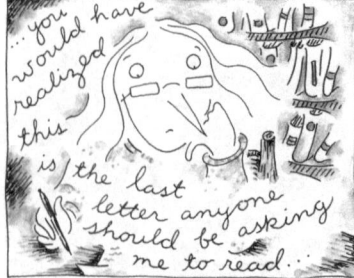

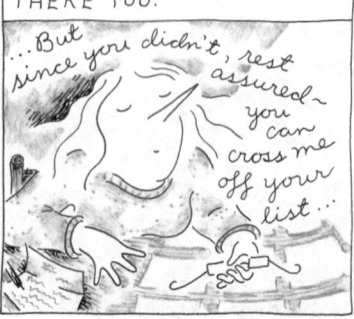

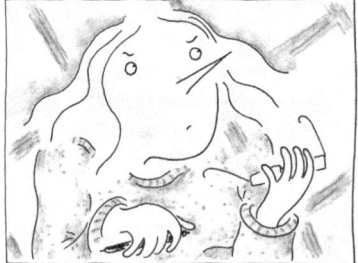

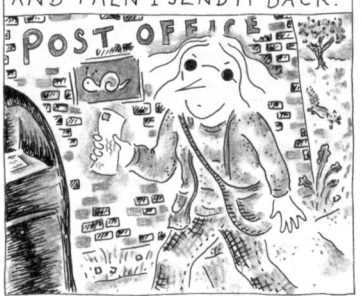

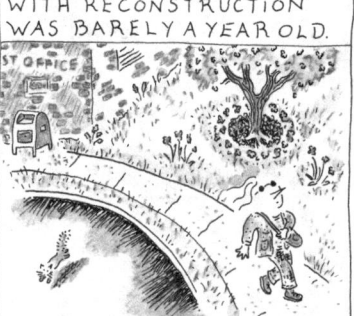

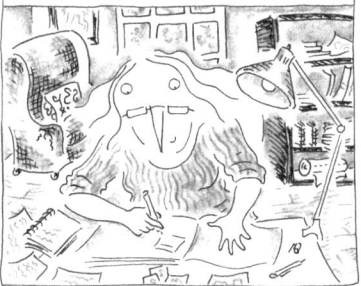
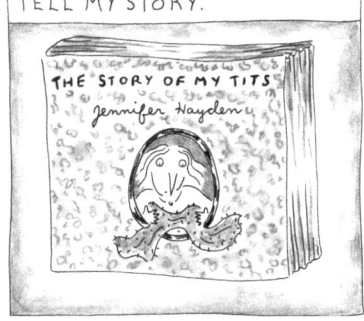
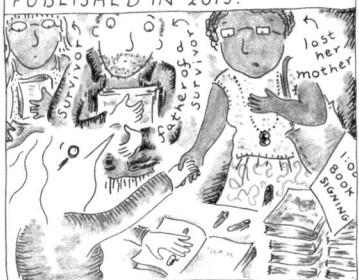
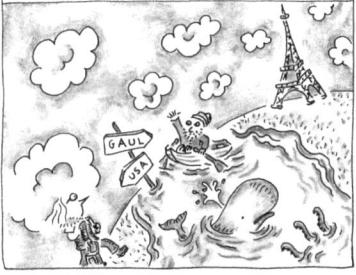
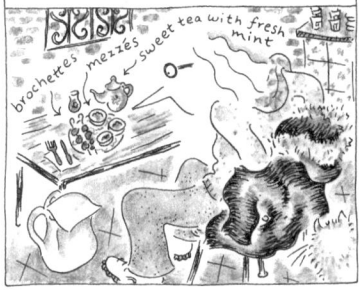
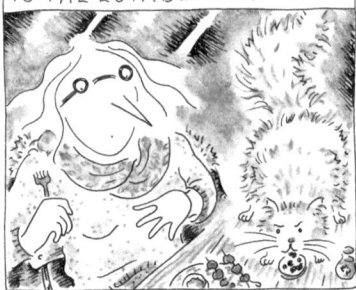

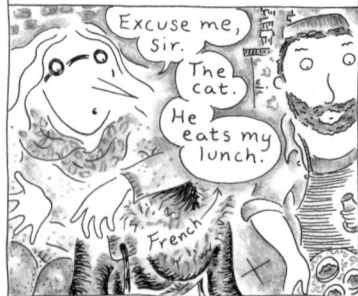
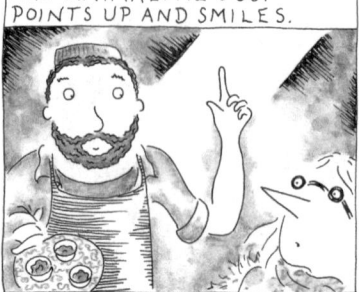
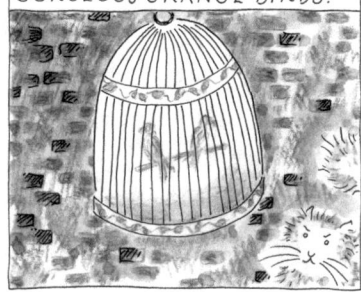
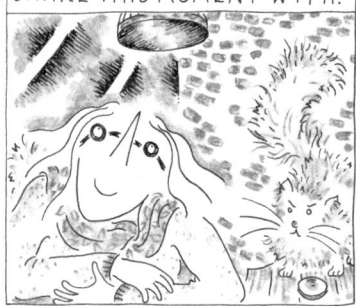
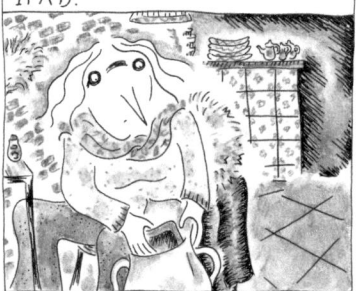

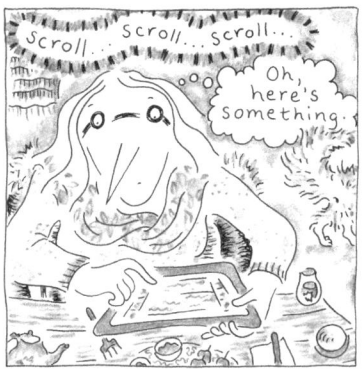
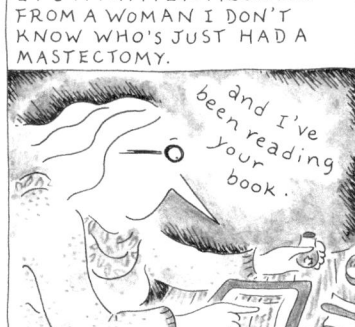
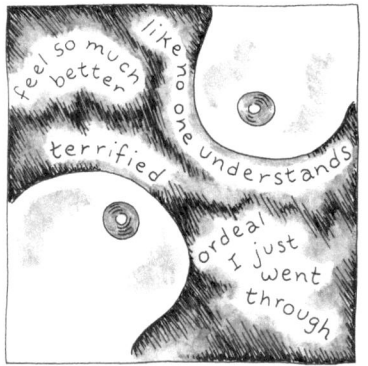
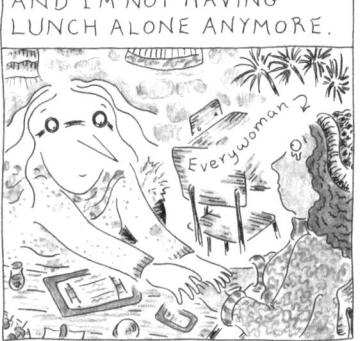
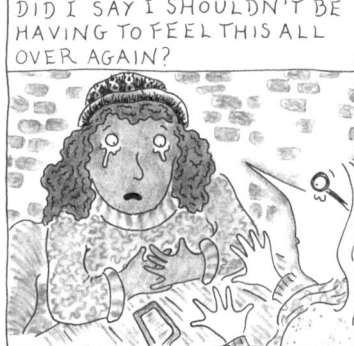
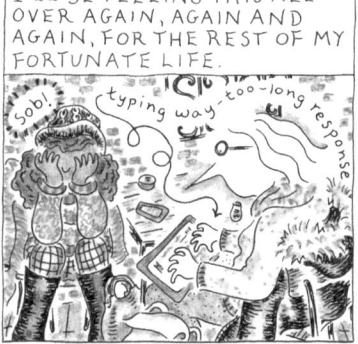

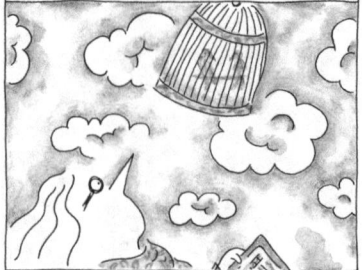
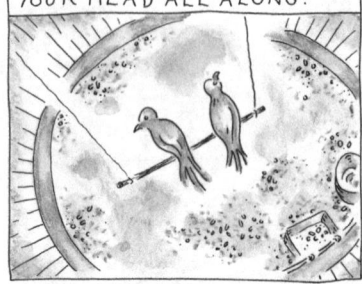
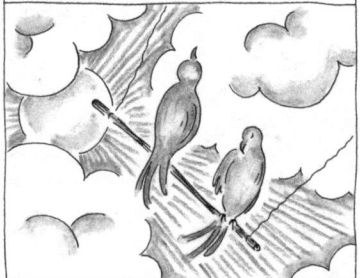
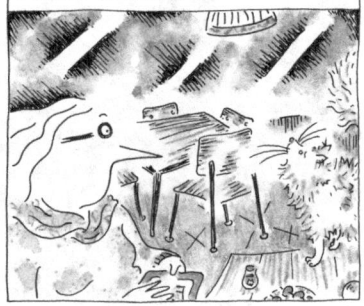
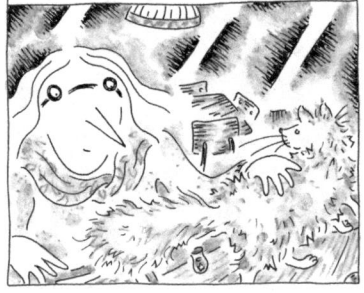
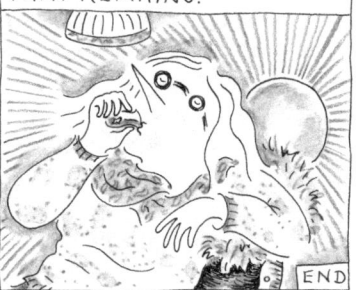

KIMBERLY R. MYERS

Breast Cancer Comics in the Classroom and the Clinic

As a medical educator, one of my main goals is to further our students' comprehension of what it feels like to live with a given disease. The theory is that if they have a firm, multifaceted understanding of the challenges, losses and perhaps gains that, say, a breast cancer patient experiences, they will be better able to empathize with that person. And while empathy might be mostly theoretical in the early stages of their training, the hope is that it will mature and flourish in their later work with the individuals in their care. The best way I know to help students understand others' lived reality is through stories. Curiously, reading patients' stories of illness (or "pathographies," as they're sometimes called) benefits medical students in another way as well: It helps them envision the kinds of physicians they want to be, the kinds of people they *are* as they practice the art and science of medicine face-to-face with another human being.

In a seminar for fourth-year medical students a few years ago, I chose breast cancer as the particular disease we would explore via stories told in different genres. Perhaps the most effective of these stories was the graphic pathography (that is, illness story told in the form of a comic) by Marisa Acocella Marchetto entitled *Cancer Vixen*. In what follows I hope to capture something of the nature of our discussions as if in real time.

One of the greatest stresses for many patients is the keen anxiety they feel while awaiting test results, and Marchetto depicts this expertly in an early sequence. (Figure 1) I begin by isolating the first panel and the final borderless panel. Looking at these together, students understand that the cell phone is the patient's sole focus, literally the only thing in her range of vision when it rings. That she receives fifty-seven calls indicates a pressing issue of some sort, especially as Marchetto can number the calls from each member of her primary support group: fiancé, best friends and mother. That

Marchetto includes "doctors" in this list indicates the weight of their significance to her in this moment; and the understated "0" Marchetto draws to indicate the number of calls she has received from these doctors depicts a glaring contrast. (Students often talk here about how they would draw the telephone from their perspective and how they would indicate the number and recipients of phone calls they make in a single day – casual comments that unexpectedly and fruitfully broaden the discussion.)

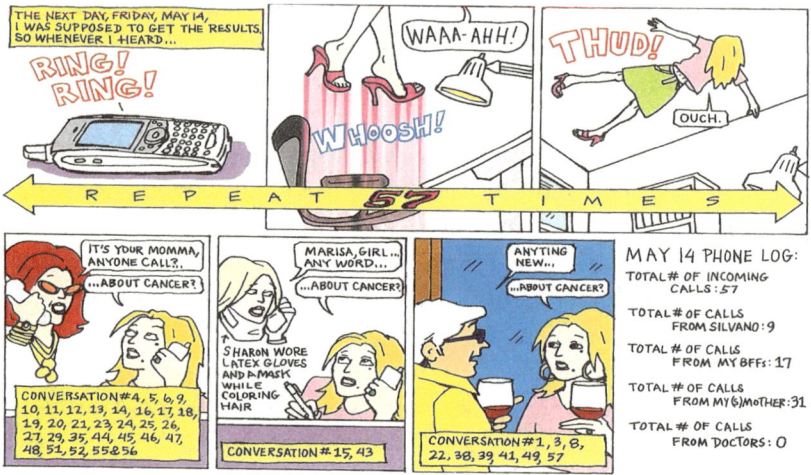

Figure 1: "Illustrations" from CANCER VIXEN: A TRUE STORY by Marisa Acocella Marchetto. Copyright © 2006 by Marisa Acocella Marchetto. Used by permission of Alfred A. Knopf, an imprint of the Knopf Doubleday Publishing Group, a division of Penguin Random House LLC. All rights reserved.

While this two-panel excerpt kindles students' understanding of what Marchetto wants to convey, it is the intervening panels that drive home her point; and we explore these together. Every time the phone rings, Marchetto is so startled that she feels as though she is sucked out of her chair into the air with a force that slams her into the ceiling. These calls are all dead-ends, false alarms that add to her discomfort ("ouch"); she has no capacity to move beyond the walls (or ceiling) of her room, metaphorically speaking, to become pro-active because she does not receive the information she needs to proceed. Again, Marchetto emphasizes this point with the yellow text arrow that spans the first three panels in the sequence: "Repeat 57 Times," the 57 in bold red font. The grinding tedium of such continually thwarted expectation is underscored by the numbers that crowd the yellow text boxes, and her growing exhaustion is evident in her eyes and mouth.

When the dreaded call finally comes, Marchetto registers, in close-up, Dr. Mills's name on the screen of her PDA; this is the name she has been waiting to see, and it fills the screen as fully as it commands her attention. (Figure 2) And then immediately, the next panel that conveys the impact of Dr. Mills's report. (Figure 3) By this point, there is no need to analyze the panel part by part. Students are attuned to the kinds of lines Marchetto uses to convey bad news: Her hair stands straight out and up, and the dialogue "bubble" is not the typical curvilinear but rather angular, "spiked" to indicate the news that will impale her.

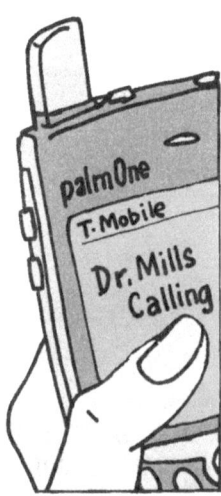

Figure 2: From CANCER VIXEN, by Marisa Acocella Marchetto.

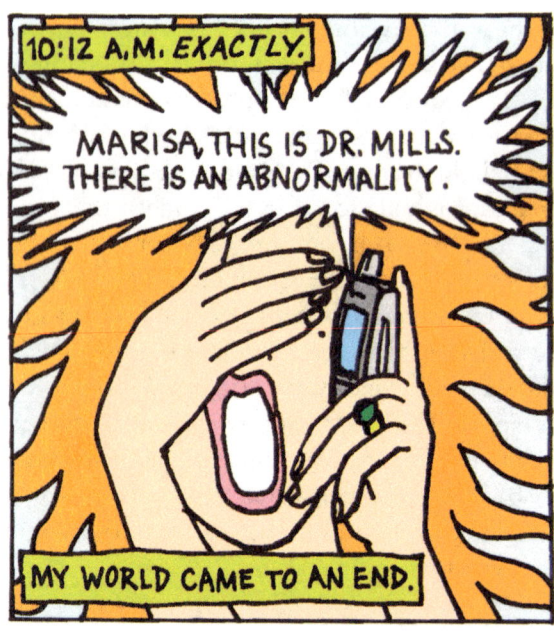

Figure 3: From CANCER VIXEN, by Marisa Acocella Marchetto.

Her precision in time – 10:12 a.m., instead of, say, rounding it off to the quarter-hour – and the italicized word "exactly" complement the green text box at the bottom of the frame: "My world came to an end."
Ironically, so would mine.

Cancer Vixen in the Clinic

Discussing this particular text in such minute detail with my students made me a bit uneasy. My annual mammogram was coming up the next day, and, as any woman might do, I couldn't help placing myself in Marchetto's position, wondering "What if?" The timing of this session on breast cancer seemed especially inauspicious in the context of other events that were, I fretted, too numerous to be coincidental: my recent presentation on breast cancer pathographies at an international conference, my husband's colleague's recent diagnosis of breast cancer, my sudden and inexplicable affinity for pageboy hats that led me to buy three of them, and the return of a dull ache in my left breast that had waxed and waned over the course of two decades. I was eerily aware of the confluence of these events, and I tried to stave off my deepening sense of foreboding with the rhetorical question, "So what are the odds that you would be diagnosed with breast cancer just when so many vectors in your life right now point toward breast cancer?" Pretty good odds, as it turns out.

Fewer than twenty-four hours after discussing Marchetto's text with my students, I was undergoing many of the procedures – and the emotions – she so memorably depicts in *Cancer Vixen*. I can't be sure if someone who casually reads a comic recalls details as vividly as one who teaches a comic, but Marchetto was my constant companion throughout the entire next day … and several of the days in the weeks and months to come. For one thing, while I was waiting in the "diagnostic room" to be called back for my imaging study, I kept thinking about various ways I would draw myself at that moment – if I had had the presence of mind to focus on drawing instead of on the anxiety that was consuming me. It might have looked something like this. (Figure 4).

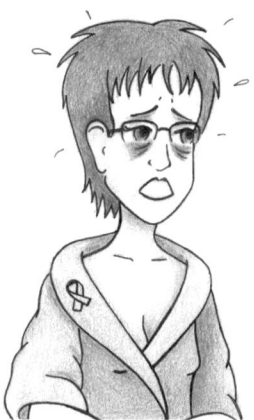

Figure 4: All original images by Pamela Wagar Smith, MD. Reproduced with permission.

While I was waiting for the mammogram, a radiologist colleague-friend of mine, Dr. Julie Mack, saw me and asked if I would like her to read my study. (Please see our co-authored essay about this experience elsewhere in this book.) I had already arranged to wait for the test results and was very pleased that she would be reading the image. When the pictures had been taken, the technician asked me to remain in the exam room while she made sure Julie had all the shots she needed. I was expecting the technician to return. Instead, Julie came into the room. (Figure 5)

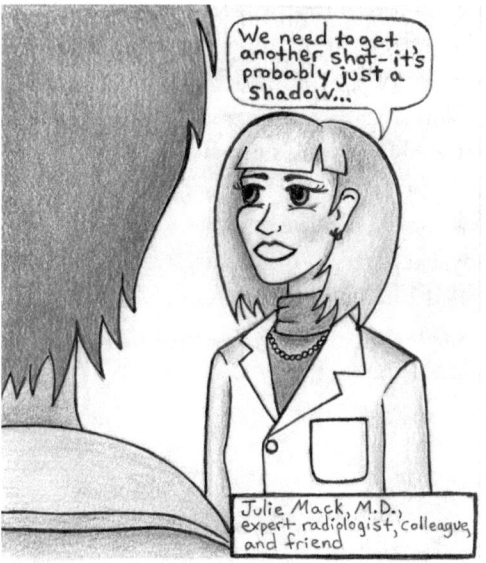

Figure 5: Original image by Pamela Wagar Smith, MD.

I knew from past experience that the need for additional images didn't necessarily mean anything bad, but hearing this – especially from the radiologist herself – fanned my fear. When I saw Julie coming down the hall after the second set of pictures had been taken, I could tell immediately that everything was not okay. (Figure 6)

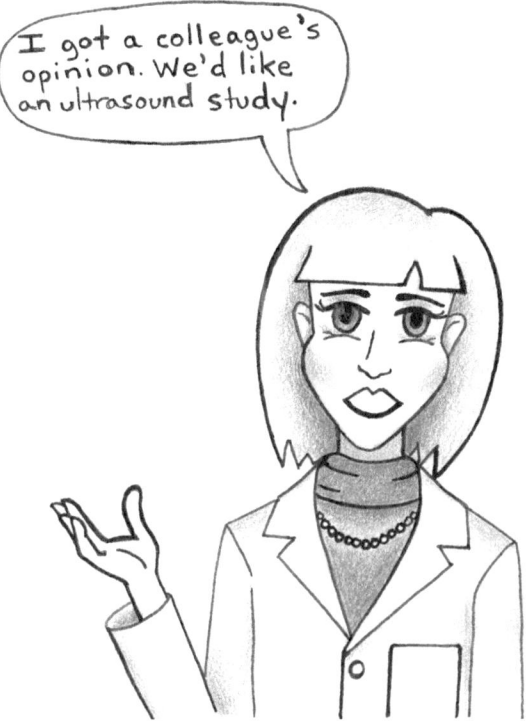

Figure 6: Original image by Pamela Wagar Smith, MD.

Following the third set of images, Julie did not return for a very long time. I sat in the diagnostic waiting room marking each second as it passed. I was keenly aware of how large and bulky the Breast Center robe was on my petite frame, keenly aware of how blank my mind was except for the overwhelming sense of terror that consumed me, keenly aware that there were two other women waiting in that room but that the only thing I could do was turn the pages of a magazine without seeing (much less reading) anything that was on them. (Figure 7)

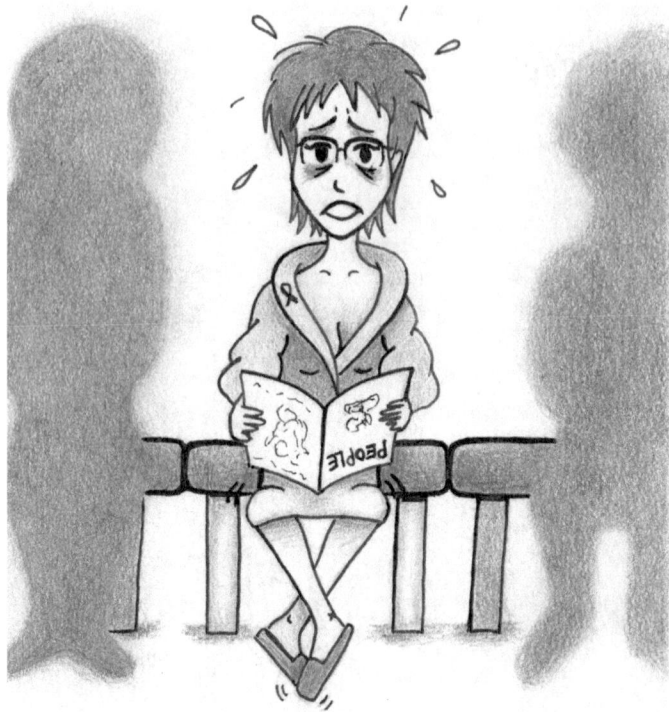

Figure 7: Original image by Pamela Wagar Smith, MD.

In the few flashes of lucidity I had, I kept returning to Marchetto's process, deciding how I would visualize and verbalize my experience in that moment. The only similarity between Marchetto's (page 4) and my sonogram was the look of terror on our faces as the probe rolled over our breasts. In my case, the room was quite dim. For a while, I stared at the ceiling, waiting almost breathlessly (literally holding my breath) for Julie to say everything was okay. Instead, (Figure 8)

Breast Cancer Comics in the Classroom and the Clinic   263

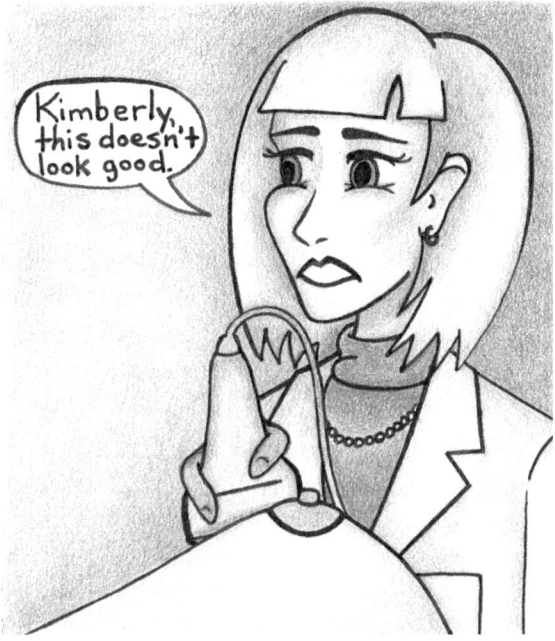

Figure 8: Original image by Pamela Wagar Smith, MD.

Because she was a friend, Julie was able to move things along all in one sitting so that I didn't have to return multiple times for multiple tests. The returning wouldn't have been so bad except that it would have entailed waiting. And waiting for procedures or the results of those procedures is my idea of hell. Just like Marchetto's panels about The Call.

Next came the core needle biopsy, and this is when Marchetto was most fully present in my own medical suite. I felt myself morph into the bug-eyed patient in Marchetto's frame on page 89 and realized that most of what I was hearing was squiggles. (Figure 9) That is, I literally couldn't hear – or recognize – the technical language used by the radiologist and technician; I couldn't make sense of it. I heard only individual words and phrases as they were performing the needle biopsy; and, because I was desperate to exchange my patient status for that of colleague – no doubt to reclaim some semblance of control – I began telling Julie about *Cancer Vixen*. I remember describing this particular panel to her and telling her how the students and I had discussed it. I believe she was glad that I was talking while she was punching out the "biopsied wormy bastards," as Marchetto calls the specimens (89).

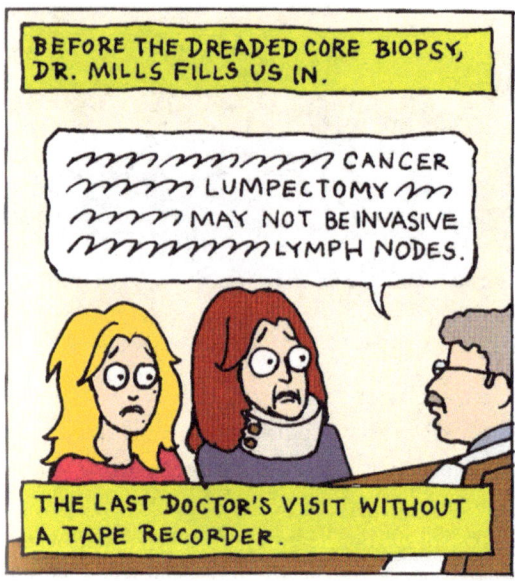

Figure 9: From CANCER VIXEN, by Marisa Acocella Marchetto.

A lot transpired on that winter Friday. Although I didn't have pathology results to confirm my diagnosis, both Julie and another friend who specializes in breast surgery for cancer patients left little room for wishful thinking. People's responses to breast cancer are as individual as their cancers themselves and the treatments prescribed to treat them. I can understand many reasons why women choose not to reveal their diagnosis, but I did not want to hide mine. For one thing, it seemed the perfect teaching/learning moment. In every course I teach, I strive to help students cultivate a real community of trust, openness and vulnerability; usually, it works. This was an opportunity to practice what I preach.

Taking Marchetto Back to Class

Still mostly numb, I went into class on Monday and carried out the activities we had scheduled, including Skyping with two people whose pathographies we would later read. When these interviews were over, I began: "Remember what we were discussing this time last Thursday? Well, last Friday was my annual mammogram, and ...."

I was initially struck by how having read and discussed the breast cancer pathographies made discussing my real-time experience so much easier, which confirmed my longtime suspicion that using pathographies in the clinic would be an excellent tool for doctor-patient communication and patient empowerment. These soon-to-be residents were eager to understand how the experiences conveyed in our texts corresponded to my recent experience. *Cancer Vixen*, in particular, gave them and me excellent points of departure. For instance, whereas Marchetto was not surprised and was seemingly untroubled when her primary care physician asks her about the lump in her breast during an exam (Figure 10), I was acutely overwhelmed, to the point I thought I would pass out on the sonogram table. The students and I returned to Marchetto's depiction of the minute her "world came to an end," and they asked me how I would convey my experience. (Figure 11) In this way, the students and I were essentially co-creating a graphic pathography, whereby tweaking the details – they asking me "Is this the right color?" and "What would you put here?" – clarified issues that would be important for our continued work that semester and, indeed, for me as well, throughout the year of treatment that lay ahead.

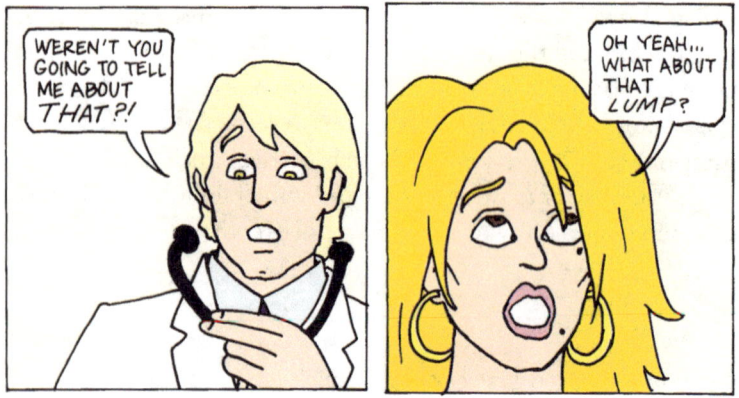

Figure 10: From CANCER VIXEN, by Marisa Acocella Marchetto.

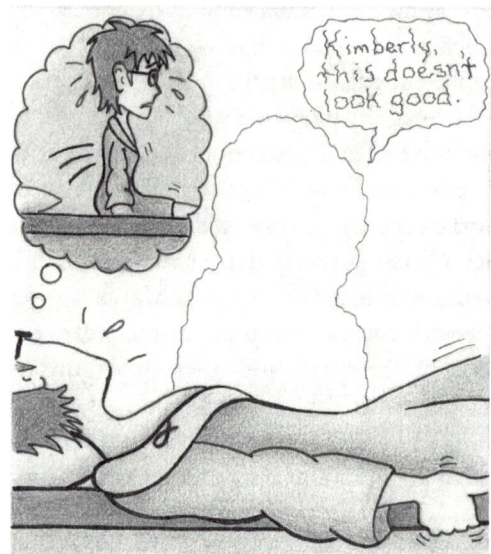

Figure 11: Original image by Pamela Wagar Smith, MD.

A second example illustrates this point. On page 68, Marchetto conveys her panic in a four-panel sequence in which water continues to rise. (Figure 12). Students had earlier identified this sequence as one of the most effective in the book, as it expertly exploits many of the conventions of the comics medium (e.g., the repetition of the image, changing in the fourth panel; the easy integration of the surreal; the effect of the initial framing caption, etc.) "Salt water fish" indicates that this water is her tears, and her avatar's gasping for breath in the final panel indicates that Marchetto is metaphorically drowning in her fear. Using this sequence as a springboard, the students and I explored how my response differed significantly from Marchetto's. After the biopsy, I shakily dressed and met another physician friend of mine, who had come to wait with me for our surgeon friend who would see me after his clinic ended.[1] I cried briefly when I first saw him. But then I got very still and was numb. I was aware of feeling incoherent as I kept circling back to the basic issue: I had breast cancer. The point was that I needed to talk about it – not call everyone close to me to let them know, but just talk until I could get my head around the shock. Unlike Marchetto, I had no outward emotion; my energy was almost entirely internal. Neither did I experience Marchetto's anger (69) or her questioning "Why me?" (71).

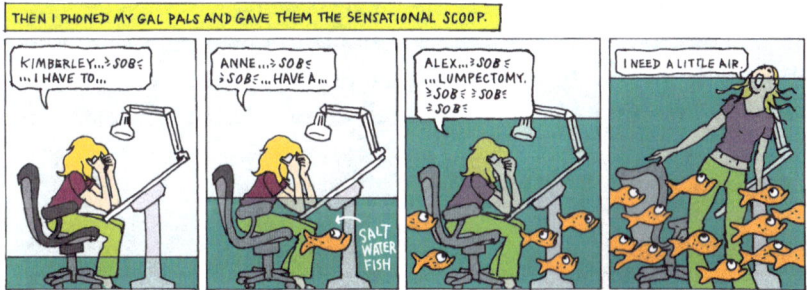

Figure 12:   From CANCER VIXEN, by Marisa Acocella Marchetto.

---

1   Throughout this experience and the treatments that would follow, I was keenly aware of how privileged I was to have excellent medical professionals who were

Talking about these contrasts empowered the students as budding clinicians. I was struck by their professionalism and maturity as the power dynamic in the classroom shifted for the day: I was a vulnerable patient who welcomed any medical information they might have, and they were eager to impart that information in case it might assuage my anxiety about what was yet unknown. Because we had discussed how my experience had differed from Marchetto's, they knew some important information about how best to care for me even as they could not cure me.

This experience created a bond between teacher and students unlike anything I had ever experienced. After that day, except for a couple of very brief updates – for example, confirmation of diagnosis and, later, stage of tumor – our work in the classroom went on in the usual way: I was their professor and they were my students. Marchetto followed me around in my private life, though, providing me a kind of virtual community and, in fact, information that proved to be quite useful.

So many times I saw myself in the midst of the panel on page 83. (Figure 13). Marchetto doesn't even need to finish the sentence she begins in the green text box. The drawing makes her message perfectly clear: Every aspect of life, no matter how pleasant on the outside, is permeated by thoughts and fears of cancer. Cancer preoccupies; it invades every inch of space. Its often unspoken presence is unchecked, haphazardly proliferating, like the erratic cell division that characterizes the disease itself.

---

also personal friends. Although my anxiety was intense, I knew it would have been far worse had I not had insiders who helped me navigate the labyrinthine medical system swiftly and efficiently. I eagerly welcomed this support, yet I also felt somehow guilty, realizing that most patients would not have such advocacy and encouragement. This realization is another reason for my commitment to work with women and men who have been diagnosed with breast cancer, helping them in whatever ways I can.

Breast Cancer Comics in the Classroom and the Clinic 269

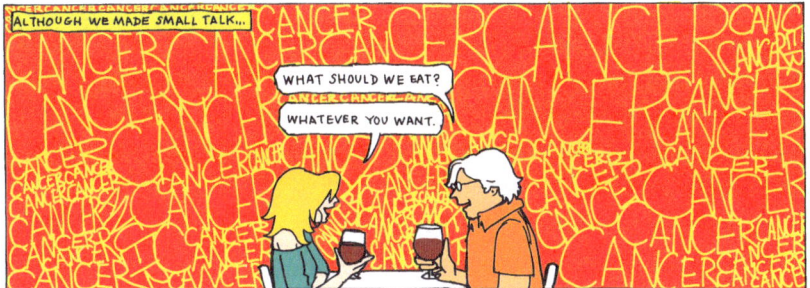

Figure 13: From CANCER VIXEN, by Marisa Acocella Marchetto.

Cancer is a world unto itself, and not even my friends who are physicians had very much to offer me in the way of information about the protocols and procedures specific to oncology. Marchetto did, though. In fact, I am convinced that physicians could use graphic pathographies to empower their patients largely because *Cancer Vixen* helped me in so many concrete ways. I was surprised at just how quickly other people took over when I was diagnosed with breast cancer. Things need to move quickly, and they certainly did for me. Appointments were set up and procedures scheduled. My calendar filled almost instantly. But especially because I was still overwhelmed by this new world I had entered, I needed to slow down so that I could think carefully. I returned to Marchetto to see what, with time and distance as she was creating *Cancer Vixen*, she had considered important enough to include. I mention only three things to illustrate the utility of this comic in the most serious of circumstances.

First, while I probably would have thought of getting a second opinion, I can't be sure, given how fast things were moving. Marchetto certainly convinced me that having a second opinion is simply a smart thing to do, though, especially when she shows how some things she had been told by one physician were factually incorrect. I set up an appointment for a second opinion at a leading cancer institute in a nearby city, which helped me understand the range of options available to me.

Second, working in medical humanities, I am well aware of how important it is for patients to have some means of capturing the information their physicians convey to them. I often advise patients to invite a friend to appointments, as two heads have a better chance remembering details than one, and disagreements over what was said lead to important requests for clarification. I believe it is safe to say that, unless I had read *Cancer Vixen*, I would never have considered taking a digital voice recorder (the equivalent of Marchetto's "tape recorder") to my appointments. Yet that turned out to be absolutely critical as I was trying to decide between two courses of chemotherapy suggested for my particular kind of cancer; I was able to listen to highly technical information as many times as I needed in order to comprehend my options and thereby act autonomously. On a more basic level, being able to replay fundamental information about how tumors are typed and staged, in what circumstances chemotherapy is and is not recommended, how oncotypes are determined, etc., facilitated discussions with family and friends. I returned again and again to listen to what various physicians had explained to me, which helped me feel knowledgeable enough to ask intelligent questions that were crucial to my care.

I chose not to re-read *Cancer Vixen* before beginning chemotherapy because I know that every person's experience is unique and I didn't want to psych myself out by projecting any particular reaction. After completing chemo, however, it was helpful to return to the comic simply to compare and contrast Marchetto's experiences with my own. For example, we both experienced the pain of Neulasta injections to boost white cells, and we both feared extravasation (I actually experienced it) and subsequent nerve damage (which I did not experience). However, while Marchetto became preoccupied with gaining weight and losing hair, those concerns seemed utterly inconsequential to me. She continued to work out regularly and maintain a vibrant social life, but I could manage neither. Perhaps most interesting was to look at our different chemo cocktails and their respective side effects, long- and short-term: The chemo she had chosen was the one I had rejected. This process provided a powerful sense of community for someone who didn't want to join a support group for fear of collective fear-mongering. Ultimately, though only in retrospect, it was helpful to see how my body's terribly unfamiliar responses were actually quite familiar to someone else.

My positive experience with *Cancer Vixen*, both professional and personal, has convinced me that graphic pathographies are excellent resources not only for teaching factual material but also for instilling in others – and reminding ourselves of – the importance of compassion and presence with one another, breast cancer or not.

Bibliography

Marchetto, Marisa Acocella. *Cancer Vixen: A True Story*. New York: Alfred A. Knopf, 2006. Smith, Pamela Wagar. Original drawings.

RACHEL O'CONNOR

A Curator's Interpretation of *Edges of Light*

The photographic and poetic collaboration *Edges of Light: Images of Breast Transformation*, by Wendy Palmer and Kimberly Myers, is a deeply personal look into Myers' journey through breast cancer. However, the series dives deeper than mere biography. It is a reminder of the human spirit's tenacity, a *memento mori* of sorts that is also simultaneously a call to life, and a shining example of art's power to aid in empathy, humility and inspiration.

Edges of Light is a narrative, one that is readily followed through Palmer's nuanced photographs. The series begins with "Lines," a tight close-up of Myers' face, cropped just above her eyebrow, along the bridge of her nose and below her lower lip. The lines on her face speak of a person who smiles often and reads for long hours, and the intimacy of the photograph can be seen as a metaphor for the body of work as a whole. This is Myers' invitation to the viewer to join her in a story: "Lines / on my face / of the song I hear in my head / of the poems I want to write / to you / about / this." What is "this," though? The accompanying artists' statement reveals that Myers had already been diagnosed with Stage 1 invasive ductal carcinoma at the time the photographs were taken, even though there is no physical indication of cancer this early in the work. The viewer would have no idea that Myers is already sick. By allowing the viewer to see the details of how physically striking Myers is in the first photograph of the series, Palmer challenges the assumption that sick people – especially those with breast cancer – look macerated, while only healthy individuals are physically attractive and vibrant. In fact, the viewer is not even visually tipped off to the looming presence of cancer until "Skew," the fourth photograph, where a faint yellowish-green bruise appears around the curve of Myers' right breast. Even with this visible injury, Myers' body looks fit and strong.

In the poem "Recognition," paired with the second photograph of the series, Myers writes, "I sense your coming / unsure of your shape / or the sharpness of your teeth. // You can be sure of mine." This is a warning sent to the cluster of traitorous cells within her body. Myers is not only physically strong, as the viewer sees in the accompanying image of toned arms and stomach; she is also strong-*willed*. The will to live is a sacred act. It hides somewhere within each of our bodies and often seems to surface with noticeable force only when we are faced with our own mortality. In these moments we must make a choice: to live or to die. If the choice is to live, then we must be present and intentional with our bodies and with our minds.

The tone of the series quickly shifts with "Bānhūs," the sixth pairing. Here we see only Myers' nude torso, ribs undulating out under her skin and lungs full of freshly inhaled oxygen. Again, the bruise on her right breast appears, this time more visible than before. Life and death are displayed in close proximity to one another. "Bānhūs" is an Anglo-Saxon kenning (a compound metaphor that is often visually vivid and serves as a synonym for a simple noun) that signifies "body" – literally "the bonehouse": "Bones(that)house / *soul*, / the me of me. // So small / these bones. / So small / the me / they house," as she writes. The term "bone house" also conjures an image of a building that holds the remains of the dead. The woman who was once sure of her ferocious bite is now questioning the size of her teeth – and her spirit. In this moment Myers reveals her fragility. The bravado seen in the last line of "Recognition" was an energetic battle cry, but self-confidence in the face of danger is not the full picture. Wariness and fear are inherent in any act of courage, and Myers is brave enough to be honest, vulnerable and human. This is where the power of *Edges of the Light* resides.

As one might expect, an element of existential reflection runs throughout the series. "Epiphany," which immediately follows "Bānhūs," is a black-and-white aerial view of Myers from behind as she lies prostrate on the floor. Her head is to the ground, arms and hands reached out in front of her with fingers widely spread as if in supplication. Both the position of Myers' body and the monochromatic tonality of the photograph speak to

Myers' surrender; she writes, "Through the dark night / St. John prayed on / understanding / the prayer / changed / him." It is obvious that Myers has realized that gripping tightly onto fear will not serve her. She cannot control the uncontrollable; and though diagnosed with cancer, she must find a way to keep living, allowing herself to be changed. This resolution is what we find in the pairings entitled "Resolute" and "Choice." These photographs and their accompanying poems specifically exemplify the freedom that comes from letting go of the uncontrollable. In "Resolute" her challenging gaze peers directly out to receive the viewer's eyes. Despite this contact, Myers appears to be looking *through* the viewer, focused only on her mission to continue living a full life. "*Let's Roll*," she writes, a spunky albeit serious statement.

Sobering as a journey with breast cancer can be, Palmer captures moments of levity and playfulness. "Excognito" reveals Myers in a long blond wig, taking her brother's advice to "Have fun with it, Sis!" and experimenting with a new look when she has lost her brunette hair after the first chemotherapy infusion. Following reconstructive surgery, she and her husband share a fun "Secret" during a moment of flirtation: "Catching my eye / as I slip by / in red lace / you arch / a brow / and wink: // 'I'd never know / if I didn't know,'" he says.

The back-and-forth between color and black-and-white; the variation of closely cropped views, meditative full-body poses, and straightforward portraiture; and the sometimes riddle-like brevity of the verbal reflections weave a tapestry of various emotions as the viewer follows Myers through chemotherapy, a double mastectomy, breast reconstruction surgery and recovery. Palmer's photographs and Myers' poems are not only of a woman living through breast cancer and all of the emotions that come with that diagnosis. They are of a human being, living through the unpredictability of life and revealing what each one of us feels in our "dark night of the soul" moments. The truth is, any of us can get sick. While our bodies are amazingly complex and high-functioning biological machines, they are also fragile. Bones break. Organs fail. Cells mutate. Masses grow. The body degenerates. Though it is at best an unpleasant thought, this rendering of truth nevertheless has its own raw beauty. *Edges of Light* confronts the viewer with her or his own mortality and thereby poses the question, "How would you face the uncontrollable?" But the series also reminds us of our own ability to be courageous, our resilience. In the end, perhaps illness is not so much a reminder of death as it is a reminder that we are still alive.

KIMBERLY R. MYERS AND WENDY PALMER

Edges of Light: Images of Breast Transformation

Artists' Statement

On an ordinary Friday afternoon in January 2012, a gifted and intuitive radiologist, Dr. Julie Mack, told me she'd just found a mass deep within my right breast, a tumor that would later be diagnosed as Stage 1 invasive ductal carcinoma. Like so many other women who've been diagnosed with breast cancer, I felt my world collapse around me.

Somehow amidst the numbness and confusion of the week between that discovery and a partial mastectomy, I realized that I would want to remember how I had looked before surgery. A friend suggested photographs by a professional photographer, and that's when I met Wendy Palmer. Our unscripted, unposed photo shoot resulted in hundreds of photographs that were far more than mere documentary; they were pieces of art in their own right – masterful in line and composition, alive with color and light, thanks to Wendy's talent and vision. Surprised by the range and nuance of emotion conveyed in the photos, Wendy and I decided to document the subsequent stages of my journey through treatment and recovery.

Three surgeries, four rounds of chemotherapy and a couple of cosmetic procedures later, my prognosis is good. "They caught it early," as we say: a gift indeed. Going through the various phases of diagnosis, decisions and treatments, one thing became increasingly clear to me: I would do whatever I could, professionally and personally, to help other women have a sense of what to expect – and to encourage them – on their own journeys with breast disease. This project is a major part of the commitment I have made.

Each of the photographs you find here is paired with an imagist poem, my reflection on the visual image itself and what I was experiencing when it was created.

Kimberly

During our initial photo shoot, all thought evaporated and the process was instinctive – for Kimberly and for me. It was the first time we met, but somehow we were catapulted into a swirl of movement and dance, poignant with the knowledge of Kimberly's upcoming surgery. We were locked in the moment of light and shadow, embracing and letting go. Three hours evaporated.

Photography is a means of telling a story through image, and so it happened with these.

Photos that were originally meant only to remind one woman of her story propelled us onward to further photographic sessions and much discussion about what it means to live. Our hope is that these images and words will empower women facing a similar situation to see edges of light along the way.

Wendy

Lines

on my face
of the song I hear in my head
of the poems I want to write
to you
about
this

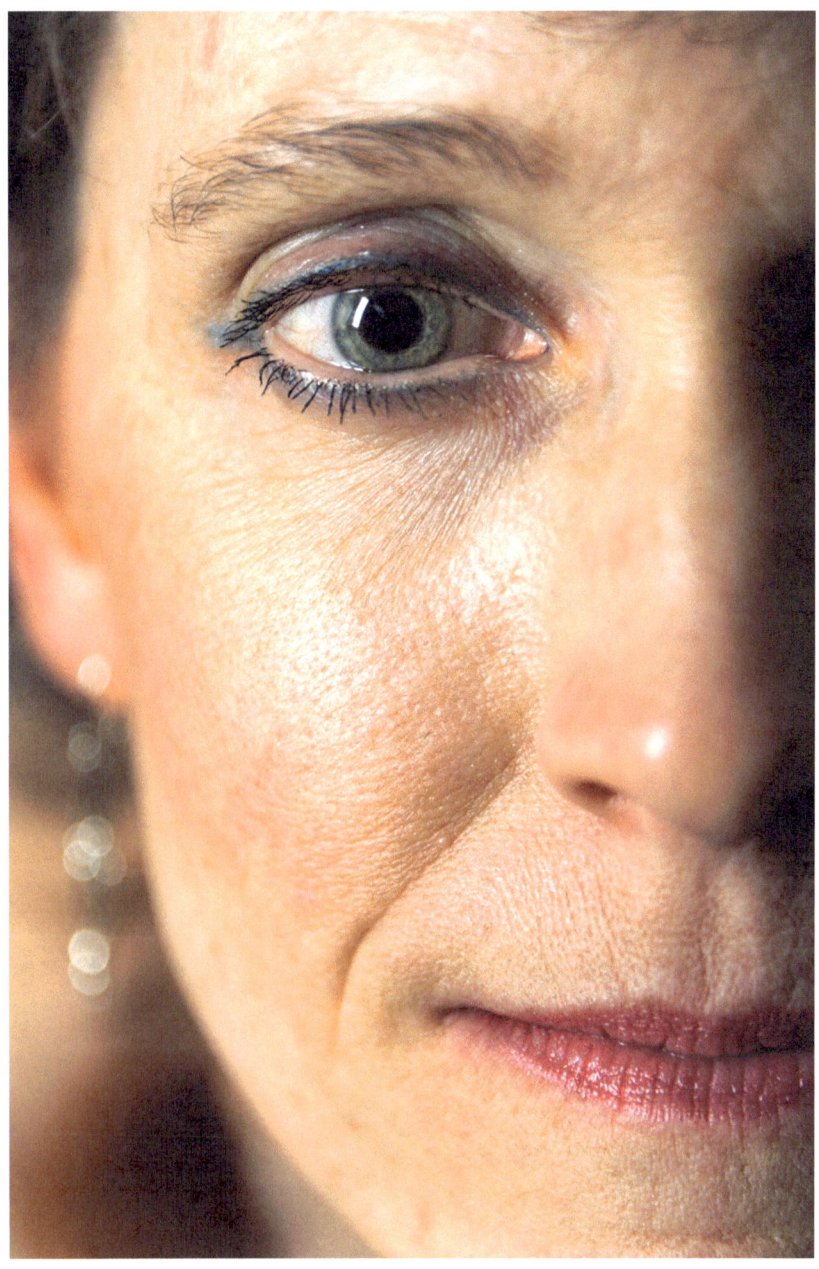

Recognition

I sense your coming
unsure of your shape
or the sharpness of your teeth.

You can be sure of mine.

Edges of Light: Images of Breast Transformation

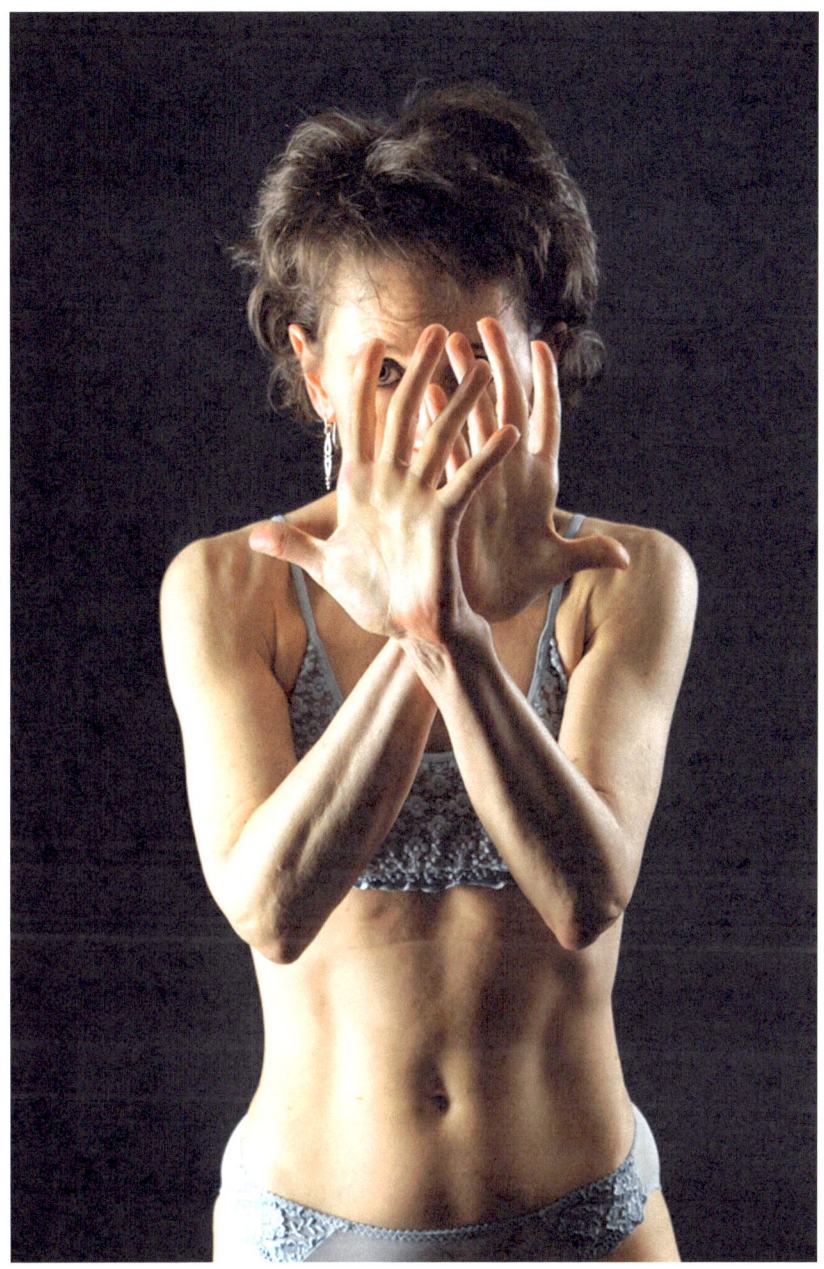

Holding

No enemy
that has betrayed me,
my body is a hurt thing
that wants sanctuary.

And so I gather all of me together.
Holding while there's still time.

Edges of Light: Images of Breast Transformation

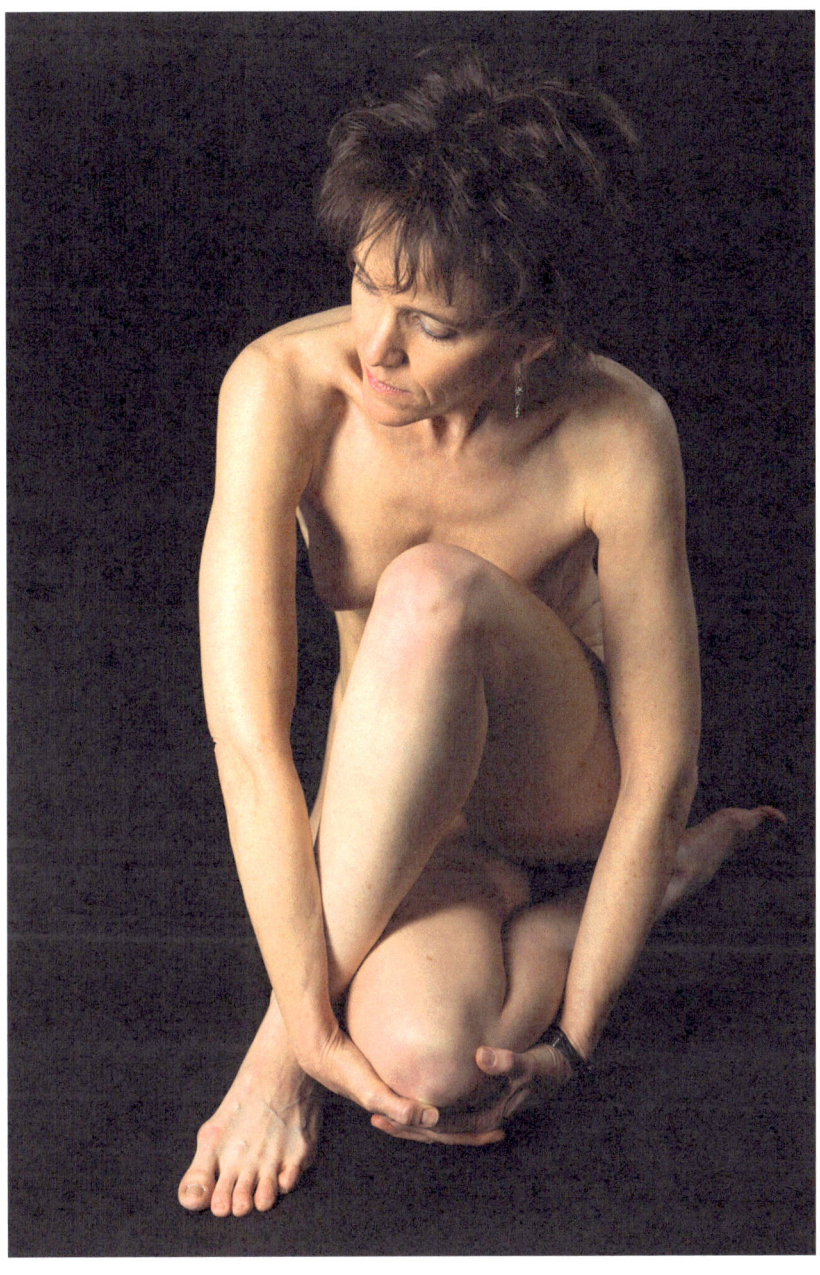

Skew

Emily Dickinson knew to
Tell all the truth but
tell it slant ...
    for
the Truth must
dazzle gradually
or every man be blind

This is truth.

Edges of Light: Images of Breast Transformation

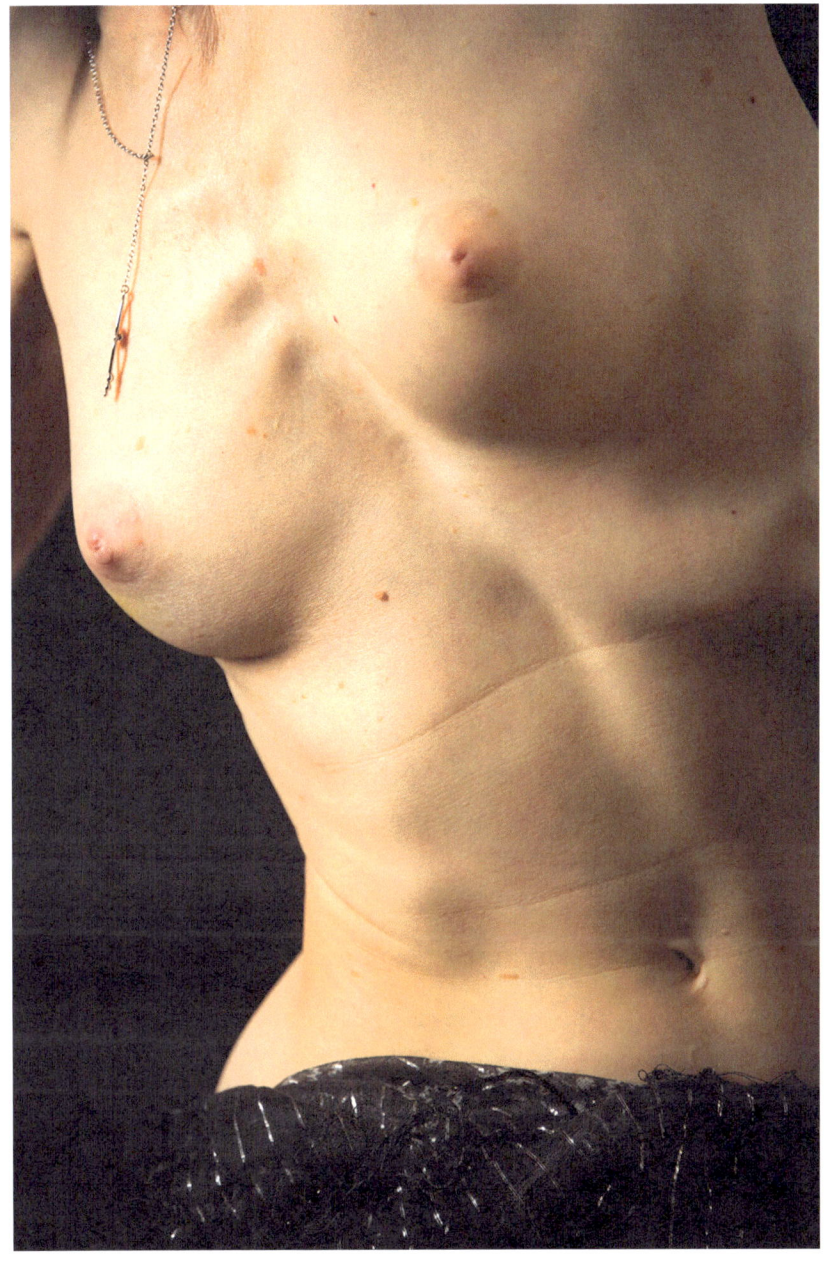

Wings

Stieglitz loved O'Keeffe
's hands into art
fingers feathered over
ample-beauti
full breasts
he caressed in the dark

In the wasteland
of scattered skulls
carrion pick my wings bare
breasts lighter than air

simply not there

Edges of Light: Images of Breast Transformation 289

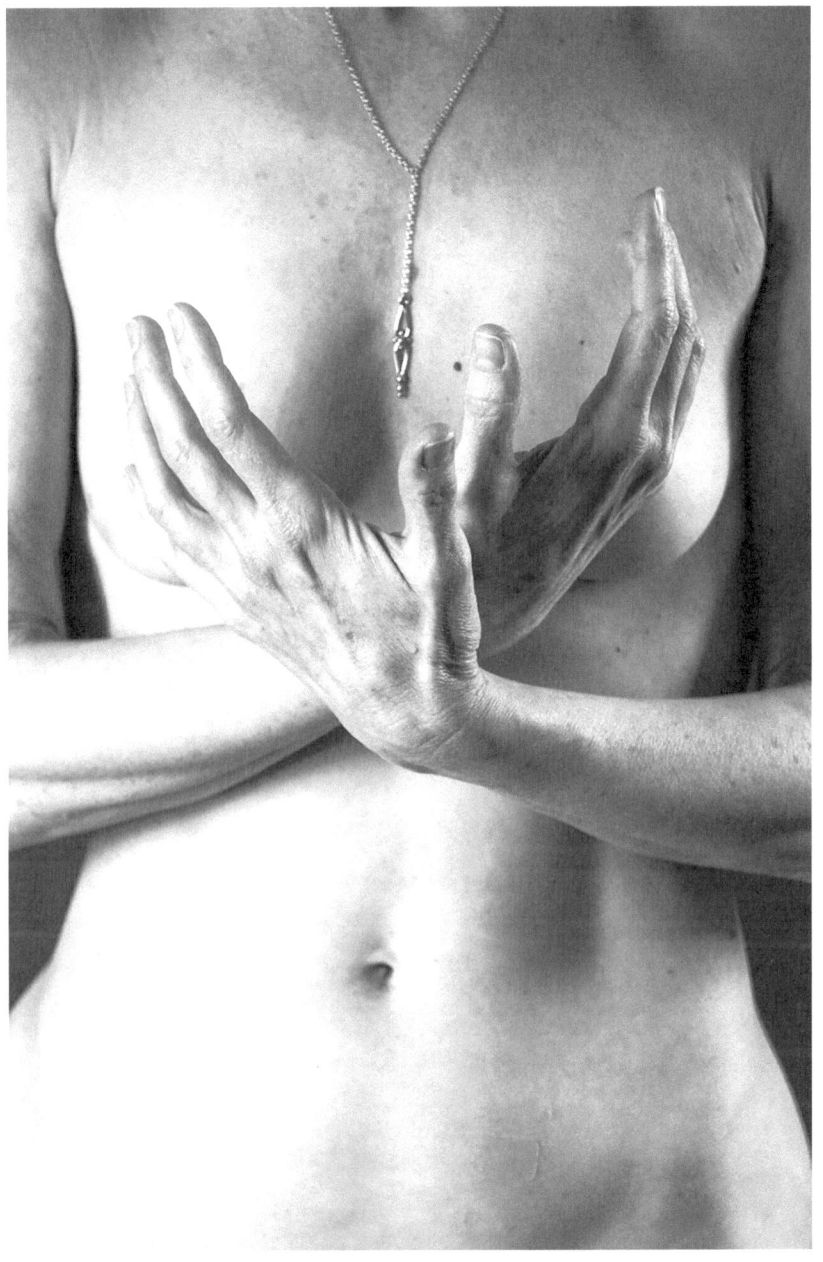

Bānhūs

"Bone-house"
the Anglo-Saxons
called it,
kenning for
body.

Bones(that)house
soul,
the me of me.

So small
these bones.
So small
the me
they house.

Edges of Light: Images of Breast Transformation 291

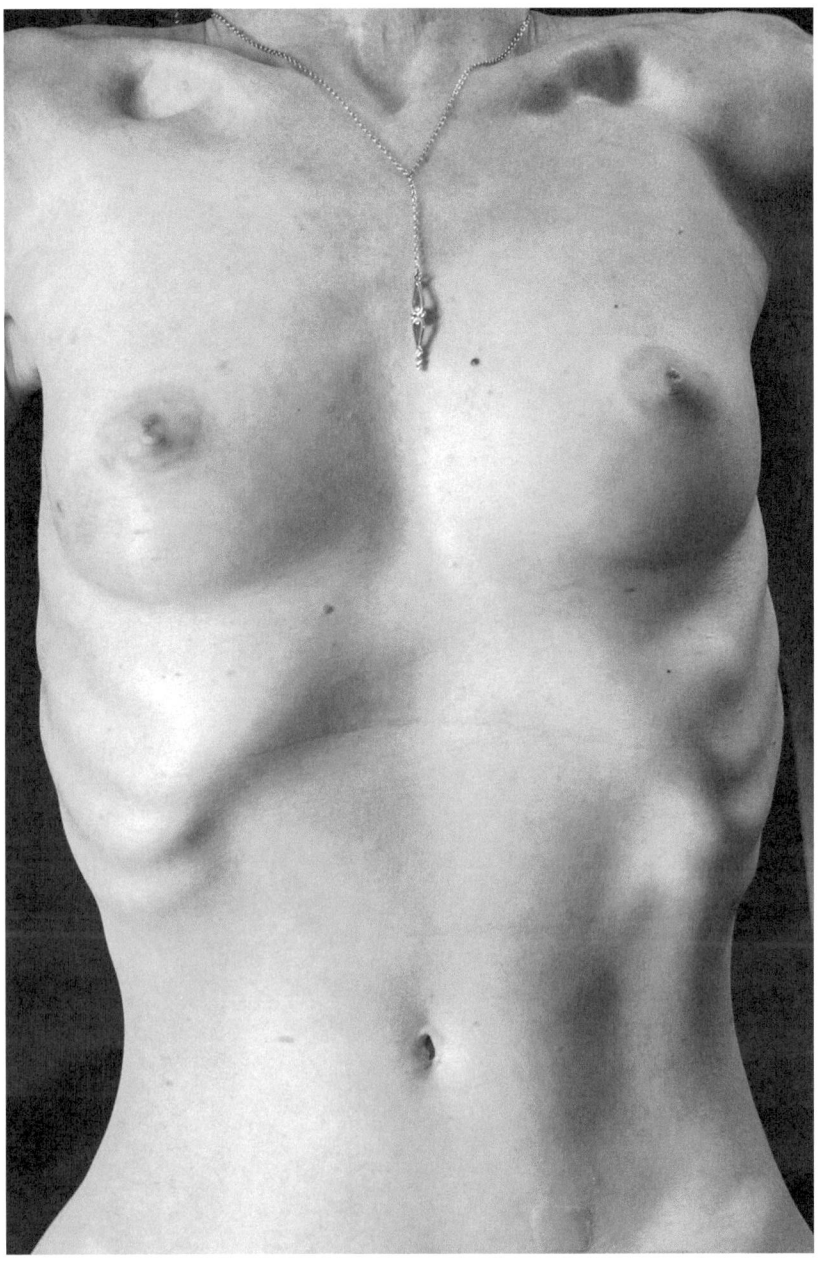

Epiphany

Through the dark night
St. John prayed on
understanding
the prayer
changed

him.

Edges of Light: Images of Breast Transformation

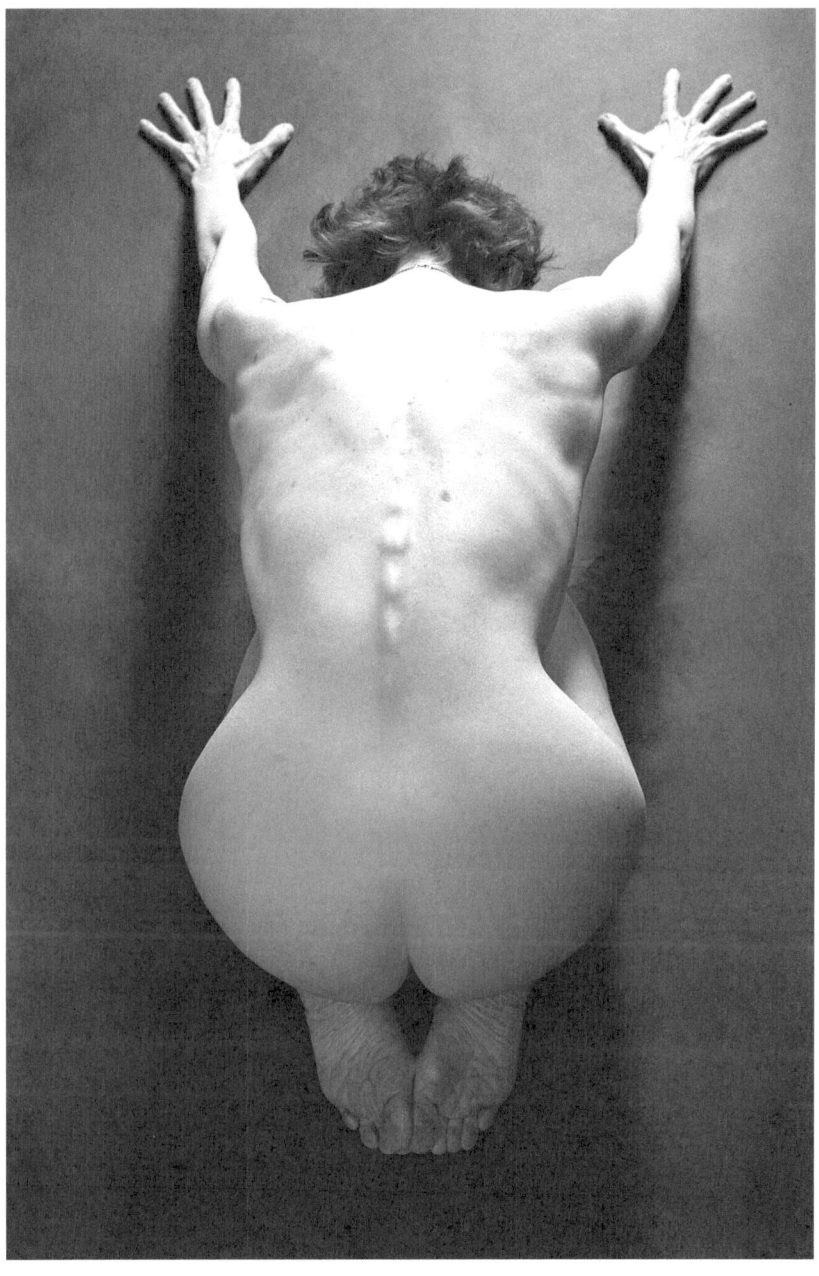

Nothing

*is worth more
than this day.*

I wonder
if Goethe too
feared something
he couldn't see.
So I send for it, a
talisman
to remind me
every time
I feel the ticking

And now
bruised and waiting
at six o'clock on
a winter Tuesday
there's
    still
      nothing
worth more
than this day.

Edges of Light: Images of Breast Transformation 295

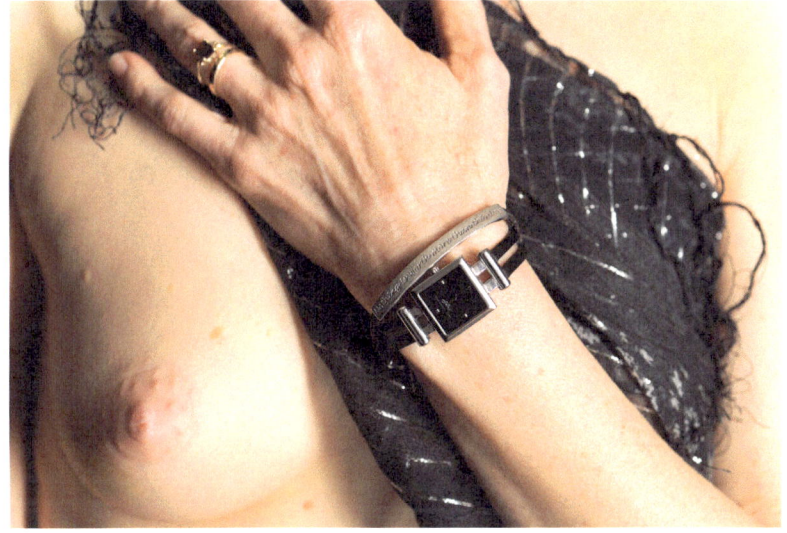

Fetal

Ribs & vertebrae
knuckles of the flesh

protection
in a
quietly furled
fist

Edges of Light: Images of Breast Transformation 297

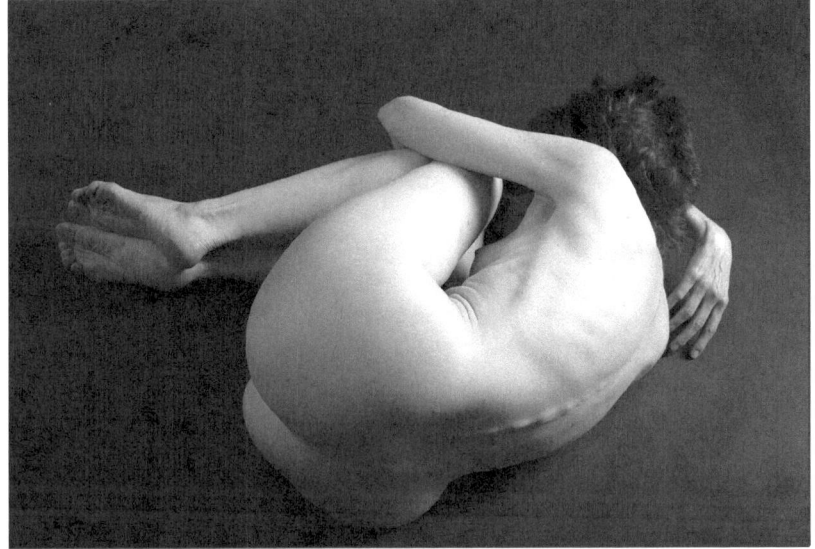

Resolute

Let's roll.

Edges of Light: Images of Breast Transformation

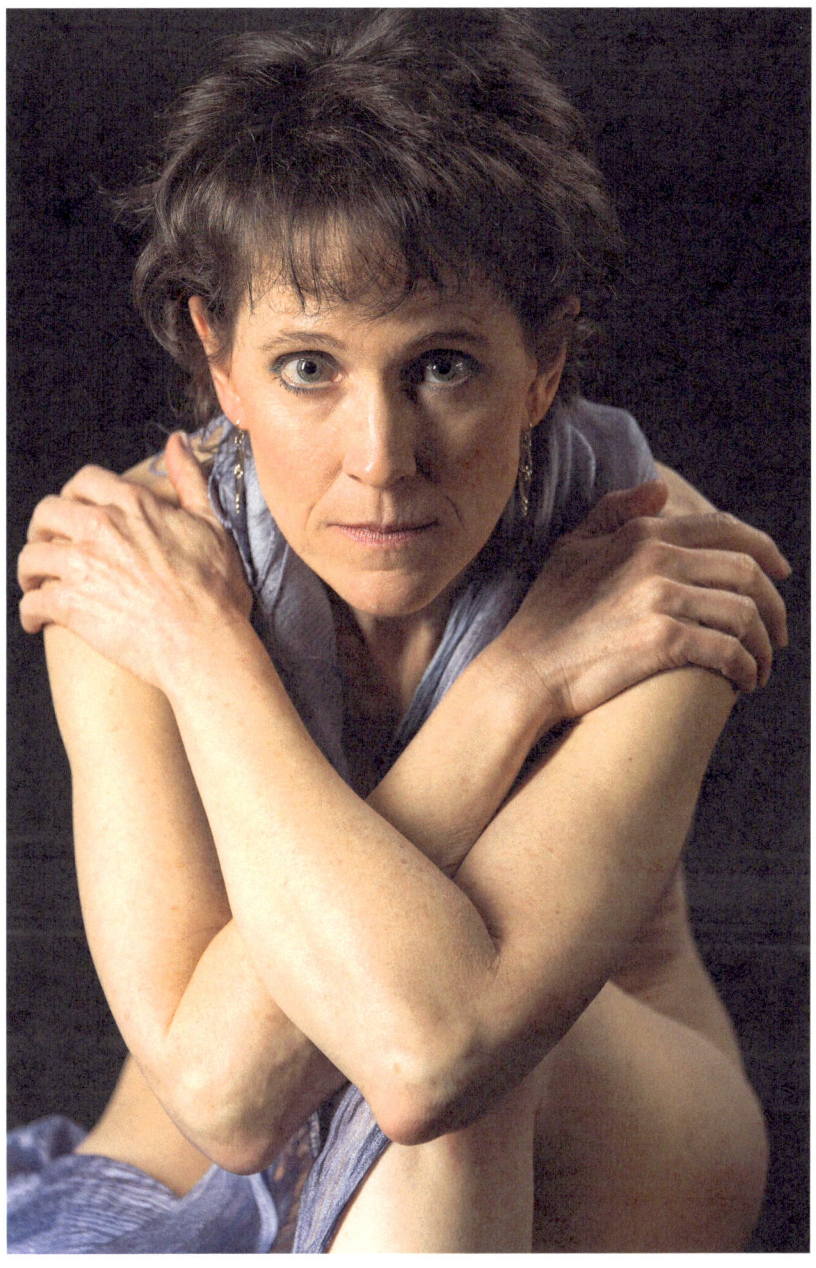

Ceremony

Those midnights
of shoji and tea
we knew
veils falling through
summer air
and starlight.
You loosed
the chignon, freed
my hair to tumble
along our pillow.

This morning
it falls too.

Edges of Light: Images of Breast Transformation

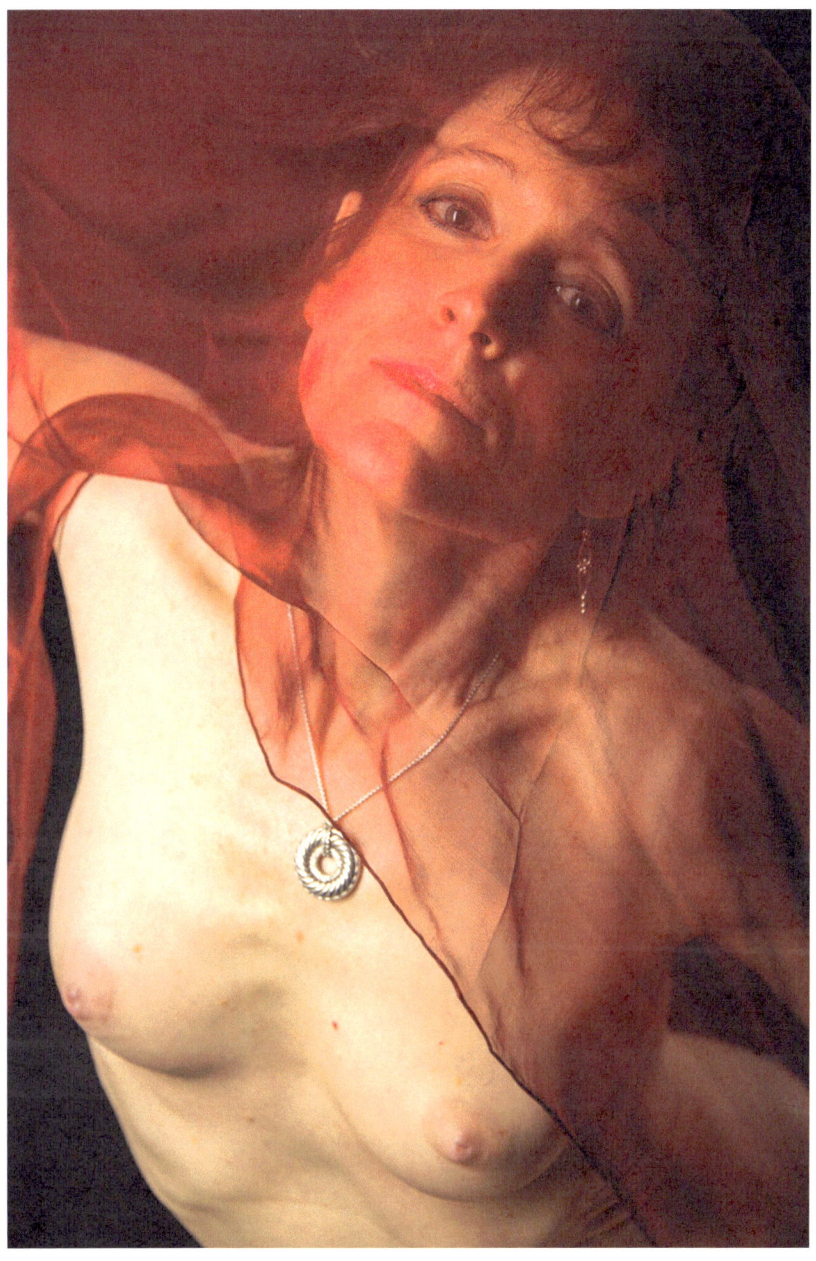

Edges of Light: Images of Breast Transformation 303

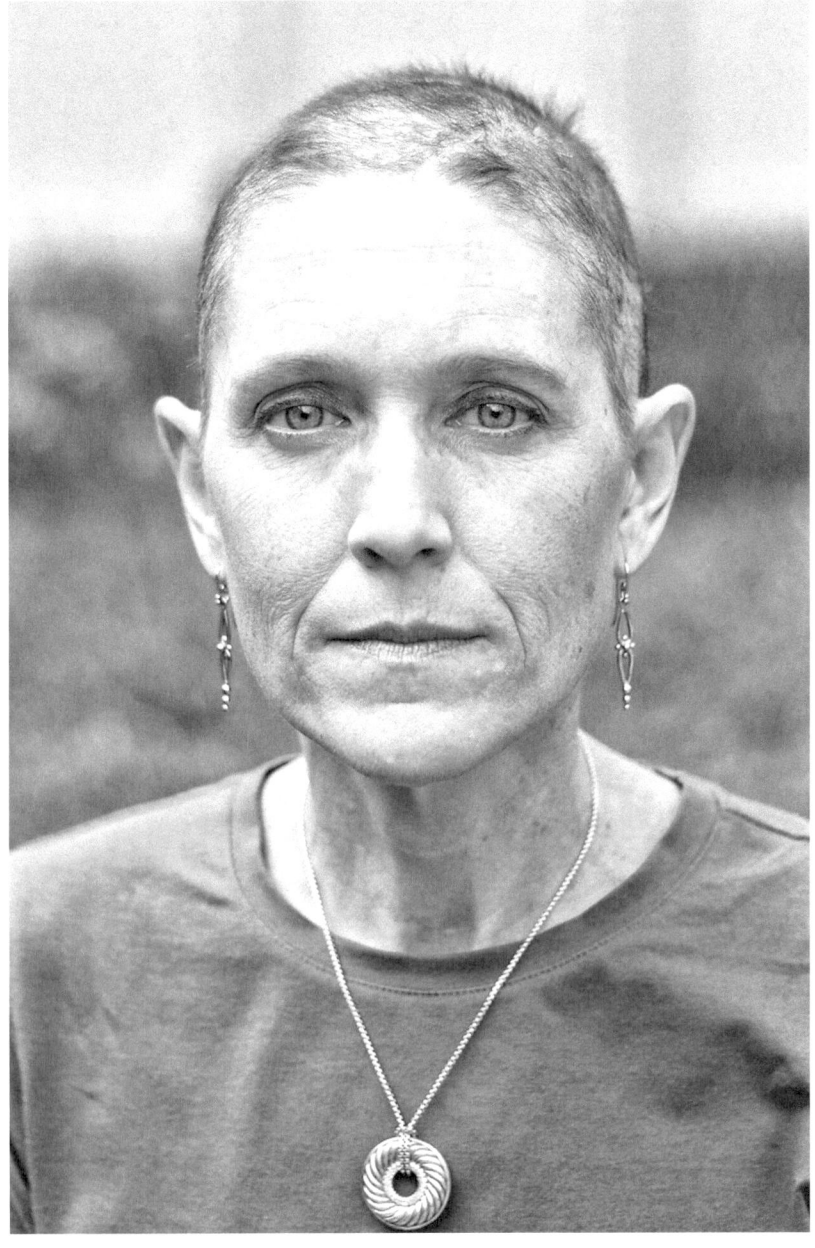

Choice

You decided
the struggle wasn't
worth it.

A shot in the dark.

I'm glad I stayed.

The violets are so
gentle
this spring.

Edges of Light: Images of Breast Transformation

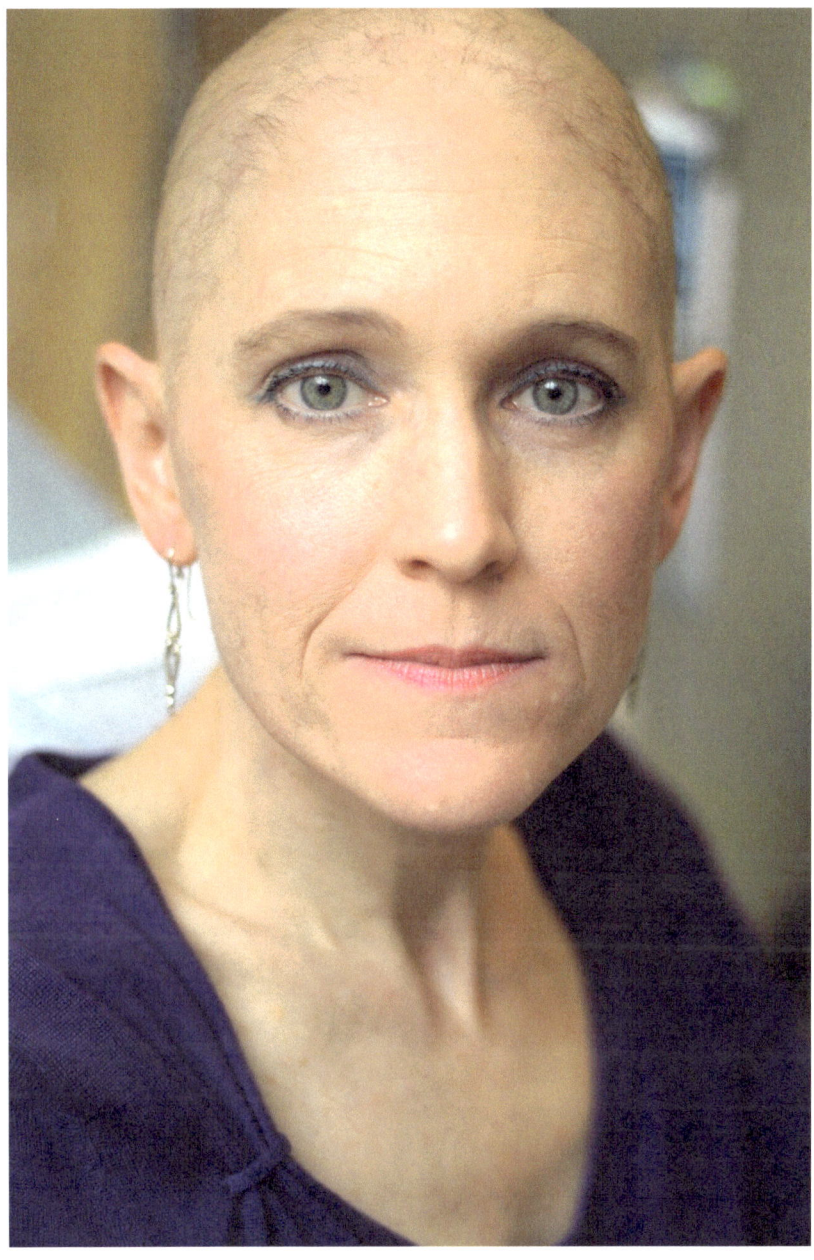

Excognito

Driving up outside the wig shop
I check my phone: brother,
uncommonly, calling.

"Have fun with it, sis!" he says.

I did.

Edges of Light: Images of Breast Transformation

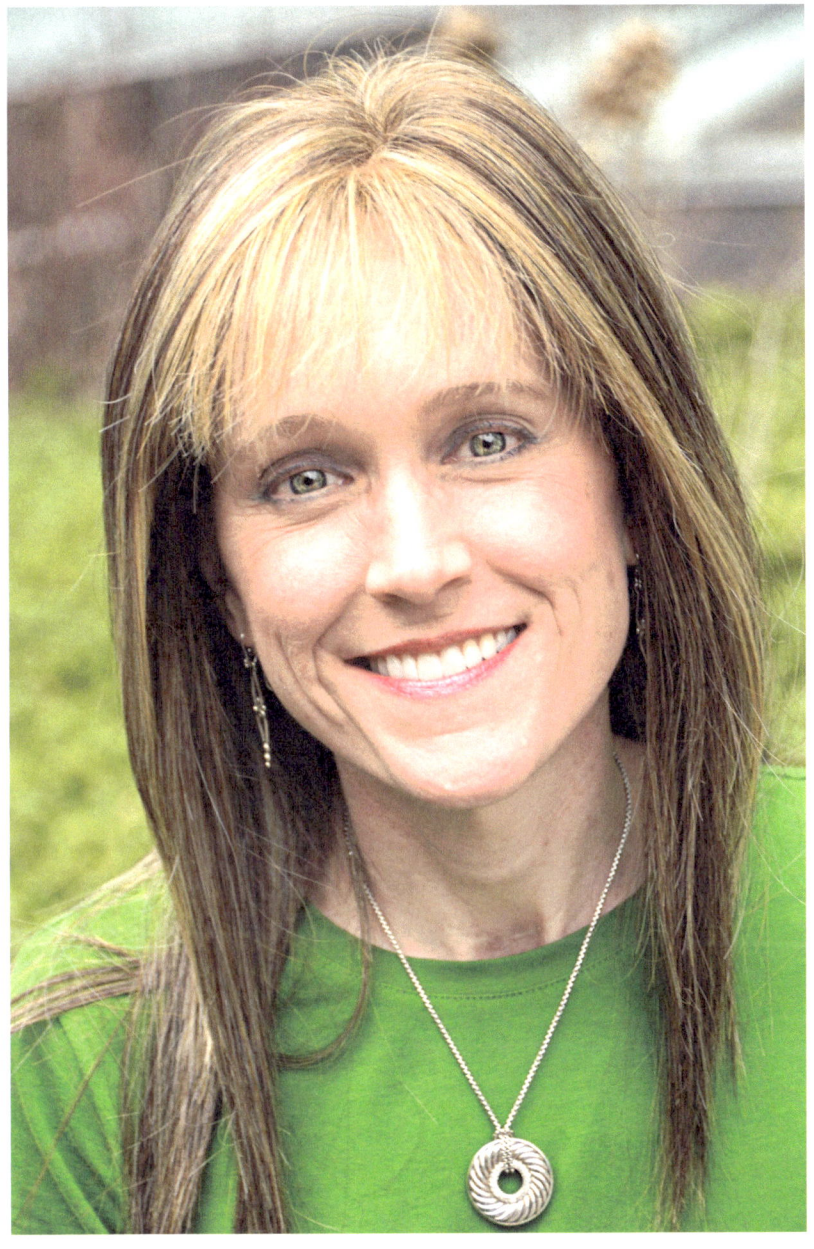

Metamorphosis

After the body blow
tongue cut out
at the root
Philomela lay
dumbstruck
   stunned
    .
     .
      .
   transmuting
    .
     .
    .
  into
nightingale
filling barren spaces
with inviolable song

Edges of Light: Images of Breast Transformation

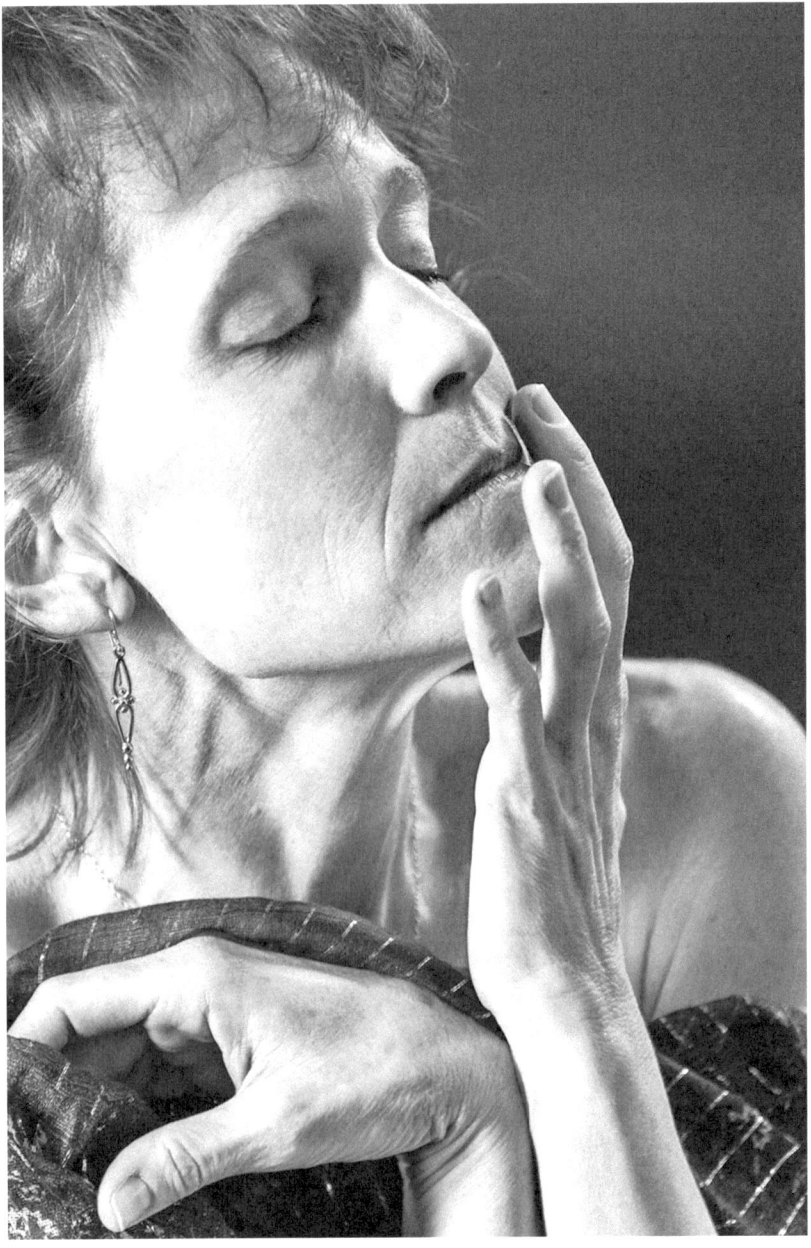

Skindraft

flesh
in
progress

Edges of Light: Images of Breast Transformation

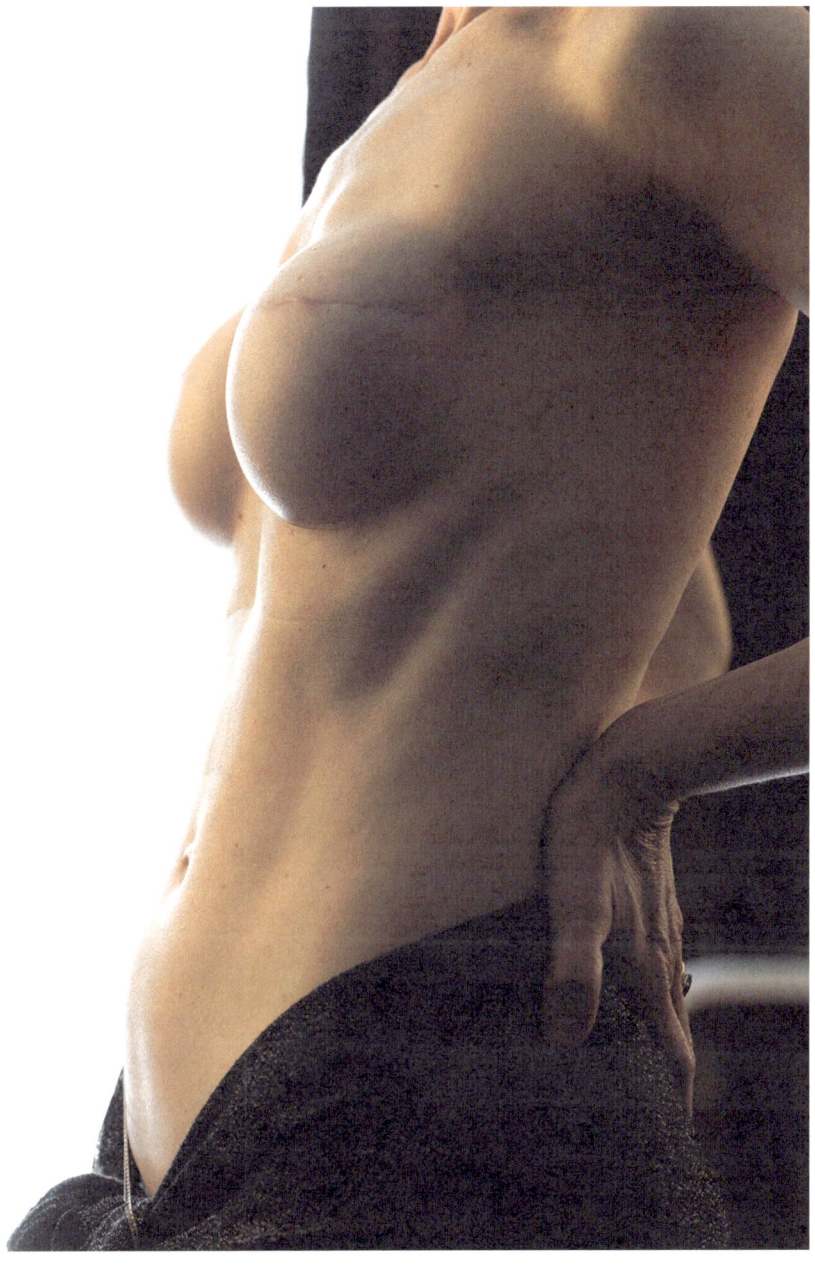

Archimedes

Planes & angles:
the geometry of hope.

Edges of Light: Images of Breast Transformation 313

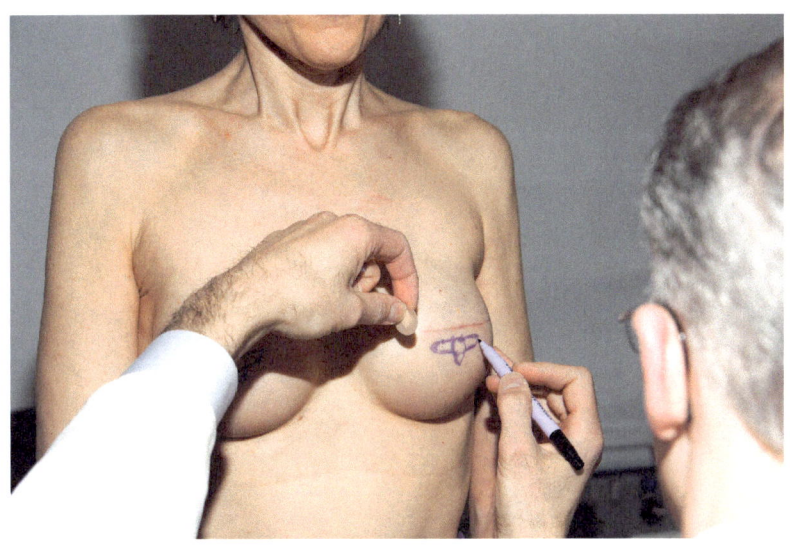

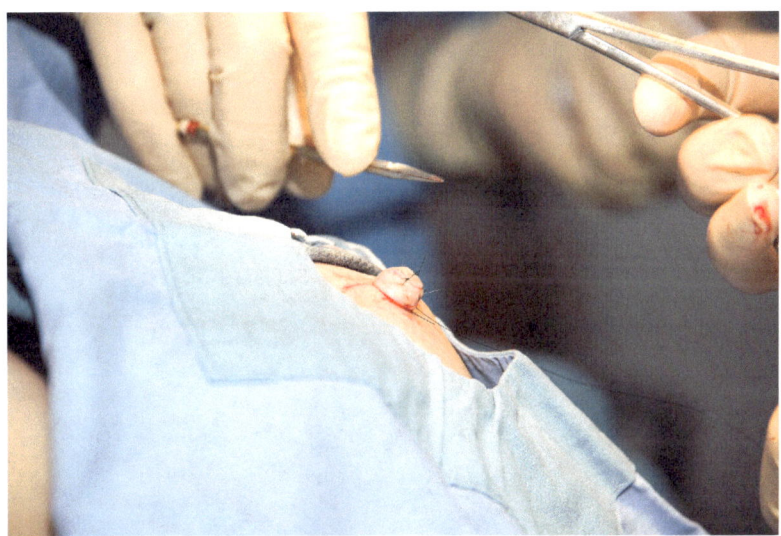

Marked

Cancer comes
with steely tips
sharp edges by the dozens:
    blood draws
    chemo infusions
    anesthesia IVs
    surgical scalpels.
Today: tattoo
needles inscribing
me one of the tribe
no one wants to join.

Through tender bodies, strong selves
cancer cuts.

Edges of Light: Images of Breast Transformation 315

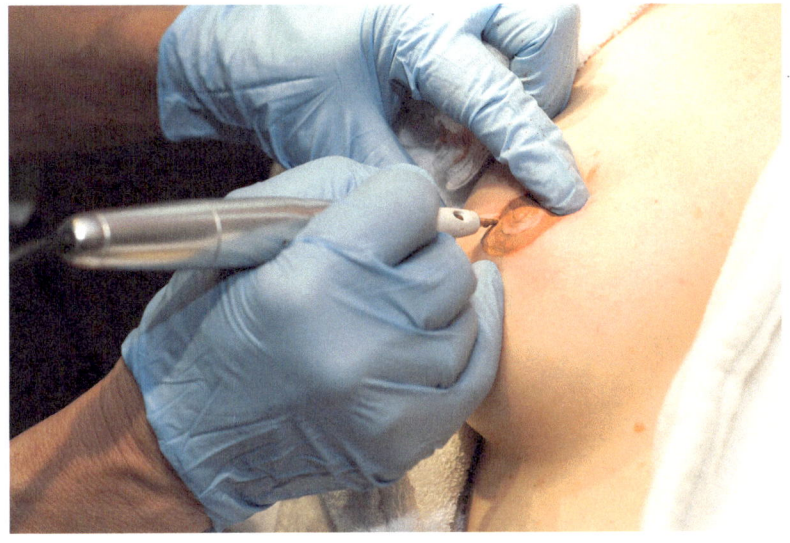

Secret

Catching my eye
as I slip by
in red lace
you arch
a brow
and
wink:

"I'd never know
if I didn't know."

Edges of Light: Images of Breast Transformation 317

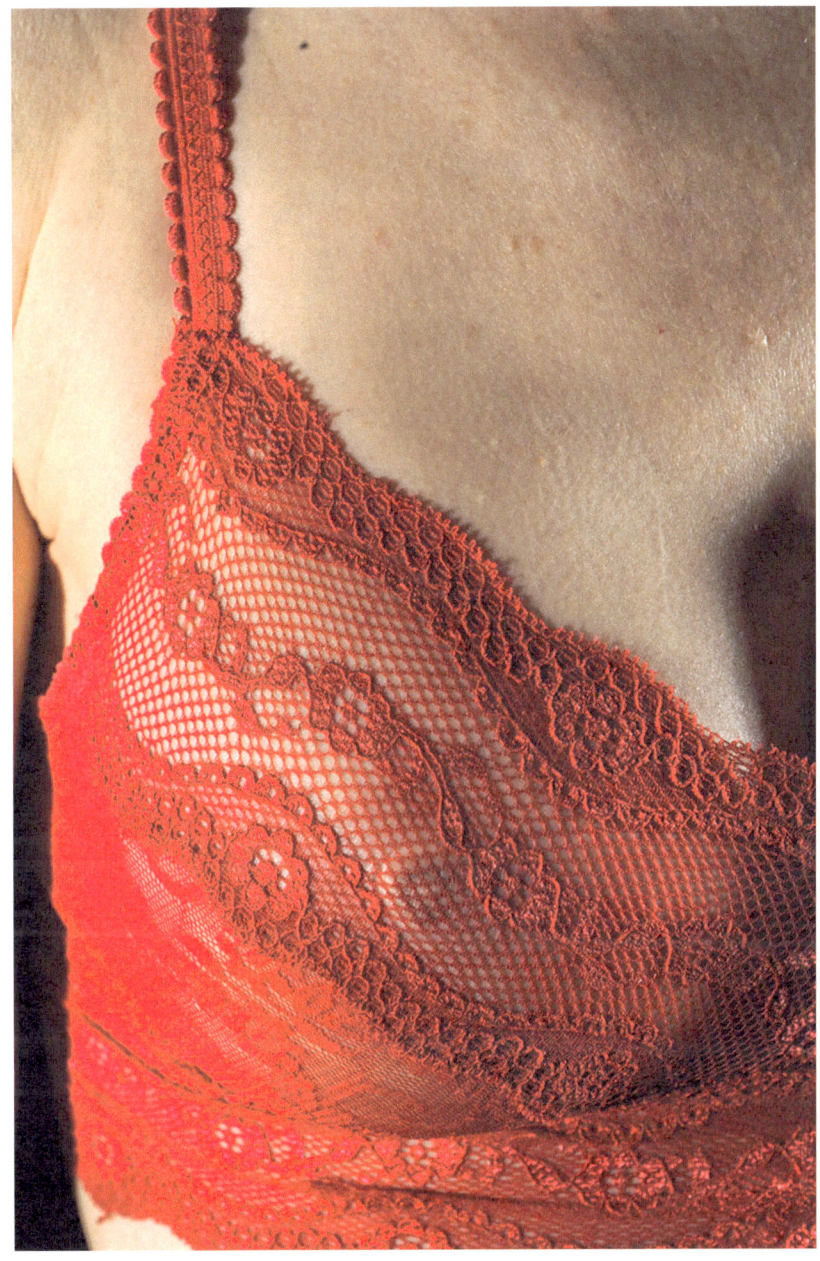

Light

Weight of the world
off my shoulders,
sheer joy
to lift
   (only)
these.

Edges of Light: Images of Breast Transformation

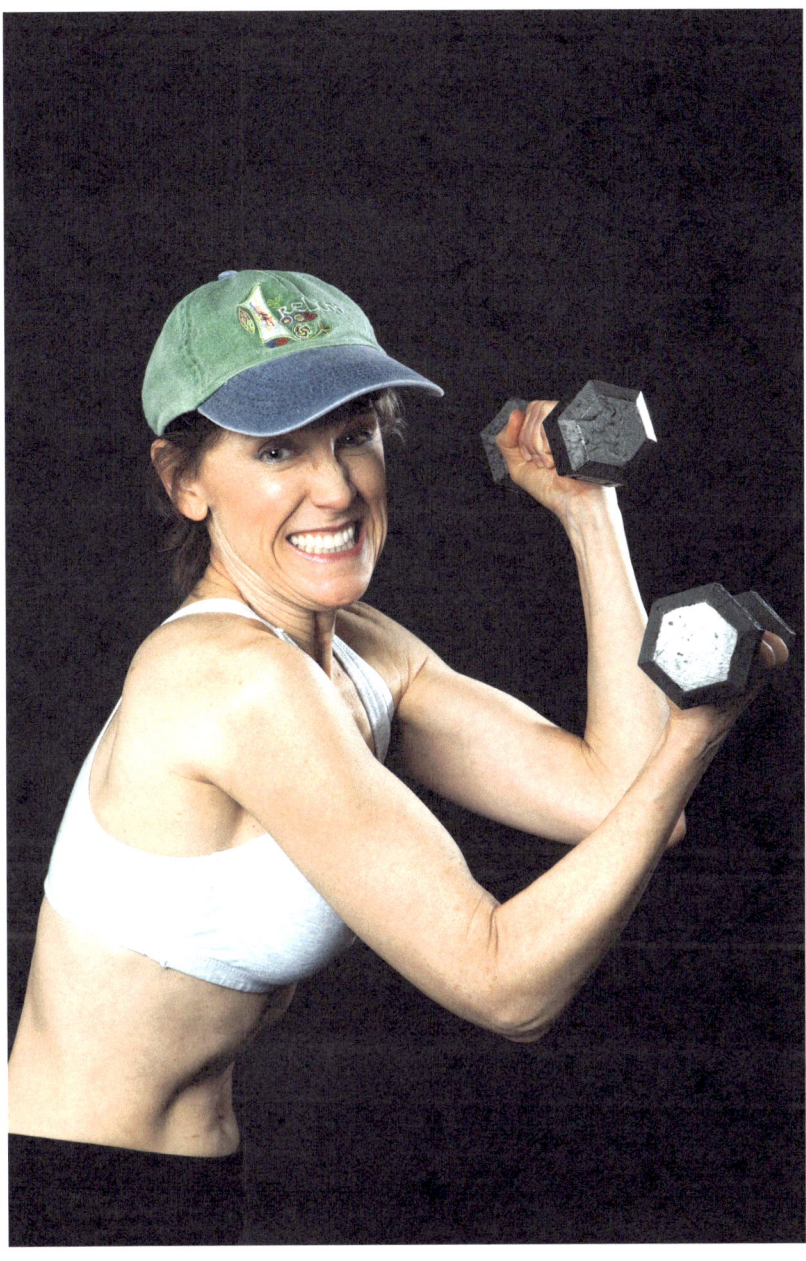

Vermont

in the fall:
a dream since I was twenty.

If not now, when?

Through
cool vermillion and
burnished gold
to the little shop
on Church Street
where I find
jewels like water
shining like stars
in the night sky.

Edges of Light: Images of Breast Transformation

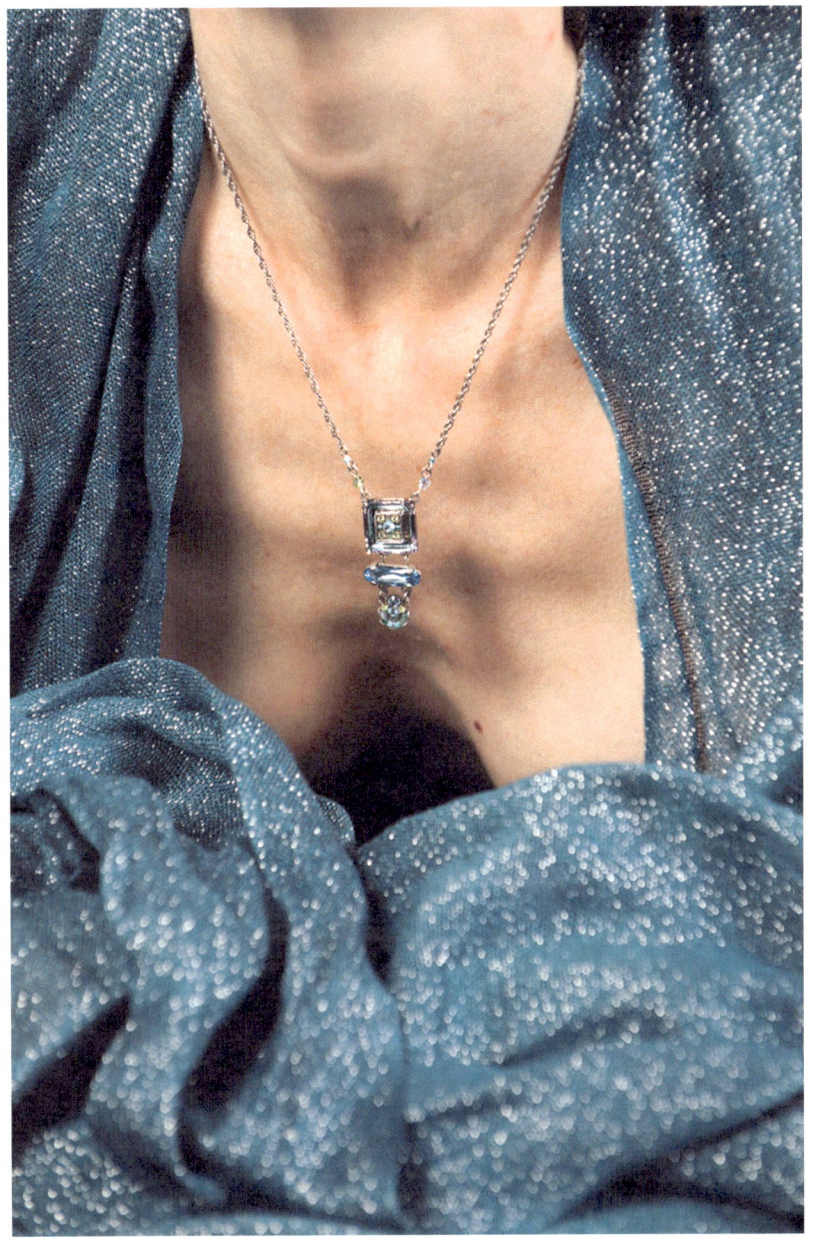

October

always my favorite
a month of
smoke and maple
    Awareness
this year
a whole new way

whole
new body
bare like the trees
our shedding leaves
celebrating
the gifts of loss.

Edges of Light: Images of Breast Transformation

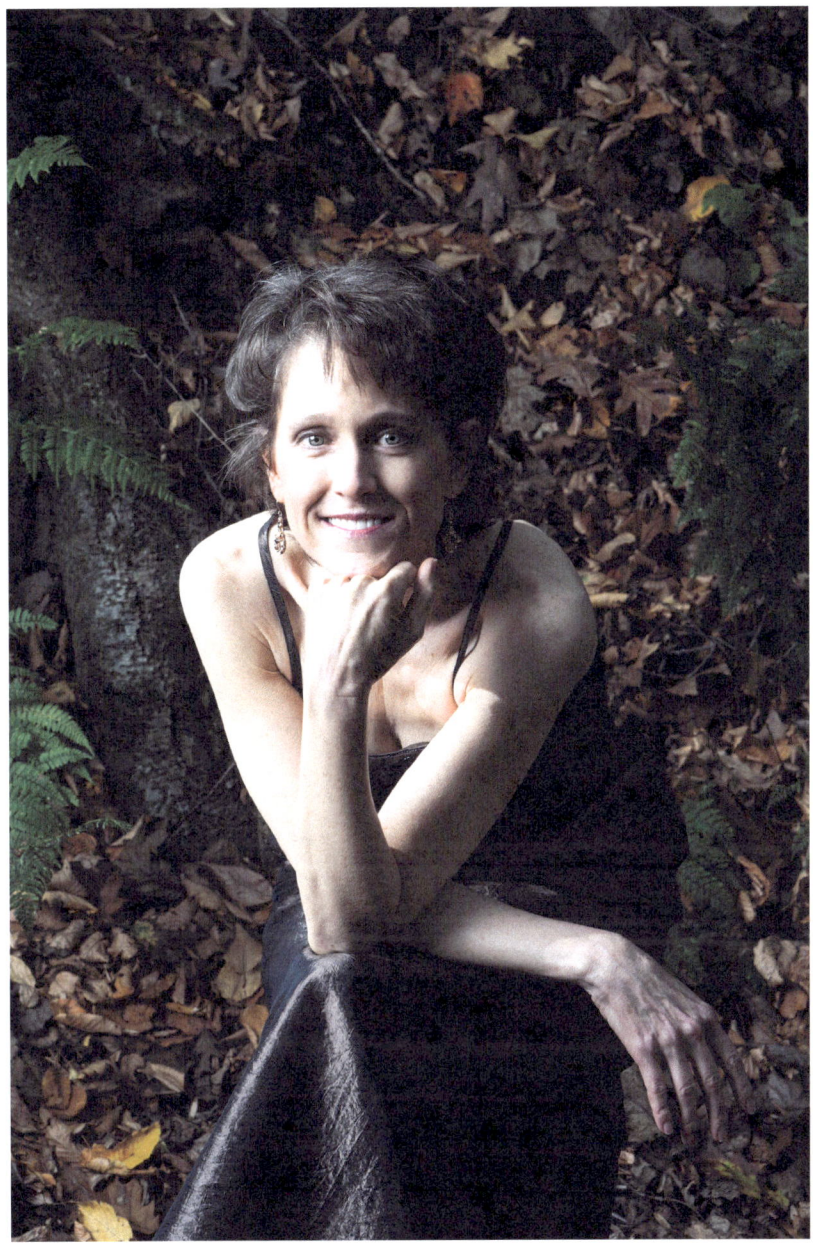

Chiaroscuro

Contours
of shadow and light
again a dancer
incandescent
in the night

Edges of Light: Images of Breast Transformation

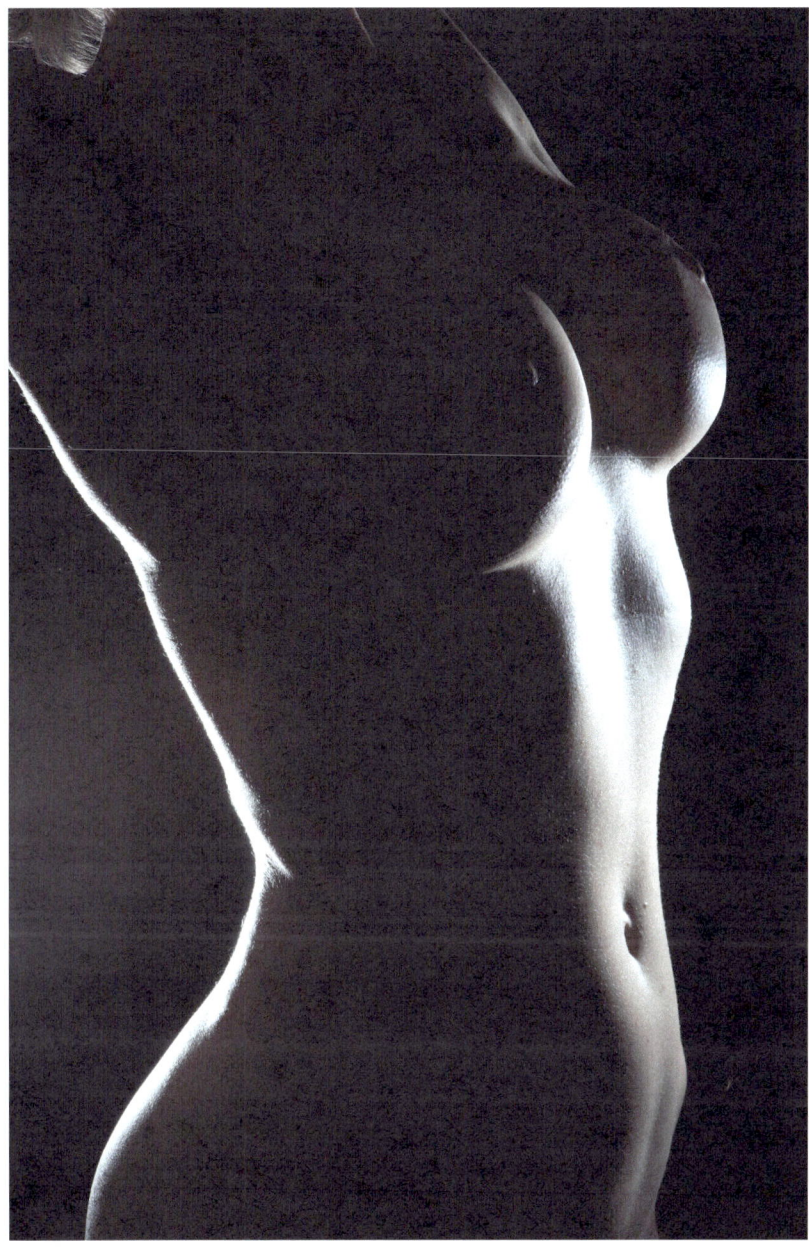

LISA KATZ

The Form

Near Kastoria,
we were four kilometers from Metamorphosis
when I began to throw masks
out of the car window,
litter the road with my clothes,
infant, girlish, and grown-up,
foreign bra with one cup filled,
the new costume
of my lopsided middle age.
You ask me
not to throw my human shape away.

Three kilometers from Metamorphosis,
when we get there I will accept
the transformation, for worse or better:
the wife into bird, the mother into stone.
Not least of all I want the story meaningful.

Two kilometers from Metamorphosis,
and though my nakedness suits me now,
it won't be easy
to wear the body I've chosen,
the flat breastplate, no silicon or salt water.

One more kilometer. I tell you
everything here will be or was
human once,
the form I pick
is absence.

PART IV

Breast Cancer over Time: Evolutions in Understandings, Representations, Tools and Treatments

SIOBHAN CONATY

Milestones in the Depiction of Breasts and Breast Cancer in Art History

> *"Breast cancer may very well be history's oldest malaise, known as well to the ancients as it is to us."* (James Olson, *Bathsheba's Breast*)

The earliest known recorded history of breast cancer appears in Egypt in what is known as the *Edwin Smith Surgical Papyrus*, c.1600 BCE, a document that is believed to be a copy of an even older document from c.3000 BCE. Since then, breast cancer has been consistently mentioned in medical history. And yet, images believed to depict breast disease are not seen in visual art until the Renaissance. To understand how and why breast cancer appears in fifteenth-century painting and sculpture, we must also examine representations of women's breasts as shifting symbols – of fertility, power, maternity, sex, sin, exploitation and illness – that serve as a mirror of the cultural norms of each era from prehistoric to contemporary times. What follows is a selective, not exhaustive, look at key pieces of western art throughout history as they reflect and inform our understanding of the cultural significance of breasts and breast cancer over time.

I begin in the prehistoric world, where artifacts suggest that women commanded power and prestige related to fertility and the creation of life – symbolized by breasts that feature prominently. An analysis of sculpture from the Greek period signals a shift toward breasts as objects of eroticism and danger in the classical world, followed by the medieval depiction of breasts to designate women as either saint or sinner. Works by Renaissance masters such as Michelangelo deepen our understanding of the cultural significance of breasts and present us with the first credible example of breast cancer in art history – a malady that becomes even more obviously rendered in a painting by Rembrandt in the mid-1600s. Works by four artists from the nineteenth to the early twenty-first century illustrate a marked contrast in the depiction of breast cancer in the modern world.

Prehistoric (c.25,000 BCE)

The *Venus of Willendorf* (<https://en.wikipedia.org/wiki/Venus_of_Willendorf>) is a tiny carved figure, roughly four-and-one-half inches tall, that reveals much about what was important to the people of the Paleolithic era. A close look tells us this is a nude woman with an enlarged abdomen and hands resting on full breasts. The artist carved deep lines in the limestone to create shadows that bring the viewer's eye to her belly button and vulva, the entrance to the birth canal. Traces of red ochre are still visible on parts of her body, perhaps suggestive of blood and the birth process. Her head and face are covered in an abstract pattern that may represent a woven hat, curls or braids. While there is no discernable face, she gently tilts her head downward, as if looking at her swollen belly.

The *Venus of Willendorf* was created when survival of the species was a critical goal. Groups of people lived as nomads, moving from one cave to another, depending on the food supply and weather conditions. We know from historians, archeologists and scientists who specialize in this era that men hunted while women gathered food and tended to the near-constant work of hearth and home. But more specifically, women birthed, fed and cared for children and were therefore viewed as keepers of the "survival" of their clan. Considering high infant and child mortality rates – along with the presumed lack of scientific understanding of the birth process – the ability to grow, birth and nourish a child with her breasts seemed to place women in the realm of the sacred and powerful. This heightened status is supported by the sheer number of sculptures of bare-breasted women with the attributes of a "fertility goddess," compared to the relative lack of sculpted male figures in various cultures and locations throughout the prehistoric era.

These small sculptures were carved out of limestone (a difficult task at a time before metal tools were invented) and were believed to be carried by women as a kind of sacred talisman to promote fertility and successful pregnancies (Ehrenberg 66). While there is no historical evidence documenting women's daily lives and experiences during this period, the fact that prehistoric people took the time and considerable effort to carve so many of these fertility goddesses points to the social value of women and to the sacred life-giving power connected to their bodies.

Classical (fifth century BCE)

Women's status and experience in ancient Greece were controlled by men from the outset. Greeks practiced female infanticide, and girls who survived infancy were fed an inferior diet. Males outnumbered females by two to one. Confined to domestic duties, women were excluded from education, denied political participation and rarely left their homes. While women could legally inherit family money and property, they were expected to marry and they had no legal rights (Slatkin 34).

In *A History of the Breast* (1997), Marilyn Yalom notes that the early Greek goddesses of fertility, such as the multi-breasted Artemis, eventually fell out of favor (Yalom 16). Often, Greek women were illustrated with bodies covered from head to toe in tunics and veils as they conducted domestic activities within the home (Yalom 19). At the same time, some women in Greek art are shown with exposed breasts in scenes of breastfeeding and beyond. This category includes women who were depicted as modest symbols of love and beauty (such as Aphrodite) as well as courtesans (*hetaerae*) who engaged in graphic sexual activities with Greek men. Also popular were scenes of gods engaged in various forms of sexual activities with earthly women, such as *Leda and the Swan* (Figure 1). These nudes were created for the male gaze, and their breasts functioned as objects for male desire. Women's "status" and "power" in these cases were directly related to how well their bodies provided an aphrodisiac effect on the male viewer.

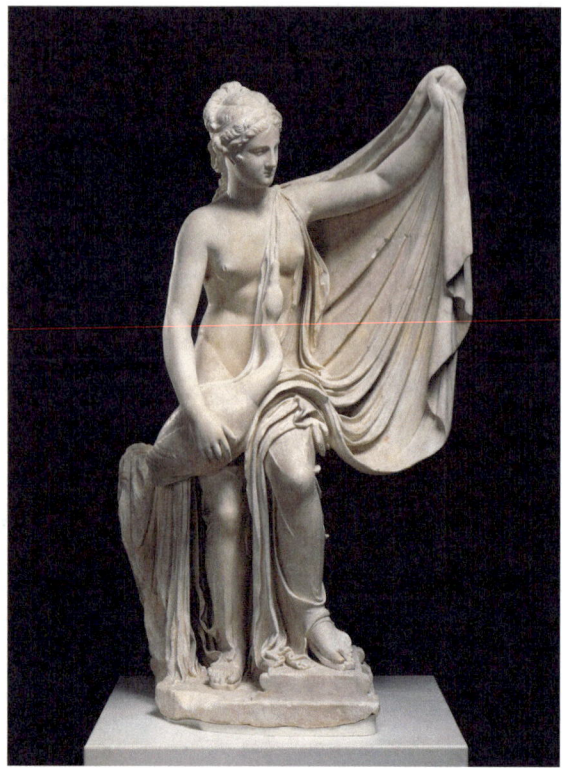

Figure 1: *Unknown, Statue of Leda and the Swan*, first century AD, Marble, Roman copy of earlier Greek sculpture, 132.1 × 83.5 × 52.1 cm (52 × 32 7/8 × 20 1/2 in.), 70.AA.110, The J. Paul Getty Museum, Villa Collection, Malibu, California.

A more interesting case of the connection between breasts and power is the legendary "Amazon" women. The *Marble Statue of Wounded Amazon* (Figure 2) is a first- to second-century CE Roman copy of a Greek original from the fifth century BCE. The sculpture of a warrior woman with a bared breast represents a form of female resistance against a patriarchal society, but it also stands as a dire warning to women who attempted to take control of their own bodies and govern themselves and thereby challenged prescribed roles in Greek culture.

Milestones in the Depiction of Breasts and Breast Cancer 335

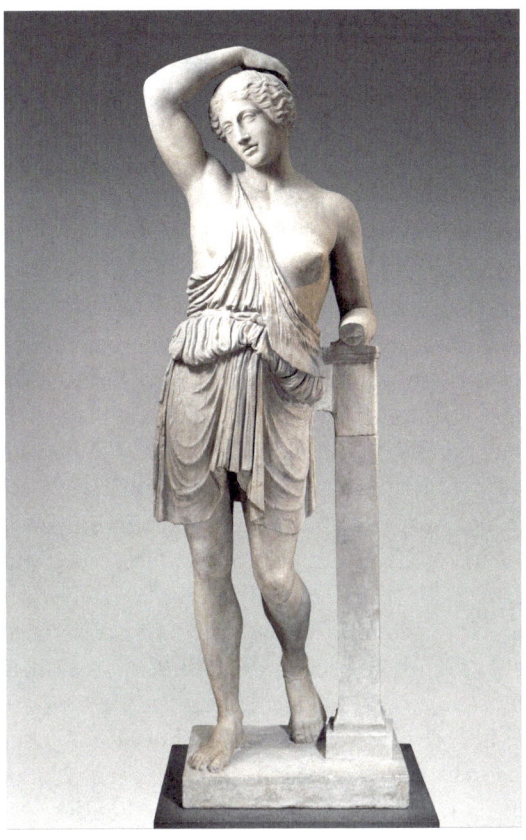

Figure 2: *Marble Statue of Wounded Amazon*, imperial period, first–second century AD, Roman, Marble, H. 203.84 cm (80 1/4 in.), Gift of John D. Rockefeller Jr., 1932, Metropolitan Museum of Art, New York.

The Greeks identified Amazons as the daughters of Ares (god of the violent and untamed aspects of war), who formed a women-only society in Asia Minor. Representing the complete reversal of the Greek ideal for women, Amazon tribes were ruled by a queen and used men only for procreation. While female children were trained as warriors, male offspring were killed, maimed or used as slaves. According to legend, Amazon women cut off (or cauterized) one of their breasts so they could more adeptly use a bow and arrow or sword in battle. This supposition is supported by one of the most common etymological interpretations of the name "Amazon," which comes from the Greek "a" (without) and "mazos" (breast) (Yalom 22-3). The Greeks condemned (and likely feared) the power of these aggressive and "unnatural" women, and thus their gods always managed to defeat the Amazons in epic battles. These victories were an important part of Greek history, and therefore art history, as evidenced by the sheer number of sculptures, pottery and shields depicting their downfall: There are over 400 surviving artworks celebrating Hercules' defeat of the Amazons alone.

The *Marble Statue of Wounded Amazon* is a perfect example of the Greek desire to demonstrate visually a narrative of defeat and domination of aberrant women. The larger-than-life sculpture is believed to have originally stood in front of a temple dedicated to Artemis of Ephesus in Asia Minor (<https://www.metmuseum.org/art/collection/search/253373>). The warrior stands without weapons, unprotected and bleeding from a wound just below her right breast. The calm look on her face, along with the languid and leaning stance with an arm casually resting on her head, implies sleep, a common symbol for oncoming death in the classical Greek iconography of the fifth century BCE (metmuseum.org). While the scale of this work (over 6 feet tall) denotes a certain level of respect for these women as enemies, the slash under her breast is a clear message about what happens to women who upset the Greek power structure. The bleeding wound brings attention to the Amazon's bare breast and to the fact that she used it to increase female power rather than using it for nourishment and male pleasure. It is no coincidence that this sculpture of a dying Amazon was placed in front of a temple dedicated to Artemis Ephesus, the multi-breasted goddess of fertility, chastity and childbirth: It clearly served as a powerful warning for women who dared to defy the Greek order of nature for women.

Medieval (fifth to fifteenth centuries)

Status for women in the western world did not improve much during the medieval period. As the dominant religion in Europe, Christianity taught that women should be subordinate, chaste and pious. Breastfeeding featured prominently, and the nourishing mother motif took on sacred status with the common Christian theme of the "Lactating Madonna." It was not unusual to see paintings of the Virgin Mary fully clothed, holding one awkwardly posed and anatomically suspect breast out of her cloak to feed the infant Jesus. At the time, breast milk was believed to be transformed blood of the mother, and church leaders made a symbolic connection between a mother's ability to feed her children and Christ, who fed humanity through his blood in the sacrament of Eucharist (Slatkin 64). This connection is evident in popular images of the twelfth-century legend of the *Lactation of St. Bernard* (1470) (Figure 3), where Bernard of Clairvaux, a Cistercian monk, was praying devoutly to the Virgin Mary when she miraculously appears with the infant Jesus and uses her breast to squeeze milk into his mouth, thereby blessing and nourishing his soul.

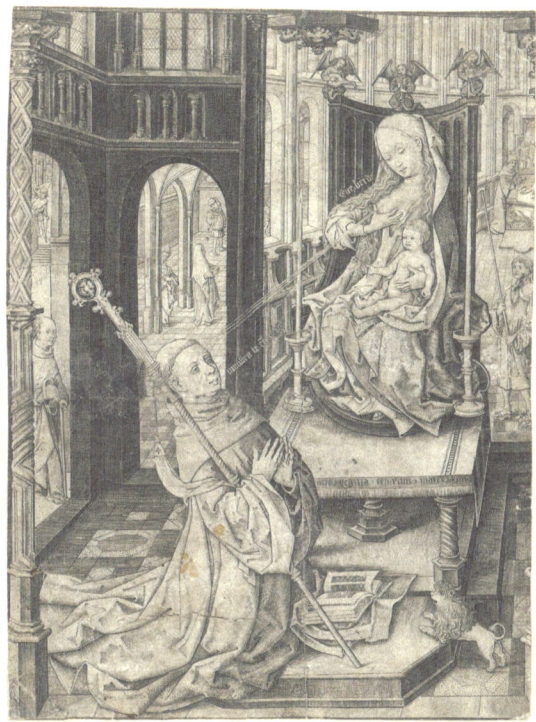

Figure 3: Master of IAM of Zwolle, *Lactation of St. Bernard*, 1480–5, Engraving, 320 × 241 mm, RP-P-OB-1093, Rijksmuseum, Amsterdam.

A darker side to the sacred dimension of female breasts in the middle ages is found in *Martyrdom of Saint Agatha* (1470–3) (Figure 4), which tells the story of one of the first female martyrs of the early Christian era. Agatha was a third-century Sicilian noblewoman who dedicated her body and soul to Christ. When Agatha rejected the sexual advances of a Roman consul and refused to make a sacrifice to what she considered pagan gods, her breasts were cut from her body. According to the legend provided in the medieval book of saints, *The Golden Legend*, St. Peter appeared in her jail cell and healed her breasts. This so infuriated the Roman consul that Agatha was put on trial (during which she defended herself) and tortured, and she died in prison. This was a popular story in both the Medieval and Renaissance periods, and Agatha was typically depicted either bound in the nude in the process of having her breasts cut off, or standing fully clothed and holding a platter with her perfectly round breasts presented to the viewer. By the fourteenth century, most images of Agatha emphasized the brutal scene of her "forced mastectomy" (Easton 99). These powerful and visceral images of faith and physical suffering ultimately led to Agatha's identification as the patron saint of breast disease (Cheney 6).

Milestones in the Depiction of Breasts and Breast Cancer 339

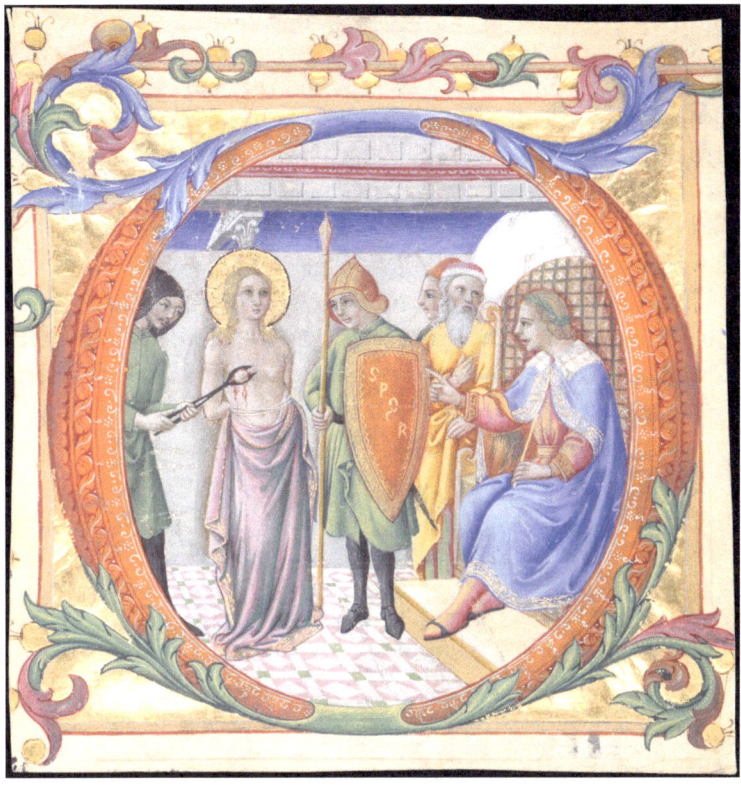

Figure 4: Sano di Pietro, *Martyrdom of Saint Agatha*, ca.1470–3, Tempera and gold on parchment, 1470–3, 10 3/8 × 10 1/8 in., Robert Lehman Collection, 1975, The Metropolitan Museum of Art, New York.

Much of the art in the middle ages was commissioned by the Christian church as a teaching tool, a visual narrative or sermon for the many church-goers who could not read. Thus, images of female nudes were used in manuscripts, sculpture and paintings to make clear the distinction between those who were saints and those who were sinners. Sinners were typically shown in the nude with body parts, often breasts, being tortured by demons as they prepared to enter hell. One example, known as the *Luxuria (Unchaste Woman)* (c.1120–35) (Figure 5), can be seen in the Romanesque Church of Sainte-Pierre at Moissac, France. The artist carved this almost life-size woman in the entry wall of the church as a warning for women who might give in to carnal desires. An emaciated, nude skeletal woman with long flowing hair is shown with snakes biting at her breasts and a toad devouring her genitals. The woman looks down at her body in horror as the demon standing next to her spits another toad from his mouth toward her. This unchaste woman's body serves as a counterpoint to the Christian ideal of the modest, pious mother who uses her breasts to nurse and nurture both body and soul. And yet, if we compare the fate of this "unchaste" woman to St. Agatha – the woman who died for her chastity – both paid a similar price: an act of violence to their breasts. As Marilyn Yalom has pointed out, these images, "whatever the didactic intent, afforded some artists the opportunity to vent their sadistic impulses on women's breasts" (Yalom 36).

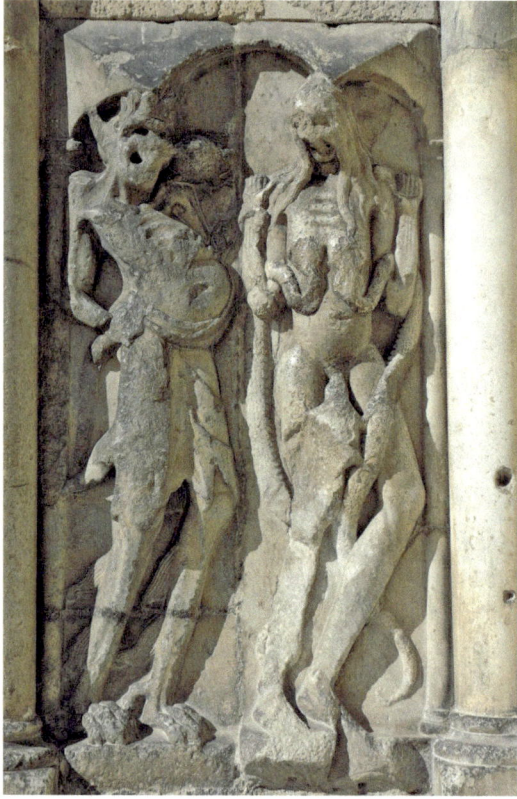

Figure 5: *Luxuria (Unchaste Woman)*, c. 1120–35, Sculpture, West Wall Porch, Romanesque Church of Sainte-Pierre at Moissac, France.

Although there is a direct line from the ancient fertility goddesses to the "Lactating Madonna" in the middle ages, the power of the breast in the medieval period is once removed. Images of the Virgin Mary and Saint Agatha taught medieval women that it was their sacred duty to be a vessel for God, and women were certainly held in some esteem for this position. But whereas ancient women were life-giving *creators*, whose bodies and breasts were critical to the survival of humanity, medieval women's bodies and breasts were relegated either to a supporting role for God as the great creator or an object of violence.

Renaissance (sixteenth century)

In the Renaissance period, instances of breast disease appear in sculpture and paintings made for public consumption. Why now – especially when we know breast cancer was a known entity and had been discussed in medical documents and treaties since the ancient Egyptian period? We've seen images of breasts exaggerated to emphasize fertility and the power to sustain life, breasts manipulated to show erotic appeal, breasts wounded as a warning against too much power for women, and breasts tortured to punish sins of the flesh. But so far, we've seen no instances of breast disease in art. The following is an investigation of some individual works and the relevant socio-historical contexts that help bring to light why Renaissance artists began to include breast disease in their work.

Before we begin analyzing breast disease in art history, it is important to note that these "diagnoses" cannot be confirmed, as they were made by physicians looking at art, and not at an actual patient. Over the last few decades there have been lively debates among physicians in academic journals about whether a piece of art depicts breast cancer or another form of disease. To complicate matters further, art historians often dismiss clinicians' observations about art, because clinicians typically lack, as the argument goes, appropriate cultural and historical contexts – particularly as they relate to an artist's creative agenda. As an art historian, I stand clear of the clinical side of this debate and respect the scientific deliberation among professionals in the medical field. Instead, I focus on the fact that visual representations of breast disease and irregularities *are* indeed visible in art in considerable numbers for the first time between the sixteenth and seventeenth centuries, and I use art history methods to add necessary depth and context to interdisciplinary discussion.

A prominent example of a visual representation of breast cancer in the Renaissance is Michelangelo's sculpture *Night* (1526–31) (Figure 6) in the Medici Chapel in the Basilica of San Lorenzo in Florence, Italy. While it may not be the first – some physicians have suggested that a cancerous tumor can be detected in the left breast of Raphael's *La Fornarina* (1518–9) eight years earlier – *Night* is one piece of art that most clinicians agree depicts abnormalities consistent with advanced breast cancer. For decades doctors have viewed Michelangelo's work and written about the signs of cancer in medical journals. In one article, art historian Jonathan Katz Nelson and oncologist James J. Stark worked together using their disciplines' skills to jointly analyze this sculpture. They identified a swollen nipple and areola, a large bulge medial to the nipple, and an area of skin retraction lateral to the nipple. These features indicate a tumor medial to the nipple, causing tethering and retraction on the opposite side of the breast (Nelson and Stark 1577). It is important to note that while oncologists look at art and identify clinical evidence of breast cancer, art historians look at these images as visual constructions chosen by an artist to communicate a message. Even in the Renaissance, when "naturalism" was the ideal, images were not always representations of reality; they were *visual strategies* used by artists to tell a story. In their letter to the *New England Journal of Medicine*, Nelson and Stark introduce the idea that Michelangelo *intentionally* included the diseased breast in *Night*. Considering the artist's visual strategy in relation to historical context and medical history may illuminate Michelangelo's possible intention.

Milestones in the Depiction of Breasts and Breast Cancer   343

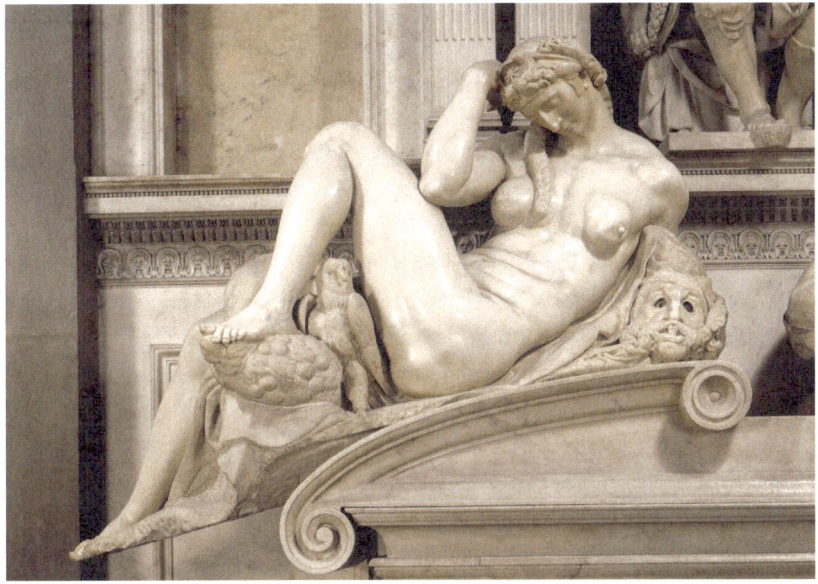

Figure 6: Michelangelo, *Night, Detail from the Tomb of Guiliano de' Medici, Duke of Nemours*, marble, 20 feet 8 in. × 13 feet 9 in., 1519–24, Medici Chapel, Basilica di San Lorenzo, Florence, Italy. Credit: Scala/Art Resource, NY.

In the early part of the sixteenth century, Michelangelo was commissioned to design a mortuary chapel for members of the Medici family. Only two tombs were completed for two minor Medici dukes, Guiliano and Lorenzo. The tombs are positioned across from each other, with larger-than-life seated sculptures of the dukes, each with a male and female reclining at his feet. These massive reclining figures, each over 6 feet in length, were allegories reflecting the passage of time – and thus life. *Night* and *Day* are in front of Guiliano's tomb (<https://www.britannica.com/topic/Medici-Chapel>); *Dusk* and *Dawn* are in front of Lorenzo's tomb on the other side of the chapel. Michelangelo sculpted *Night*'s left breast with visual abnormalities associated with cancer, while the other female nude, *Dawn*, was shown with nonsymptomatic breasts. Why? A close look at *Night* reveals that Michelangelo surrounded the sleeping woman with obvious symbols of night: the owl, and the stars and moon on the woman's crown. But he also included a bunch of poppy seeds (a medicinal plant from which opium is extracted to relieve pain) and a theatrical tragedy mask – both symbols of death in art history.

Most art history studies of Michelangelo's *Night* do not address the irregularities of the left breast, and the discipline frowns upon medical diagnosis applied to works of art without stylistic and cultural context. Doctors writing on this topic, however, tend to suggest that Michelangelo was sculpting what he actually saw and that therefore the model must have had breast cancer. Perhaps neither perspective is entirely accurate. Michelangelo, like other Renaissance artists, was by no means tied to a literal rendition of "what he saw." Note, for example, the elongated torso of the female figure of *Night* and the anatomically unfeasible length of Giuliano's neck. These breaks from naturalism were intended constructions by the artist to portray ideals: a graceful elongation of the female body and the nobility of Guiliano's neck. Considering clinical analyses alongside this art historical context, I agree with Nelson and Stark that Michelangelo intended to include breast disease in the female figure *Night*, whether the model presented with symptoms or not (343). This choice is most likely an attempt by Michelangelo to suggest death even more directly, through disease. Michelangelo had an avid interest in anatomy, biology and dissection, and he certainly would have been aware of this common pathology of the time. He also would have been aware that a model presenting with these symptoms would eventually die from this illness. Did his model for this particular sculpture "happen" to have breast cancer? We don't know for sure, but it is likely that Michelangelo used various model sources to create a hybrid figure for his ideal final product.

Renaissance artists were well educated and pointedly connected art to science and medicine. In fact, artists and doctors and shared the same patron saint, St. Luke, and the same working guild. The sixteenth century was a revolutionary period for medical practice, including treatment for breast cancer. In the sixteenth century, Michael Servetus (1511–53) presented for the first time the concept of mastectomy and suggested extended lymph node excision (Konstantinos et al. 4); and Barthélémy Cabrol (1529–1603), surgeon to

England's King Henry IV, recommended mastectomy "including the removal of the pectoralis muscle and the axillary lymph nodes that appeared to be affected by the disease. His approach paved the way to 'radical mastectomy' that William Halsted would perform three centuries later" (Bianucci, et al. 166). Most women, however, did not opt for this surgery for a number of reasons: the lack of anesthesia, postoperative infections and bleeding that often led to death and finally, but perhaps equally important, the social and cultural symbol of the breast as fertility, femininity and beauty. This type of surgery was considered inhumane by Renaissance standards (Bianucci, et al. 167), so it is reasonable to assume that most women with breast cancer died with the diseased breast intact. It is believed that Michelangelo was performing his own (likely "private") dissections in the early sixteenth century, which enabled him to produce remarkably accurate anatomy drawings decades before Andreas Vesalius published the groundbreaking *Fabric of the Human Body* in 1543 (Park 78). Given his exacting knowledge of the human form and his connections with physicians of the time, Michelangelo would have knowingly and perhaps cunningly included these breast abnormalities as part of his visual strategy in a sculpture that symbolized death.

Baroque (seventeenth century)

Baroque (taken from the Portuguese word *barroco*, meaning irregular) art tended to be more dramatic, theatrical and emotional than Renaissance art. Baroque painting styles and subject matter varied among the different cultures and religious persuasions in Europe at the time. In this section I will focus on the seventeenth-century Dutch artist Rembrandt van Rijn, whose style falls under the general category of "Northern Baroque." Baroque art produced in the new Dutch Republic came out of a free commercial market – unlike in Italy, where the Catholic church remained a primary patron. The result was a significant change in the kind of art being made (landscapes, still-lifes and "genre painting" with scenes of everyday life) for a different kind of customer (upper- and middle-class citizens, art dealers and commercial groups). Though post-Reformation

Protestant (iconoclastic) churches were not a source of funding for the arts, religious and moral subjects made specifically for viewing in private homes were popular.

One of the paintings made for private consumption was Rembrandt's *Bathsheba at Her Bath* (1654) (Figure 7), a work that has been the subject of intense scrutiny in both the art historical and medical fields. In addition to extensive commentary throughout the history of Rembrandt scholarship, Ann Jensen Adams dedicated her book *Rembrandt's Bathsheba Reading King David's Letter* to this painting alone. With similar enthusiasm, physicians have been diagnosing, debating and publishing opinions on *Bathsheba's* breast from the clinical side since 1970. I present the following analysis as a case study that highlights both the conflict between – as well as the interdisciplinary possibilities for – the art history and medical fields as they seek to provide a robust analysis of this pivotal work.

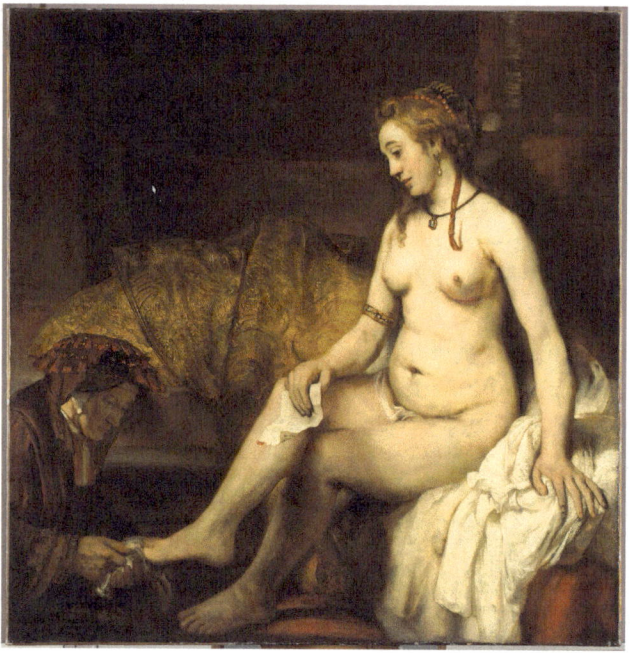

Figure 7: Rembrandt van Rijn, *Bathsheba at Her Bath*, 1654, Oil on Canvas, 142 × 142 cm, Inv: M1957. Photo: Mathieu Rabeau, Musee du Louvre, Paris, France. Credit: © RMN-Grand Palais/Art Resource, NY.

The Old Testament story of Bathsheba would have been well known to the seventeenth-century viewer, as it was a popular theme in art as one of the few justified female nudes (along with Eve and Susannah) from the Bible. In summary, Bathsheba was the wife of Uriah, a heroic military captain in King David's army. King David was walking on the roof of his palace in Jerusalem one evening when he observed Bathsheba bathing outdoors, and he immediately desired her. He sent messengers "and took her; and she came in unto him, and he lay with her" (KJV Bible, 2 Samuel 11:4). Bathsheba became pregnant, and King David had Uriah sent to the front lines of battle, whereby he would surely meet his death. King David then married Bathsheba, who gave birth to a son. The infant's death shortly thereafter was considered a punishment from God for the sins committed by the couple. Bathsheba and David were eventually forgiven, however, as evidenced by a second son, Solomon, who became a leader in the church.

In visual art, Bathsheba typically appears in the foreground, depicted as a sensuous nude with full, eroticized breasts. Rembrandt's earlier *The Toilet of Bathsheba* (1643), for example, portrays Bathsheba as alluring, thereby positioning her as a willing participant in the sin of adultery with King David. In the later *Bathsheba at Her Bath*, however, Bathsheba is depicted as a woman with little choice in this power dynamic. Many art historians believe that this later Bathsheba is possibly based on Hendrickje Stoffels, Rembrandt's lover, who was hired as a nurse for his son Titus after his wife's death. There is no documented evidence that this is the case, but other images of Hendrickje indicate that Rembrandt modeled Bathsheba's body – or her perhaps just her face – after his lover at the time (M. D. Carroll, qtd. in Adams 167).

Here, Rembrandt plays with the narrative a bit, inserting into the story a message sent from King David to Bathsheba, calling for her presence at his side. Bathsheba looks down while she considers the letter. A master of depicting psychological emotions, Rembrandt captures Bathsheba's face with flickering emotions of sorrow, resignation and fortitude as her strong hand grips the letter. She is a woman burdened with a decision that will determine her fate and her faith. Margaret D. Carrol has argued that Rembrandt painted Hendrickje as Bathsheba in this way to suggest similarities between the two women. Hendrickje and Rembrandt were not married, and when Hendrickje became pregnant in 1652, she was called before the church authorities "for acting like a harlot" (Adams 5) with the artist. She chose to continue to live with Rembrandt, even at the cost of ostracism from her religious community and seventeenth-century Dutch society. While that pregnancy was not successful, Hendrickje did become pregnant again and gave birth to a daughter in 1654, the same year *Bathsheba at Her Bath* was painted (Carroll, qtd. in Adams 167–8).

An Italian surgeon, T. C. Greco, was the first to publish, in 1970, speculations about breast cancer in *Bathsheba at her Bath*. He noted asymmetry in Bathsheba's left breast, swelling or fullness near her left armpit, some discoloration and a section of *peau d'orange* – a portion of the skin that looks like the texture of an orange peel – all of which are signs of breast cancer (Olson 9). When Greco learned that the woman believed to be the model, Hendrickje Stoffels, died after a long illness, he concluded that she died of breast cancer. Two similar independent analyses were published in English by Braithwaite and Shugg in 1983 and in Russian by Dymarskii in 1984. Braithwaite and Shugg argued that, taken together, the lack of symmetry, discoloration, axillary fullness and *peau d'orange* texture of the left breast indicated that the painting "could not be anything but a deliberate depiction of what he [Rembrandt] saw. They are clinical signs of breast cancer" (Braithwaite and Shugg 337).

For decades, these studies were cited and generally accepted as conclusive in both medical articles and the popular press, until surgeons in the 2000s provided "second opinions" of the diagnosis. In 2000, R. G. Bourne cited Dymarskii's prior research that Hendrickje Stoffels had given birth in 1652 – two years before the painting – and that she died at the age of 37 after a long illness, nine years after the painting was completed. Bourne challenged the prior diagnosis of breast cancer, arguing that it was highly unlikely for a woman to live beyond two or three years while presenting with the symptoms observed in Bathsheba's left breast. Even with surgery, there would have been little hope for that kind of survival rate in the seventeenth century (Bourne 231). Bourne concluded that if the model were in fact Hendrickje, it was more likely that she had a chronic breast abscess, possibly tuberculous mastitis. Only if it were an unknown model with an unknown fate would breast cancer have been a viable possibility. In 2006, Hayakawa, Masuda and Nemoto combined their knowledge of infectious disease, surgery and pathology to propose that Hendrickje (modeling as

Milestones in the Depiction of Breasts and Breast Cancer   349

Bathsheba) suffered from lactational breast abscess and mastopathy resulting from her 1652 pregnancy. The pregnancy was believed to have ended in miscarriage or neonatal death, which could have induced lactation; without feeding, breast inflammation and infection could result. While this illness can be resolved by antibiotics today, the authors submit that in the seventeenth century her condition likely progressed to an acute phase that produced the areas of redness and swelling that Rembrandt observed and painted (Hayakawa, Masuda and Nemoto 1241).

But again, art historians generally disregard physicians' attempts to use art to diagnose illnesses, since we are trained to recognize that art is most often not a literal representation of reality. A visual image may tell a story and it may be depicted in a naturalistic manner, but it is a story that is constructed by the artist nonetheless. Indeed, renowned Rembrandt scholar Ernst van de Wetering dismissed Bathsheba's breast cancer diagnosis in the following manner:

> From time to time, one reads an occasional medical diagnosis that explains some painter's distinguishing characteristics or choice of subjects ... In the case of *Bathsheba*, it was the sensational "news" that Rembrandt's companion, Hendrickje Stoffels, who is usually (but probably wrongly) considered to be the model for this painting, died of breast cancer. (624)

Van de Wetering continues with a science-based explanation to debunk the purported diagnosis of breast cancer. Using x-rays and ultraviolet photographs, he notes that a 1950 restoration left thick layers of varnish on top of prior yellow layers of varnish, which caused discoloration on the darker, shaded part of Bathsheba's left breast. He describes the surface *peau d'orange* as an "uneven abrasion" in the fragile dark paint which is more easily damaged over time due to the chemical makeup of its binding medium (Van de Wetering 624). That is, perhaps the *peau d'orange* was merely chemical and not created intentionally by Rembrandt.

So, what to make of this dispute between two disciplines so uniquely positioned to enrich each other? Art history and the health sciences share a relationship bound by the need to observe and understand the particularities of a given body or object in light of environment and context. Both disciplines must also be able to acknowledge uncertainty while conducting an analysis. Do we know that Rembrandt used Hendrickje Stoffels as his model for Bathsheba? Do we know if Hendrickje had breast cancer? In both cases, the answer is no, but I argue that we can proceed with the following questions using skills from both fields: Did Rembrandt intentionally include what clinicians deem some form as breast disease as part of his visual strategy for this story? Do these clinical observations connect to or amplify the artist's narrative in any way?

Taking into account the similarities in the stories of the two women, why *might* Rembrandt include elements of disease in Bathsheba's breast? I suggest that Rembrandt included some kind of diseased breast in this second, more personal Bathsheba as a kind of private *memento mori* or *vanitas*, two closely related cautionary themes prevalent in seventeenth-century Dutch art. The Latin phrase *memento mori* means "remember death"; it is a reminder of the inevitability of one's death. *Vanitas* means "empty," referring to the excesses and overindulgence in life that have no value in the afterlife. These paintings, greatly influenced by the Calvinist church, served as a reminder to the faithful to eschew their vanities in life and instead focus on attitudes and behaviors that lead to rewards in the afterlife. Typically, symbols of plentiful food, expensive glassware, silks and silver represented excess; and skulls, decaying flowers and dead insects were inserted into scenes to remind viewers of their behavior on earth and of inevitable judgment at the time of death. Rembrandt's *Bathsheba* of 1654, with her diseased breast, was a corporeal version of the *memento mori* and *vanitas*. Breast cancer – a well-known and incurable pathology at that time – became a subtle but visible symbol of Rembrandt's and Hendrickje's excesses and his contemplation of the ultimate price for their sinful behavior. (Still, I argue that, like Bathsheba, Hendrickje had very little agency in her relationship with Rembrandt.)

Realism (mid- to late-nineteenth century)

Many artists of this time were interested in a kind of scientific realism that demonstrated in-depth knowledge of anatomy and celebrated advances in science, but I will take a moment here to make clear the difference in

Milestones in the Depiction of Breasts and Breast Cancer

mission and meaning of medical illustration and medical scenes in art history. Art historian Martin Kemp describes medical illustration as an attempt "to provide a surrogate experience" to practitioners who did not have access to an actual body. Medical illustration documents anatomy and disease useful to clinical studies. By contrast, artists who create medically oriented work depict their own personal observations of health and illness, providing a perspective that illustrates the cultural and political contexts and biases of the era (Kemp 1–3). Thomas Eakins' *Agnew Clinic* (1889) (Figure 8) serves as a really good example of what may at first look like a clinical scene but in fact provides a much deeper view into nineteenth-century views on women, illness and breast cancer.

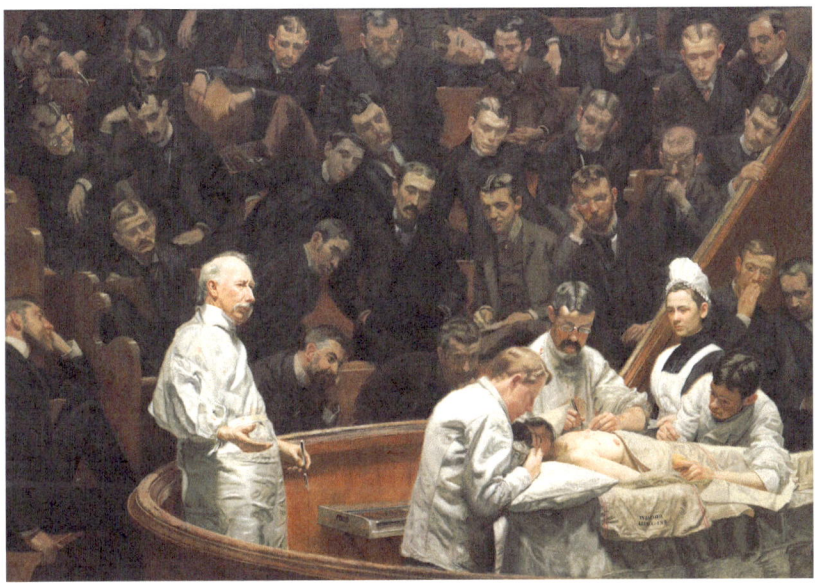

Figure 8: Thomas Eakins, *The Agnew Clinic*, 1889, Oil on Canvas, 214 cm × 300 cm, University of Pennsylvania Art Collection, Philadelphia, PA.

While studying painting at the renowned Pennsylvania Academy of Fine Arts (PAFA) in Philadelphia in the 1860s, Eakins attended medical lectures and anatomy and dissection demonstrations at the nearby

Jefferson Medical College, where he became so interested in the subject that he considered becoming a surgeon (Canaday 96). He ultimately choose art, however, and became a pivotal figure in nineteenth-century American Realism, a style that attempted to show the "truth" of the subject, however unpleasant, while at the same time incorporating scientific and anatomical precision. Eakins' close association with the medical world in Philadelphia brought about a commission by the Penn Medical Class of 1889 to paint a portrait of Dr. D. Hayes Agnew before he retired from the faculty. Agnew's surgical specialty was gunshots and abdominal battlefield wounds, skills he honed while serving as a consulting surgeon during the American Civil War. His expertise was such that he was brought in to tend to President James A. Garfield's wounds when he was shot in 1881.

In *The Agnew Clinic*, Eakins chose to honor the esteemed surgeon not by depicting Agnew performing abdominal surgery but, instead, mastectomy (for reasons discussed below). It is impossible to see exactly what type of mastectomy it was, but this operation predates Halsted's radical mastectomy that became the norm just a few years later in 1894. Eakins used a large (seven-by-ten-foot) canvas to present an unfolding narrative: Agnew has just removed the patient's breast and stands back to lecture the medical students (shown in various states of attention) as his assistants complete the procedure. Agnew leans against the railing, scalpel still in his (remarkably unbloody) hand, his head and white surgical clothing bathed in radiant light against the contrasting dark-suited students. His second in command, Dr. William White, completes the operation, while one surgical assistant provides ether and the other holds a sponge and anchors the patient's lower body to prevent sudden movement. Two women appear in this portrait: the patient, who lies unconscious with one non-diseased breast exposed; and the nurse, Charlotte V. Clymer. Nurse Clymer's presence demonstrates the new possibilities for women in the late nineteenth century while at the same time making clear her subordinate, servile role to the men in the clinic. The doctors are shown in active or intellectual modes; Clymer stands inactive, at attention and waiting dutifully to respond to a command. Nursing historian Susan Reverby has noted that the ideal nurse at this time embodied many of the same qualities as the ideal wife (Goodbody 40).

Eakins' *Agnew Clinic* was not received well either by the public or the artistic community. He had been promised it would hang in upcoming PAFA exhibit, but it was rejected by the selection committee upon its completion. An art critic at the time claimed "it was repulsive to the public and not cheerful for the ladies to look at" (Barker 41). Eakins had gone through a similar situation fifteen years earlier with the reaction to his *Gross Clinic* (1875): It was considered much too gory for most people and even unrealistic. In fact, art historian David Lubin challenged the idea that Eakins was a "Realist," describing the figure of Dr. Gross as a "towering, bloody-fingered Mephistopheles looming out of the black shadows" and noting that the scene's style was like a combination of Mary Shelley and Caravaggio. Lubin maintains that Eakins painted a "melodrama of life and death, light and darkness, knowledge and despair" disguised as scientific realism (Lubin 512). Something similar happens with *The Agnew Clinic*: Thomas Eakins certainly honors the retiring doctor, but by no means does he produce a literal representation of the surgical scene.

How did Eakins manipulate the scene to suit his purposes? One could say the subject of a mastectomy was the first example of the artist making a selection that suited his own interests, as this was not Agnew's specialty; in fact, the surgeon had little faith in the operation itself. Agnew stated in a lecture that he performed mastectomies for "moral effect" and believed it shortened rather than prolonged the patient's life. He further estimated that one in ten patients died from blood loss alone during surgery (Goodbody 43). The grim prognosis at the time led one of Agnew's colleagues, Dr. S. Weir Mitchell, to note that despite scientific advances, surgeons were doomed to be "defeated by a woman's breast" (Goodbody 43). A mastectomy did, however, allow a scene through which Eakins could demonstrate his anatomical knowledge and his skill in depicting the female nude.

In light of Agnew's statistic of blood loss and death during mastectomy, the woman's body and the surrounding surgical site are remarkably free from blood – which is perhaps the most obvious indication of a lack of realism in the painting, especially given the absence of surgical clips that would have prevented some of the excess blood. We know that Eakins was burned by the criticism of "blood and gore" in his first clinic painting, and we also know that Dr. Agnew made him remove some of the blood from the surgeon's hands in this second clinic, which Eakins reluctantly agreed to do. The patient herself seems relatively young, given that the average age for mastectomy at this time was forty-eight (Goodbody 47); and her healthy breast is left uncovered, highlighted and exposed. We know this was not normal procedure from Nurse Clymer's own surgical class notes, where she makes clear that a mastectomy patient's healthy breast was always concealed (Goodbody 45). Indeed, Dr. Agnew's own instructions in *Principles & Practices for Surgery* (1873) stipulate that a light blanket cover the healthy breast during a mastectomy (Agnew 715).

Though Eakins did create a narrative that celebrated Dr. Agnew, medical education and scientific progress, he also distorted the surgical scene while providing a gratuitous view of the healthy nude breast for the viewer. And while this painting is considered one of the greatest examples of nineteenth-century American Realism, we should also understand the nature of an artist's choices and "the fiction of *The Agnew Clinic's* realism" that does not accurately portray the disease or the violence of breast cancer surgery at the time (Goodbody 49).

Postmodern (late twentieth- and early twenty-first centuries)

In the early part of the twentieth century, breast cancer was a private and somewhat taboo subject that, although clinically prevalent, seemed to operate under a veil of silence except in medical settings. While this lack of representation was mirrored in early twentieth-century art history, there was a dramatic shift in the late twentieth and early twenty-first centuries – notably after the sexual revolution and second-wave feminism. It is important to note here that while breast cancer was not visibly present in early twentieth-century art, healthy women's breasts were certainly depicted, marketed, eroticized and exploited in popular culture and commercial media. The following section illustrates the shift in representations of breast cancer in art during the postmodern era.

This journey begins with Hannah Wilke, who was born and raised in New York City, attended Tyler School of the Arts in Philadelphia and later taught sculpture and ceramics at the School of Visual Arts in New York City. Her wide-ranging corpus includes drawings, photographs, sculptures, installations, video art and performance art. In self-portraits of the 1960s and 1970s, Wilke used her own body to counter feminine stereotypes. These works were often criticized and at times dismissed as narcissistic, in part because she happened to be "pin-up girl" beautiful. Wilke's anatomical content – that included vaginal and vulva imagery – challenged traditional ideas of sexuality and asserted power for women, though critics of the time argued that her work was "politically ambiguous" and "ends up reinforcing what it intends to subvert" (Watlington).

Detractors notwithstanding, Wilke's life and work embodied second wave feminism's mantra "the personal is political." In *Portrait of the Artist with Her Mother, Selma Butter* (Figure 9), Wilke juxtaposed portraits of herself and her mother, both posing nude from the waist up. Her full frontal pose, with a gaze that meets the eyes of the viewer, presents a powerful and moving contrast of her health and beauty to her mother's mastectomy-scarred body on the right. Using exaggerated makeup on her face and placing a "toy gun and other metal paraphernalia" (Skelly) on her breasts, Wilke complicates the idea of "the feminine" and plays with the idea of the "the body politic" by portraying the female body as a battleground. In creating a diptych – a dual-frame format typically used in churches as images for prayer and veneration – Wilke reclaims and honors the female body in a loving, almost spiritual manner that includes and enriches the status of both sick and well women in the postmodern era. Moreover, she effectively removes the veil of silence, shame and repulsion surrounding breast cancer.

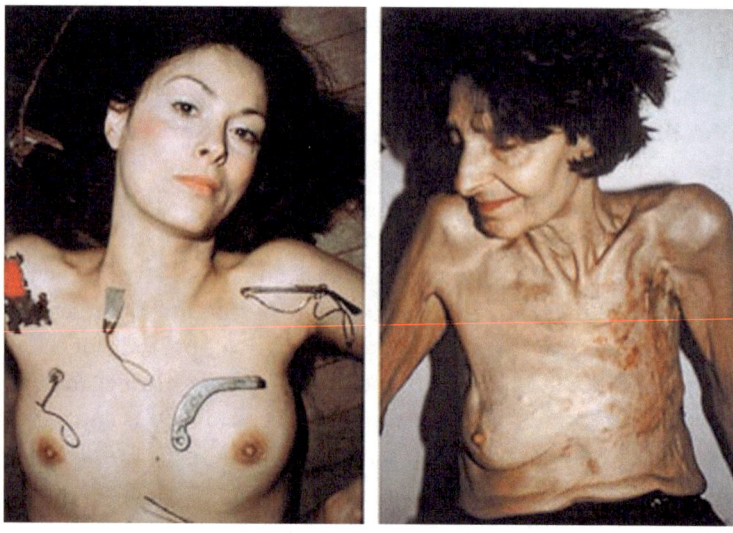

Figure 9: Hannah Wilke, *Portrait of the Artist with Her Mother, Selma Butter*, 1978–81, cibachrome photographs, framed size: 42 × 31 3/4 inches. each. © 2020 Marsie, Emanuelle, Damon and Andrew Scharlatt, Hannah Wilke Collection & Archive, Los Angeles/Licensed by VAGA at Artists Rights Society (ARS), NY.

When Wilke was diagnosed with lymphoma about five years later, she documented her hair loss and dramatically changed body throughout treatment in her *Intra-Venus Series* (1992–3) before her death in 1993. While Wilke's powerful images of female bodies ravaged by cancer have gained critical acclaim, this is in stark contrast to her earlier, more overtly sexual work. Art critic Emily Watlingston aptly gets to the root of the problem that still exists for women today, noting that Wilke's "images serve as a reminder that there may be a greater cultural comfort with the naked body of a dying woman than of one who is exercising her agency fully" (Watlingston).

Another late twentieth-century artist breaking similar ground in the UK was Jo Spence, a commercial photographer who eventually shifted to documentary photography with feminist themes. Using role-play, humor and subversion in her early photos, Spence attempted to liberate women from outdated societal stereotypes. When she was diagnosed with breast cancer in 1982, she began to explore through her work the politics of the disease. This was a time when there was little room for discussion of alternative treatments or for counselling to support a woman through the process. And when Spence refused the prescribed treatment plan by requesting a lumpectomy instead of a mastectomy, "her doctors were dismissive and patronising – though in the end they did as she asked" (Smith).

Spence asked photographer Terry Dennett to collaborate with her on the *Picture of Health?* series (1982–6), documenting her experience living with cancer. The night before her operation she had Dennett take a portrait of her with "Property of Jo Spence" (1983) written in bold black letters on her diseased breast (Figure 10). Using a bit of humor, Spence made it clear to the operating room clinicians that although they had temporary control, it was she who ultimately made the decisions for her body. Post-surgery, Spence and Dennett created *Crash Helmet Portrait* (1983) (Figure 11) in which the artist poses topless, wearing a motorcycle helmet and goggles with her arms over her head in a sensual "odalisque" pose – but in this case, to showcase her imperfect, scarred breast (Smith). Tamar Tembeck has noted in *Selfies of Ill Health* that in the late twentieth century there was "a recurrence of the subject shown in a frontal pose with a gaze directed straight toward the viewer, consistent with the willful intent to show oneself as being ill or in treatment .... Particularly in the context of breast cancer activism, being seen as sick (or as having been sick) was in part the very purpose of the self-portrait image" (Tembeck 3–4). In *Crash Helmet Portrait*, Spence makes fierce eye contact in order to connect with the viewer; she is battle ready with her helmet and goggles. Because it was important for the artist to get people to *see* and *talk* about this socially taboo illness, Spence had this series made into laminated posters that could be loaned out in libraries for community discussion.

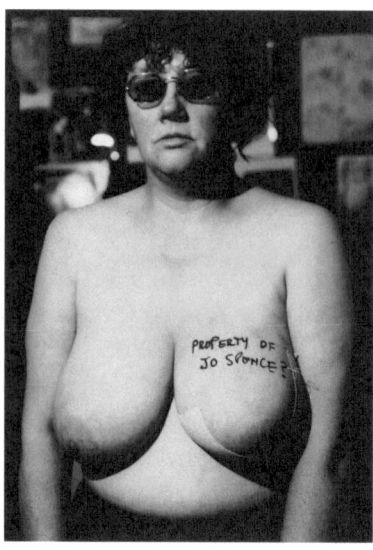

Figure 10: Jo Spence, (British, 1934–92) *Property of Jo Spence?* From The Picture of Health Series, a collaboration with Terry Dennett, Maggie Murray, and Rosy Martin, ca. 1982, The Wellcome Institute, London, England.

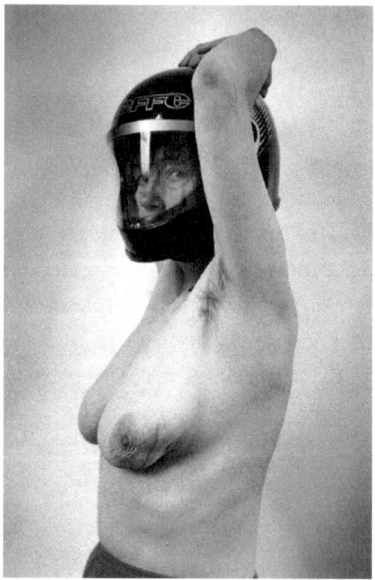

Figure 11: Jo Spence, (British, 1934–92) *Crash Helmet Portrait?* From The Picture of Health?, a collaboration with Terry Dennett, Maggie Murray, and Rosy Martin, ca. 1982 (printed 1994), Chromogenic print. Jo Spence Memorial Archive, Ryerson Image Centre (AG03.2010.5002:0002).

Wilke and Spence reflect the changes in breast cancer images in the late twentieth-century western world. Indeed, their works serve as a perfect foil to Thomas Eakins' late nineteenth-century *Agnew Clinic*, where men and medicine are highlighted and the patient with breast cancer is reduced to a young, faceless woman with one healthy breast exposed and diseased breast hidden. In *Mammographies: The Cultural Discourses of Breast Cancer Narratives*, Mary K. DeShazer makes a connection between the work of Wilke and Spence in their ability to find pleasure and power in challenging both misogyny and medicalization in their cancer photographs, as they unflinchingly expose diseased breasts, whether the art world was ready for it or not (93).

Wilke and Spence set the stage for early twenty-first-century women and artists to continue to reclaim the conversation about the experience of breast cancer by interpreting their own journey through images and text. The following section presents an interesting study of how one woman, British poet Clare Best, used the creative arts to share her personal story in the first two decades of the twenty-first century, a time of corporatization (e.g., Susan G. Komen Breast Cancer Foundation), commercialization (e.g., a sea of pink merchandise for "Pinktober," breast cancer awareness month) and, some might argue, trivialization (e.g., "Save the Boobies" signs and incessant pink tutus) of breast cancer.

Best first confronted breast cancer as a teenager when her mother was diagnosed in 1972 and then again in 1977, resulting in two radical mastectomies. She makes it clear that her multimedia project, *Breastless* (2007–17), is a response to the shame and powerlessness her mother experienced in the 1970s. Best recalled that at the time, all cancers were taboo, but it was even more difficult with cancer of the breast, the organ so closely associated with feminine identity and sexuality. (Best, *Breastless,* This body is yours, this body is mine) Best shared that in all her years of adult friendship with and nursing of her mother, her mother allowed Clare to see her breasts only two or three times; she was too ashamed to let her daughter see the scarring which was "brutal, purple and puckered in terrible ridges under the arms" (Bolaki 10–1). Best grew up with an intense awareness of the danger in her own maturing body. Her aunt and cousin were also diagnosed with breast cancer, and she felt the anxiety that came with her twice-a-year screenings. After her cousin died from the disease, Best looked into prophylactic methods for beating her genetic odds, as her doctors gave her 50–85 percent chance of getting breast cancer. She ultimately made the difficult decision to have an elective double mastectomy, acknowledging the "strangeness" of the decision while at the same time recognizing that she was taking control of her body to disrupt the cycle of anxiety that surrounded her health (Bolaki 6). Best described her family's and friends' responses to her choice as varied and including horror and fear. Best's choice for elective surgery was also clinically controversial, with some casting her as "a pawn of statistical rhetoric" and other recognizing her "empowered decision to prevent an almost certain destiny" (Bolaki 1).

As Best began to prepare for her surgery, she was shown pictures of different types of reconstructed breasts. When she asked, "What would I look like with a totally flat chest?" she was met with silence; no one could show her a picture of a woman who had chosen not to reconstruct after a bilateral mastectomy. Best writes that *Breastless,* which includes photographs, body casts, poetry, journals and a short film, aims to answer that question for other women. She considers *Breastless* to be a creative and informative source for both patients and doctors – one that contributes to ongoing discussions about options for breast cancer prevention, treatment and reconstruction. (Best, *Breastless*: Introduction) Contemplating her choice to remain "flat" after surgery, Best stated, "I unconsciously took a major step towards liberating myself from dwelling in the expected body, the body that in some ways had belonged to others – parents, friends, peers, lovers, born and unborn children. Even doctors." (Best, *Breastless*, This body is yours, this body is mine)

Best collaborated with a photographer to create a visual record of her body and her journey before and after surgery. She also made "before" and "after" casts of her chest, which she incorporated into her multimedia project. In Figure 12 (2008), photographer Laura Stevens captures Best eighteen months post-operation: Scars of her double mastectomy have healed into soft, silken lines on her chest, and she holds the cast of the breasts that have been removed. They are preserved and they are a part of her story, but they are no longer dangerous. Stevens captures joy in this image: Best smiles as she regains power over her body and her health. Indeed, this image provides a visual counterpoint to the expectations and assumptions she experienced as a patient, noted in her poem "Breast care nurse":

Milestones in the Depiction of Breasts and Breast Cancer 361

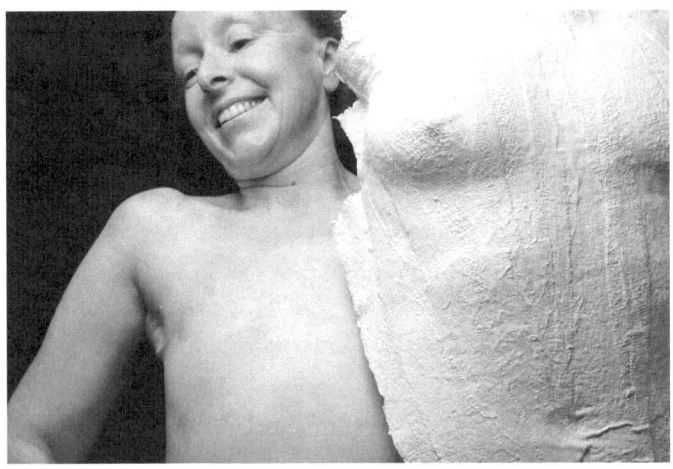

Figure 12: Clare Best photographed by Laura Stevens, from *Breastless – Encounters with risk-reducing surgery: Photographs Part Four*, 2007.

>She whistles in--flat shoes, primary colours,
>wide smile:
>*Remember to take some softies when you leave--*
>*use them as soon as your wounds are closed,*
>*wear them with a comfy bra, baggy top,*
>*nobody'll guess. Then call and make a date*
>*for silicone ones, any size you fancy, they'll look good*
>*under a T-shirt or vest. Try different brands*
>*till you find what suits--so many kinds,*
>*even stick-ons for nights.*
>I want to tell her
>I am my own woman-warrior,
>heart just under the surface. I let go of pretence
>weeks before the surgeon drew
>his blue arrows on my chest.
>(Best, *Breastless, Self-portrait Without Breasts*)

Best's cycle of poems on the subject, "Self-portrait Without Breasts," first published in full in *Excisions*, Waterloo Press 2011, and then included in the full *Breastless* project, is richly illustrated with historical references to lost breasts – from the martyred St. Agatha to the female Amazon warriors so feared and despised by the Greeks. In the opening stanza of "Amazons," Best identifies with these women who choose to remove a breast for increased power and strength: "We are warriors, women marked by a lack of breast–– / bows crafted from elm, sinew and bone, / axes double-edged."

Best repurposed her "after" cast, covering the newly flattened chest with collaged snippets of text from popular magazines that range from the humorous ("I risked my life for new boobs – would you?" and "The one that got away") to the more thought-provoking ("Would you buy an umbrella if it didn't keep you dry?" and "How to stay alive") (Figure 13). In taking a cast – rich in art historical tradition for the study of the ideal body – and juxtaposing modern headlines that span the ridiculous to the profound, it feels in some way that Best is giving us a frank and honest view of the jumble of perceptions, worries and mirth that occupied her mind and body throughout this journey.

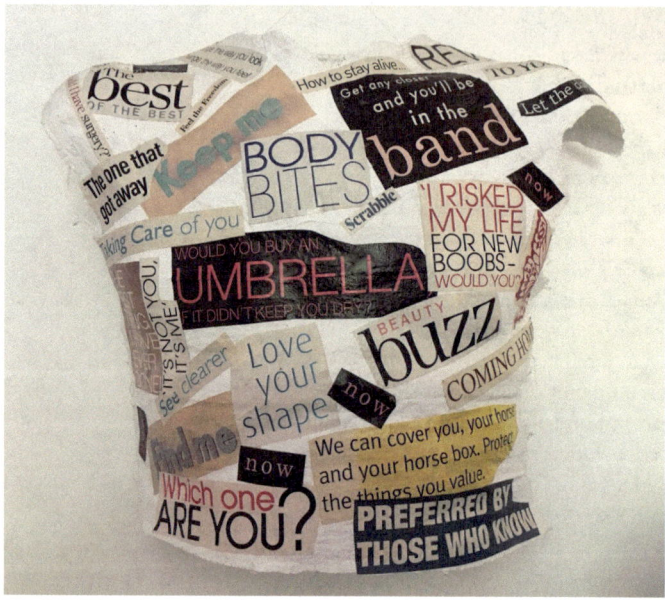

Figure 13: *Collaged body cast* by Clare Best from *Breastless – Encounters with risk-reducing surgery: Various selves*, 2017.

In a 2017 interview, Louise Kenward asked Best if this project served as an antidote to her mother's shame and powerlessness. Best replied that her mother's experience "was all about covering things up," while hers had "been about stripping away those coverings." She noted that when she began to read her poems in public, she realized that she had become a voice for the women in her family (Kenward). In *Breastless,* Best extends this voice and the experience of her body to all women who need it, stating, "I bring my body to the page, to this project, and it is at once both mine and yours. Here, it belongs to everybody and to nobody. My body and I have things to say, stories to tell." (Best, *Breastless,* This body is yours, this body is mine)

A common theme in postmodern examples of breast cancer in art is the need to open up visually and verbally, to share, to create, but most of all, to not be silent. Note the shift from prior examples in art history: These works are no longer a male artist's perspective on breast cancer; these are individual women documenting their individual experiences with the disease. Women make the clinical decisions relevant to their body, and they decide how to depict their body and the illness. In short, women are the subject – not the object – of their story, and they share their art, their voices and their stories for the other women who will come after them – for those who need it.

Conclusion

In the Renaissance, Michelangelo's *Night* is not seen primarily as the depiction of an individual woman suffering from breast cancer, but as just another layer of symbolism representing the inevitable end of life on earth. In the Baroque period, Rembrandt's *Bathsheba at Her Bath* tells a more personal story of breast disease but one nonetheless told from the (male) artist's perspective, not from his lover's point of view. Under the guise of nineteenth-century Realism, Thomas Eakins painted breast cancer surgery in *The Agnew Clinic* primarily to honor Dr. Agnew and to showcase his own skills as a painter. The nameless, faceless woman who is having the surgery is not important; she is not even secondary in the long list of recognizable physicians, students and nurse depicted in the image. By the late twentieth century, dramatic social and cultural changes and a consciousness engendered by feminism brought us artists like Hannah Wilke and Jo Spence who not only reclaimed from centuries of male-dominated representation the female body in art, but also depicted breast cancer assertively from a woman's point of view, unflinchingly showing the ravages of the breast cancer and surgery. Clare Best's more recent multimedia project demonstrates her desire to respond, document and share her own experience with breast cancer. Just as Jo Spence provided laminated copies of her breast cancer photographs to share with local libraries, Best chose to publish her project online, thus making it public, free and available to all. In doing so, Best carries on the tradition of postmodern artists who strive to remove the veil of silence and shame for women dealing with breast cancer, offering creative outlets and options that simply did not exist for women generations before them.

Inspired by Donna Haraway's idea that bodies "are like time-slices" that reveal stories of an era (73) and Rosemary Betterton's assertion that cultural production is a form of knowledge that can offer a deeper understanding of the body (9), I have traced this path of images throughout art history to shed light on the shifting power narratives of women's breasts. Analyzing selected works from prehistoric to postmodern periods, I have demonstrated that images of women's breasts, both healthy and sick, have consistently elucidated the social, political and medical histories of their era. Perhaps more importantly, these images of women's breasts also serve as visual reminders of the fluctuations of women's abilities, agency and authority over time. Understanding positions of power becomes more important and complex when looking at images of women and illness. In the end, two critical questions remain: Whose story is being told? Who has the power to tell it?

Bibliography

Adams, Ann Jensen. *Rembrandt's Bathsheba Reading King David's Letter.* Cambridge: Cambridge University Press, 1998.
Agnew, D. Hayes. *Principles and Practice of Surgery.* Philadelphia: J. B. Lippincott & Co., 1883.
Barker, Clyde F. "The Jayne Lecture: Thomas Eakins and His Medical Clinics." *Proceedings of the American Philosophical Society* 153.1 (March 2009): 1–47.
Best, Clare. *Breastless.* Brighton: Pighog Press. 2011.
———. Breastless (2007–2017) <https://reframe.sussex.ac.uk/lifewritingprojects/body/breastless-encounters-with-risk-reducing-surgery-by-clare-best/>. Accessed February 15, 2020.
———. *Excisions.* Hove: Waterloo Press. 2011.
Betterton, Rosemary. *An Intimate Distance: Women, Art, and the Body.* New York: Routledge, 1996.
Bianucci, R., A. Perciaccante, P. Charlier, et al. "Earliest Evidence of Malignant Breast Cancer in Renaissance Paintings." *The Lancet Oncology* 19 (February 2018): 166–7.
The Bible. Authorized King James Version, Oxford: Oxford University Press, 1998.
Bolaki, Stella. "The Absence Doubled? Photo Narratives of Prophylactic Mastectomy." *Literature and Medicine* 35.1 (Spring 2017): 1–26.
Bourne, R. G. "Did Rembrandt's Bathsheba Really Have Breast Cancer?" *Australian and New Zealand Journal of Surgery* 70.3 (2000): 231–2.
Braithwaite, P. A., and D. Shugg. "Rembrandt's Bathsheba: The Dark Shadow of the Left Breast." *Annals of the Royal College of Surgeons of England* 65 (1983): 337–8.
Canaday, John. "Thomas Eakins: Familiar Rruths in Clear and Beautiful Language." *Horizon* 6.4 (Autumn 1964): 88–105.
Carroll, Margaret D. "Uriah's Gaze." *Rembrandt's Bathsheba Reading King David's Letter.* Ed. Ann Jenson Adams. Cambridge: Cambridge University Press, 1998. 159–75.
Cheney, Liana De Girolami. "The Cult of Saint Agatha." *Woman's Art Journal* 17.1 (Spring-Summer 1996): 3–9.
DeShazer, Mary K. *Mammographies, the Cultural Discourses of Breast Cancer Narratives.* Ann Arbor: University of Michigan Press, 2013.

Dymarski, L. U. "The Secret of Rembrandt's Painting Virsavia." *Voprosy. Onkologii* 30 (1984): 90–101.
Easton, Martha. "Saint Agatha and the Sanctification of Sexual Violence." *Studies in Iconography* 16 (1994): 83–118.
Ehrenberg, Margaret. *Women in Prehistory*. Norman: University of Oklahoma Press, 1989.
Ekmektzoglou Konstantinos, A., Theodoros Xanthos, Vasilios German, et al. "Breast Cancer: From the Earliest Times to the End of the 20th Century." *European Journal of Obstetrics & Gynecology and Reproductive Biology* 145 (2009): 3–8.
Goodbody, Bridget L. "'The Present Opprobrium of Surgery:' *The Agnew Clinic* and Nineteenth-Century Representations of Cancerous Female Breasts." *American Art* 8.1 (Winter 1994): 32–51.
Greco, T. "Rembrandt e il cancro della mammella." *Ospedali d'Italia Chirurgia* 22 (1970): 141–4.
Haraway, Donna. "Contested Bodies." *Gender and Expertise*. Ed. Maureen McNeil. London: Free Association Books, 1987. 62–73.
Hartnell, Jack. *Medieval Bodies: Life, Death and Art in the Middle Ages*. London: Profile Books, 2018.
Hayakawa, S., H. Masuda, and N. Nemoto. "Rembrandt's Bathsheba: Possible Lactation Mastitis Following Unsuccessful Pregnancy." *Medical Hypotheses* 66.6 (2006): 1240–2.
The Heilbrunn Timeline. "Marble Statue of Wounded Amazon." <https://www.metmuseum.org/toah/works-of-art/32.11.4/>. Accessed February 15, 2020.
Kemp, Martin. "Medicine in View: Art & Visual Representation." *Western Medicine: An Illustrated History*. Ed. Irvine Louden. Oxford: Oxford University Press, 1997. 1–22.
Kenward, Louise. "Breastless: Reflecting on Creativity in the Face of Surgery." *BMJ Medical Humanities Blog*. (October 3, 2017) <http://blogs.bmj.com/medical-humanities/2017/10/03/breastless-reflecting-on-creativity-in-the-face-of-surgery/>. Accessed February 15, 2020.
Keuls, Eva. *The Reign of the Phallus: Sexual Politics in Ancient Athens*. Berkeley: University of California Press, 1985.
Lubin, David. "Projecting an Image: The Contested Cultural Identity of Thomas Eakins." *The Art Bulletin* 84.3 (September 2002): 510–22.
Nelson, Jonathan Katz and James J. Stark. "The Breasts of *Night*: Michelangelo as Oncologist." *The New England Journal of Medicine* 343.21 (November 23, 2000): 1577–8.
Olson, James. *Bathsheba's Breast: Women, Cancer, & History*. Baltimore: The John Hopkins University Press, 2002.

Park, Katherine. "Medicine and the Renaissance." *Western Medicine: An Illustrated History*. Ed. Irvine Louden. Oxford: Oxford University Press, 1997. 66–79.

Skelly, Julia. "Mas(k/t)ectomies: Losing a Breast (and Hair) in Hanna Wilke's Body Art." *Third Space: A Journal of Feminist Theory* 7.1 (Summer 2007) <http://journals.sfu.ca/thirdspace/index.php/journal/article/view/skelly/48>. Accessed February 15, 2020.

Slatkin, Wendy. *Women Artists in History: From Antiquity to Present*. Upper Saddle River New Jersey: Prentice Hall. 2001.

Smith, Giulia. "Pain, Politics and the Power of Photography." *Wellcome Institute for the History of Medicine*. (August 21, 2019) <https://wellcomecollection.org/articles/XVqudxMAACEAxxLK>. Accessed February 15, 2020.

Tembeck, Tamar. "Selfies of Ill Health: Online Autopathographic Photography and the Dramaturgy of the Everyday." *Social Media + Society* (January–March 2016): 1–11.

Van de Wettering, Ernst. *A Corpus of Rembrandt Paintings VI: Rembrandt Research Project Foundation*. New York: Springer, 2014.

Watlington, Emily. "A Survey of Hannah Wilke's Work Traces Her Engagement with Bodily Vulnerability." *Art in America* (November 21, 2019) <https://www.artnews.com/art-in-america/aia-reviews/hannah-wilke-ronald-feldman-illness-vulnerability-body-1202668693/>. Accessed February 15, 2020.

Yalom, Marilyn. *A History of the Breast*. New York: The Ballantine Publishing Group, 1997.

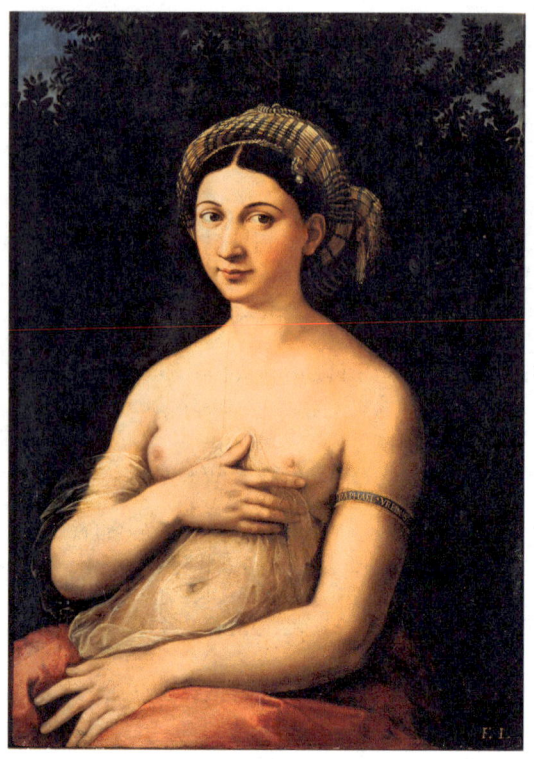

Raphael, *La Fornarina (The Baker Girl),* c.1518, Oil on canvas, 85 × 60 cm. Galleria Nazionale d'Arte Antica, Rome, Italy. Credit: Scala/Art Resource NY.

LISA KATZ

Breast Art

Raphael's *La Fornarina* lives in a Roman palace now,
touching her left breast, holding it between thumb and forefinger
like a fruit she wants to prod in the market.
Perhaps the artist asked her to demonstrate
beckoning a lover
plumping up the smaller breast
showing off in front of the mirror.
You think she's coy.
Perhaps she wanted to touch
the lump she noticed yesterday.
Her eyes look surprised.

MICHAEL BAUM

An Historical Overview of Breast Cancer and Its Treatments

The first time I guessed that something was wrong with my mother was when I noticed her clasping her lower back in pain whilst climbing upstairs in front of me. This was in about 1972 on one of my rare visits home during my period of living in Cardiff, and the image is burnt in my memory as a result of what was to follow.

My mother was extremely stoical and never complained about ill health. Following on my enquiry, she claimed that it was her "rheumatism" playing up. I thought no more about it until about three months later when she was admitted to hospital to have her gall bladder removed because of stones and increasing pain in the region just below the ribs on the right. This was in no way alarming or for that matter surprising, as she fitted the stereotype: female, overweight and over 40. In addition, she was constantly munching antacids for heartburn, presumably due to reflux esophagitis (a condition I inherited with a vengeance), that tends to co-exist with gallstones.

The operation went all right and she did indeed have gallstones; however, in the postoperative phase she developed agonizing pain spreading round from her mid-lumbar region to the upper abdomen. X-rays of her spine showed a crush fracture of the first lumbar vertebra and suspicion of skeletal secondaries from an unsuspected cancer. A rapid and more thorough clinical examination revealed an advanced cancer in her right breast. She was told not to worry as this was only "chronic mastitis," but my father was contacted immediately and told the grim news. My dad then contacted his five children, three of whom were medically qualified, and begged us not to let on to mum that she had cancer that had spread round the body. To my lasting shame, I concurred with this charade, even as she began treatment. Opiates were the only way of controlling her pain in the short term, although radiotherapy to the spine provided more lasting benefit. The chemotherapy was harsh, causing nausea, vomiting, fatigue and the permanent loss of her long, glossy black hair. I was not aware of any benefit from this cruel cocktail.

After about twelve months, the pains started up again and became more and more difficult to control. It reached the point when, according to erroneous belief at the time – that adequate analgesia would suppress her breathing and accelerate her demise – escalating doses of opiates were denied her. At this point the family gathered in London and my opinion was sought. I couldn't bear the sight of her in pain and yet the Jewish teaching was clear on this point: As life is of infinite worth and as you cannot split infinity, then every moment of life is of equal value. She therefore continued to suffer until neither she nor the family could take any more, and she died within six hours of a dose of morphine that adequately controlled her pain. It was my thirty-seventh birthday, May 31, 1974.

The Jewish tradition has it that the dead must be buried within twenty-four hours and until then the body must not be left alone. I spent the nightlong vigil with my father and had plenty of time to confront my conscience, firstly for not having done enough to help control her pain and secondly for not initially having been honest about her diagnosis.

One evening, twenty years after my mother's death, I received a phone call from my sister Linda, then aged 48. She explained that she had just noticed a lump in her right breast. Her general practitioner (GP) had referred her to the local surgeon, who had reassured her but arranged for a biopsy in about two months' time. By then I was Professor of surgery at the Royal Marsden Hospital in London, the most prestigious specialist cancer center in the UK. I swallowed hard and suggested that she get a second opinion from Mr. Nigel Sacks, a man I trusted because, as his student, I had witnessed his care and skill firsthand. It has to be understood that I couldn't examine my own sister or trust my own judgment, in part out of decorum and in part out of emotional involvement.

Mr. Sacks saw her the next day and completed the "triple assessment": clinical examination, X-rays and a needle biopsy. Within the hour her cancer was diagnosed. Within the week she had surgery that consisted of a lumpectomy and partial excision of the lymph nodes in her right axilla.

She was home in two days and, happily, the pathology was favorable. The margins of excision were clear of disease, the tumor was low-grade and hormone receptor-positive, and the lymph nodes were declared free of malignant deposits. She was started on tamoxifen, which she took without side effects for five years and underwent a six-week course of radiotherapy to the breast. She remained well and symptom-free for twenty-five years but then developed bone metastases six months ago. I'm happy that she has responded well to treatment and is once again symptom-free and full of energy.

Without wishing to over-dramatize the case, I feel that to some extent I've expunged a little of the guilt I felt over my failure to help my mother. I transferred my sister's care to a top specialist and expedited her diagnosis and treatment. Most of all, I have to take some satisfaction in having led the team that first demonstrated that the drug tamoxifen could prolong progression-free survival.

Two years ago Linda's oldest daughter came to see me for advice. I'm sure she wouldn't mind my describing her as theatrical in all senses of the word, but on this occasion I felt that her anxieties were legitimate. Her mother and grandmother had had breast cancer, and the circumstances of her great grandmother's death also gave rise to concern. In addition, we are of Ashkenazi extraction. All this hinted at the possibility of a germ-line mutation in the BRCA gene pool which, if present, could lead to an 80 percent lifetime chance of developing breast cancer. I referred her on to my friend Ros Eeles, a leading cancer geneticist at the Royal Marsden Hospital, who agreed that the family pedigree did suggest a risk of carrying a breast cancer predisposition gene. With counseling and agreement from the whole family, my sister was tested for the "Ashkenazi" mutations on BRCA 1 and BRCA2. To everyone's relief, Linda was not found to be a carrier.

This story of three generations of my family encapsulates the evolving story of progress in the fight against breast cancer over the forty years since I got involved in the campaign. My mother was too ignorant and/or modest to be aware of the disease. Cancer, the "big C," was not talked about and was considered almost a stigma, similar to "a spot on the lung," the euphemism for tuberculosis. Euphemisms for breast cancer were legion, including "chronic mastitis," "neoplasia," "mitotic lesions" and, at worst, a "tumor," which literally means nothing more than a swelling. As a result of all this dissembling, most cancers presented in a late stage, either already inoperable or with overt distant spread (metastases). Even if operable, the surgery would be a mutilating Halsted radical mastectomy. With no malice intended, women were considered too emotionally fragile to handle the truth, so the diagnosis and treatment were discussed with the husband and sons. (I still encounter this cultural mindset with some of my private patients from Pakistan, Saudi Arabia and the Gulf states). Additionally, palliative care and symptom control were poorly developed, and patients suffered unnecessarily. The myth that adequate opiate analgesia shortens life has now been exploded; in fact, the opposite is true. Too little and too late has been replaced by adequate and in good time.

By the time my sister presented with breast cancer, the subject was no longer stigmatized, and breast cancer awareness campaigns were making their mark. Diagnosis was available in a "one-stop shop" within the hour, matching "Kwikfit" car exhaust replacement for efficiency. Now, in most cases surgery can provide breast conservation with a decent cosmetic outcome without compromising the chance of cure; and adjuvant systemic therapy can prolong life or even provide a cure. The development of clinical nurse specialists and the subject of psychosocial oncology have enhanced quality of life, and the developments in palliative care and the hospice movement have improved the "quality of dying."

The experience with my niece provides a pointer to the future. The genetic code for the rare familial predisposition to breast cancer has been cracked. The mechanism that explains why a faulty gene can lead to cancer is understood, and opportunities for prevention are opening up. Within a few years I expect the genetic explanation for sporadic breast cancers will be understood and, along with that, smart ways of preventing the disease will be discovered. In the immediate future we can expect more effective systemic therapy tailored to the individual cancer with specific molecular targets in its aim. Tamoxifen, the gold standard for thirty years for postmenopausal women, has been replaced by a new class of compound (the aromatase inhibitors) that are not only more effective but carry fewer side effects. However, although promising in theory and in animal experiments, "personalized medicine" has yet to live up to its promise.

Looking Back to Look Forward: A Brief History of Breast Cancer and Its Treatments

Each October is designated as breast cancer awareness month. This annual event involves an intense campaign using billboards, leaflets and the sale of pink promotional ribbons and wristbands to persuade women to be alert to changes in the texture or contour of their breasts, possible early indications of breast cancer. The unspoken assumption is that if women "catch it early" they will save their breast and save their life. If only it were that simple! As the American humorist H. L. Menken once put it, "For every complex problem there is a simple solution, and it's wrong."

It is not the object of this essay to dissuade women from being breast-aware in the conventional sense, but to open up the subject in such a way as to teach women – and for that matter men – about the extraordinary complexity of the disease, its extraordinary history and the extraordinary progress we have made in our understanding that has led to the dramatic decline in breast cancer mortality in the United Kingdom that has nothing to do with "catching it early." To achieve this understanding, it is necessary for the lay person to join me first on a journey from the time of the Ancient Egyptians to the present in order to learn how false assumptions about the nature of breast cancer gave rise to cruel and futile interventions that added to the sum of human suffering. Next, it is necessary to try and understand the "natural history" of the disease – that is, what would happen if cancer were left to its own devices. It is also imperative to understand the exquisite mechanisms by which normal human tissue maintains its anatomical and functional integrity, in order to understand what goes wrong during malignant transformation. Only with this understanding at the cellular and molecular level can we start putting things right with rational biological approaches that started paying dividends from the mid-1980s and have led me to believe that we are at a crossroads in the history of the subject. In order to make deaths from breast cancer a thing of the past, we need the collaboration of the lay public to join in clinical trials and to keep faith with the scientific process.

Ancient Egypt

A few years ago one of my brightest medical students joined my tutorial almost breathless with excitement, knowing my interest in breast cancer and the history of medicine. She had recently returned from an elective attachment in Egypt and had taken the opportunity of visiting the temples at Karnak. There she noted and photographed a low-relief statue of a woman who appeared to have only one breast. This find convinced her that the ancient Egyptian woman must have undergone a mastectomy for breast cancer. I do everything in my power to maintain the enthusiasm and powers of observation of my students but on this occasion, with much regret, I had to inform her that she was wrong. In what follows I provide snapshots of theories and practices that serve as milestones to trace the evolution of thinking about and treating breast cancer. I invite the lay person to join me on a journey from the time of the Ancient Egyptians to the present in order to learn how false assumptions about the nature of breast cancer gave rise to cruel and futile interventions that added to the sum of human suffering.

We actually have documentary evidence that the ancient Egyptians recognized breast cancer but specifically counseled against mastectomy:

> If thou examinest a man/woman having bulging tumours of his/her breast and thou findest that the swellings have spread over his/her breast; if thou puttest thy hand upon his/her breast upon these tumours, and thou findest them very cool, there being no fever at all herein when thy hand touches him/her; they have no granulations, they form no fluid, they do not generate secretions of fluid and they are bulging to thy hand, thou shouldst say concerning him/her, there is no treatment. (Breasted 403–6)

This translation of the Edwin Smith surgical papyrus (3000 BCE – 2500 BCE), by J. H. Breasted, was published in 1930, and the papyrus itself can be seen in the Chicago Institute of Art. Perhaps this the first example of breast cancer awareness.

Many scholars have suggested that the ancient Egyptians are here distinguishing breast cancer from inflammatory mastitis. I would go further and suggest that having excluded inflammation, lactational mastitis and cysts, the ancient Egyptian has defined a new class of disease that only gets worse with surgical interference. As the swelling described has spread over the breast, the writer must be describing locally advanced breast cancer. We have learnt to our cost that in this stage of the disease, surgery makes things worse. The wisdom of this ancient was lost for over 4000 years as generations of surgeons and physicians made futile attempts to cure advanced breast cancer with unimaginably cruel consequences. Apart from describing breast cancer, this papyrus was perhaps the first expression of the old medical maxim, "There are many conditions that you cannot help, but there are none you cannot make worse."

The Greco-Roman period

Around 400 BC, Hippocrates, the great-grandfather of modern medicine, went even further when he wrote, "It is better to give no treatment in cases of hidden cancer (referring to non-ulcerating breast cancer); treatment causes speedy death, but to omit treatment is to prolong life." *Primum non nocere.* [First do no harm.] Hippocrates went on to develop his ideas concerning the "natural humors" (fluids) of the body and to suggest that cancer, like most other disease processes, resulted from an imbalance of these humors; but as far as I can judge, he never described how these humoral imbalances could be corrected to the advantage of patients with breast cancer.

Perhaps at this point a short digression is necessary to explain the concept of the natural humors promoted by Aristotle and Hippocrates that were central to medical beliefs right up until the early nineteenth century – and have enjoyed a return to fashion as "ancient wisdom" in the promotion of alternative medicine. Central to the Hippocratic teachings was the belief that health was a state of equilibrium and sickness the result of an imbalance of bodily fluids or "humors." At that time, these fluids were linked to the four elements (blood/air, yellow bile/fire, black bile/earth, phlegm/water), but these connections were entirely metaphysical: They bear no relation to what we recognize today as blood, bile and phlegm. (The fourth, "black bile," has no modern equivalent.) The humors were also linked to the personality of the patient, utilizing descriptive terms that are still in use: "sanguine," "choleric," "melancholic" and "phlegmatic." Blood made the body hot and wet (e.g., fever), choler made the body hot and dry (e.g., eczema), phlegm cold and wet (e.g., tuberculosis) and black bile cold and dry (e.g., cancer). Diagnosis for the balance of the humors was made by examining the patient's urine, held up to the light, and by noting the volume of her pulse.

It is interesting to note that women with breast cancer were said to be of a melancholic type because they were often depressed – another condition attributed to an excess of black bile. Of course, this was an early example of confusion in the direction of causality. In other words, depression doesn't cause breast cancer, but the disease can make women depressed.

Approximately 400 years after Hippocrates, during the flowering of the Greco/Roman period of medicine, Celsus made what was likely the first attempt to describe, classify and stage carcinoma of the breast. He suggested four stages, (1) Early malignancy (2) Cancer without ulcer (3) Ulcerating cancer and (4) Fungating (literally looking like a fungus) cancer (Retief and Cilliers 514). In contrast to the teachings of Hippocrates, Celsus felt that treatment, although contraindicated in the three late stages, might be of some value in the earliest stage – though what treatment he had in mind remains obscure. In approximately 200 AD, Galen, who studied in Alexandria and practiced in Rome, became the most influential physician of the then-known world. He extended the Hippocratic humoral theory of disease and taught that cancer was related to the accumulation of an excess of black bile (melancholia) that coagulated in the breast. He supported this view by postulating that women's bodies clear black bile during their monthly periods and therefore, after menopause, they are no longer cleansed. This conveniently explained the increasing incidence of breast cancer amongst women in their fifth and sixth decades. If such were the case, it would appear logical to cleanse the women again by repeated purgation and bleeding, coupled with diets with a low capacity of producing black bile. Although breast cancer was considered a systemic disorder, it didn't stop physicians and proto-surgeons from using topical applications for ulcers, and breast amputation for the smaller tumors. It is darkly comic to read how those ancient surgeons who hazarded amputation of the breast were encouraged not to stop the bleeding. So rapidly did Galen's teachings become orthodoxy that for almost 1200 years no one dared challenge his doctrine. The dark ages must have been very dark indeed for women with breast cancer.

The Renaissance

The Renaissance is usually remembered as the rebirth of interest in the arts and culture of ancient Greece. This newfound freedom of enquiry encouraged developments in anatomy and pathology but at the same time led to some bizarre and infertile pathways in the treatment of cancer. For example, Ambrose Paré (1510–90), the great French military surgeon, advised women against gossip in order to avoid breast cancer and recommended treating ulcerated cancer with puppy dogs or kittens freshly split into two with the warm viscera applied to the lesion. However, to his credit he did recognize that swelling of the lymph glands in the armpit was a bad sign and advocated the use of ligatures (stitches) to staunch the bleeding after surgery to remove the breast. (Mastectomy in those days was a simple guillotine amputation with cautery – using red hot irons, to control the hemorrhage.) Wilhelm Fabry (1565–1634) also known as Fabricius, who practiced in Germany, believed that cancer was caused by milk curdling in the breast (De Moulin 18).

Gabriele Falloppio (1523–62), professor of anatomy and surgery at Padua, modified Galen's humoral theory and introduced a non-natural bile which was a combustion product of other humors. He suggested that cancers consisted of a blend of blood and "burnt" melancholic humor with the degree of malignancy related to the relative proportions of these two substances. He was the first to describe fixation of the tumor to the underlying pectoral muscles of advanced breast cancer and used this physical sign as evidence of inoperability. Unfortunately, he persisted in advising bloodletting (venesection) to rid the body of burnt black bile.

The seventeenth and eighteenth centuries

By the seventeenth century, the influence of the humoral theory of cancer began to wane in favor of particular theories of disease due to mechanical defects or hydrodynamic processes. These attitudes were no doubt brought about by William Harvey's description of the circulation of the blood in 1628, together with the adoption of the Cartesian view of the body as a perfect machine. Thomas Bartholin (1616–80) first described the lymphatic system, allowing both humoral and mechanical theories of cancer to coexist. The tumors, it was suggested, were clotted tissue fluid (lymph) resulting from blockage of lymphatic vessels. Perhaps the most important development of this period that would in time allow a revolutionary approach to the understanding of cancer was the description of the first microscope by Antonie van Leeuwenhoek (1632–1723). With greater and greater powers of magnification, the cellular nature of human organs could be studied, and ultimately the cells forming cancers could be distinguished from normal healthy tissues. This is but one example in the history of science where the invention of an instrument that extended the human powers of observation also extended the human capacity for the generation of hypotheses.

During this time physicians were also speculating about psychological trauma and contagion as causes of cancer, whilst still not capable of understanding how the patients died of secondary spread (metastases). For example, Nicholaes Tulp (1593–1674), the famous Dutch anatomist and surgeon, believed that patients died from autointoxication from their ulcerated cancers. As a result of being called to treat both mistress and servant of the same household for cancer of the breast, Tulp was also responsible for the single anecdote that convinced generations of doctors that breast cancer was a contagious disease.

In the early eighteenth century cancer was still considered a combination of local (breast) and general (systemic) causes. The local causes included trauma, tight clothes and curdled milk, whilst the systemic factors were related to blood components – for example, "yellow bile" from serum; "phlegm" from stagnant serum; "black bile," the clot of extruded red blood cells and *materia phlogistica*, the component of blood thought to develop into pus. Most physicians favored the theory that malignancy resulted from *materia phlogistica* that coagulated internally. Other theories about cancer's etiology abounded, including ingestion of poisons, excess of acidity or alkalinity in the blood, bad diet and failure to bear children (nulliparity). Nulliparity is recognized as a risk factor to this day and was first described by Ambrose Paré, who noted a high incidence of the disease amongst the nuns in a convent he attended.

Perhaps the two most important conceptual advances of this period can be attributed to the French surgeons Le Dran (1685–1770) and Petit (1674–1750), who explained the nature of metastases as either blood born (hematogenous) or lymphatic spread of the disease to the armpit (axilla) and distant organs. Unfortunately, treatment still lagged far behind conceptual advances: guillotine amputation in rare cases of early disease; and disgusting topical applications, diet, purgation and bleeding for most other cases. However, for the first time we can see the adumbration of the controversy of conservative versus radical surgery that was to dominate the debate in the mid-twentieth century, when William Cheseldon of St. George's Hospital London (1688–1752) started advocating just the removal of the malignant lump (lumpectomy) whilst Louis Petit of Paris was advocating the more radical approach of total mastectomy.

The nineteenth century

Perhaps there is no better way of entering the nineteenth century than by quoting from the diary of Fanny Burney, a noted authoress and diarist of that time, with an entry from the year 1811:

I mounted the bed stead, he placed me upon the mattress and spread a cambric handkerchief upon my face. It was transparent however and I saw through it, that the bed stead was instantly surrounded by seven men and my nurse. Through the cambric I saw the hand held up while his forefinger first described a straight line from top to bottom of the heart, secondly a cross and thirdly a circle; intimating that the whole was to be taken off.

When the dreadful steel was plunged into the heart cutting through veins-arteries-nerves, I needed no injunctions not to restrain my cries. I began a scream that lasted during the while time of the incision and marvel that it rings not in my ears still.

When the wound was made and the instrument withdrawn the pain seemed undiminished, for the air that suddenly rushed into those delicate parts felt like sharp and forked poniards that were tearing the edges of the wound.

Again, I felt the instrument describing a curve cutting against the grain, while the flesh resisted in a manner so forcible to oppose and tire the hand of the operator. I concluded the operation over. Oh No! The terrible cutting was renewed and worse than ever. I felt the knife crackling against the breastbone- scraping it! To conclude, the evil was so profound that the operation lasted twenty minutes. (Burney)

Thus was the experience of a mastectomy before the days of anesthetics, so it can easily be understood that the majority of women kept away from surgeons and favored folk remedies.

At the same time the medical establishment were asking themselves some very pertinent questions about the nature of cancer. In 1802 a meeting took place in Edinburgh at which a committee of anatomists and surgeons discussed the question, whether cancer be regarded at any period or under any circumstances merely as a local disease or, by contrast, whether the existence of a clinically detected primary cancer signals the existence of distant disease that is merely occult at the time of diagnosis. The result of their deliberations was published in July 1806 in the *Edinburgh Medical and Surgical Journal* and, to some extent, foreshadowed the debate that started in the 1950s. In spite of all these esoteric ruminations, breast cancer was, by now, assumed to be a localized disease requiring radical extirpation if cure was to be attempted. A beautiful and heart-breaking description of James Syme (Professor of Surgery in Glasgow and Lord Lister's father-in-law) performing a mastectomy in 1830, appears in the story "Rab and His Friends," by John Brown:

> The operating theatre is crowded; much talk and fun, and all the cordiality and stir of youth. The surgeon with his staff of assistants is there. In comes Ailie: one look at her quiets and abates the eager students. That beautiful old woman is too much for them; they sit down, and are dumb, and gaze at her. These rough boys feel the power of her presence. She walks in quickly, but without haste; dressed in her mutch, her neckerchief, her white dimity short-gown, her black bombazine petticoat, showing her white worsted stockings and her carpet shoes. Behind her was James and Rab. James sat down in the distance, and took that huge and noble head between his knees. Rab looked perplexed and dangerous; forever cocking his ear and dropping it as fast. Ailie stepped up on a seat, and laid herself on the table, as her friend the surgeon told her; arranged herself, gave a rapid look at James, shut her eyes, rested herself on me, and took my hand. The operation was at once begun; it was necessarily slow; and chloroform - one of God's best gifts to his suffering children - was then unknown. The surgeon did his work. The pale face showed its pain, but was still and silent. Rab's soul was working within him; he saw that something strange was going on, - blood flowing from his mistress, and she suffering; his ragged ear was up, and importunate; he growled and gave now and then a sharp impatient yelp; he would have liked to have done something to that man. But James had him firm, and gave him a glower from time to time, and an intimation of a possible kick; all the better for James, it kept his eye and his mind off Ailie. It is over: she is dressed, steps gently and decently down from the table, looks for James; then turning to the surgeon and the students she courtesies, and in a low, clear voice begs their pardon if she has behaved ill. The students – all of us – wept like children; the surgeon happed [sic] her up carefully, and, resting on James and me, Ailie went to her room, Rab following. (Brown 26–8)

The courageous woman survived this procedure only to die of septicemia in the following week. James Syme could hardly be blamed for this outcome in the era before Lister's revolutionary discoveries led to the development of antiseptic techniques. Indeed, Syme is to be credited as the first to make the association between involved axillary nodes and the systemic nature of the disease. In 1842 he wrote, "The result of operations for carcinoma when the glands are affected is almost always unsatisfactory however perfectly they may seem to have been taken away. The reason for this is probably that the glands do not take part in the disease unless the system is strongly disposed to it" (Syme 48).

Improvements in the microscope in the mid-nineteenth century furthered the study of the cellular aspects of cancer and laid the foundation of cancer histology as a science. However, problems with the interpretation of artefacts – that is, something observed under the microscope that is not naturally present but occurs as a result of the preparative or investigative procedure – due to the poor preparation of specimens limited progress. It is likely that these artefacts led to the "Blastema" theory of cancer promoted by Karl Rokitansky (1804–78) and Sir James Paget (1814–99). The "Blastema" was considered to be a primitive form of cell seen as a solid amorphous substance under the microscope, capable of giving rise to cancers at any site within the supporting structures of healthy organs. (That is, the Blastema might have been viewed as itself pre-malignant.) This view was attacked by Rudolf Virchow (1821–1902), who suggested that cancers arose from normal cells in reaction to abnormal stimuli – a singularly modern viewpoint.

The late nineteenth century and early twentieth century

The late nineteenth century marked the transformation of surgery by the twin developments of anesthesia and antisepsis. In 1867, twenty years after the first anesthetic (ether) was given by Dr. William Thomas Green Morton in Boston, Massachusetts, a 44-year-old Londoner called Isabella Pim discovered a large lump growing in her breast. She first went to see Sir James Paget of Wimpole Street, but he explained that the dangers of surgery were too great because the cancer was at an advanced stage. Unwilling to accept this advice, she travelled to Edinburgh to see James Syme, her brother's father-in-law, for a second opinion. He also advised that the risks of surgery outweighed the benefits.

Finally, she went to her brother, Joseph Lister, professor of Surgery at the Glasgow Royal Infirmary. Shortly before her visit he had published a series of articles in *The Lancet* that would revolutionize the practice of surgery. In them he had described how he had improved the chances of survival for patients with compound fractures of the bone (that is, fractures where the sharp ends of the broken bone had punctured the skin). Whilst previously about half of such patients would die of hospital diseases, ten out of eleven of Lister's survived. Lister's breakthrough was dependent on a new understanding of the mechanism of infection. Two years earlier, he had read the publications of Louis Pasteur that laid the groundwork for the bacterial theory of postoperative infection. Lister applied these principles to prevent infection in the operating theatre that had resulted from bacterial contamination in the air, on the clothes of the surgeon and on the surgical instruments that were usually covered in a patina of blood and fat from previous patients. A dilute solution of carbolic acid was to be sprayed in the air of the operating theatre, soaked into the lint of dressings and used to clean the scalpel and forceps. When his sister sought his advice, the method had so far been used only to treat abscesses and compound fractures. One can easily imagine Lister's torment. Although he was convinced of his own method, most other surgeons were deeply skeptical. What if his sister died under his knife? How could he then live with his conscience, and what would that do for the future of his experimental technique? So, he too travelled to Edinburgh to consult his father-in-law and mentor James Syme, who gave him the courage to proceed. In the days that followed her mastectomy, the wound did not turn septic.

With the developments of anesthesia and antisepsis, surgeons were at last released from their shackles; provided that blood loss was adequately controlled, almost any surgery outside the chest and skull was possible. Of course, whether it was desirable was another question!

Radical Mastectomy

The development of the classical radical mastectomy in the latter part of the nineteenth century is usually credited to William S. Halsted, of the Johns Hopkins Hospital, Baltimore (Halsted 297), though it must be remembered that the operation was designed on the basis of the pathological teachings of Virchow. Virchow maintained that a cancer spread in continuity from its origin as columns of malignant cells; these passed along the lymphatic channels until they were arrested temporarily in the first group of regional lymph nodes, which were thought to act as filter traps. It was further assumed that when the filtration capacity of these lymph nodes was exhausted, they acted as a focus for tertiary spread to more distant lymph nodes and then via the tissue planes to the skeleton and the vital organs. Halsted even went so far as to suggest that there was no skeletal involvement unless the original cancer had spread to overlying skin; only then would skeletal malignancy occur.

Given these beliefs, it seemed quite reasonable that a radical surgery that included all the lymph channels and their nodes/glands in the axilla, would cure more patients than local amputation of the breast alone. Furthermore, it stood to reason that the operation had to be completed *en bloc* (as a single specimen with tumor, lymphatic channels and lymph glands intact) in order to prevent the spillage of cancer cells into the wound by cutting across lymphatic channels. For a short period in the early 1920s, some surgeons were taking this matter to the logical conclusion and advocating amputation of the arm at the shoulder together with radical clearance of the breast when the disease had spread locally into the upper arm. Though this seems monstrous today, it must be remembered that the extent of surgery advocated in the mid-twentieth century (circa 1940–60) included lifting up the sternum like a trap door and dissecting out the lymph glands that ran down the front of the chest cavity.

Radiotherapy

In 1898 Marie Curie discovered the extraordinary properties of the unstable element radium and was awarded the Nobel Prize for this discovery in 1911. By that time, a primitive form of radiotherapy was already in use for the treatment of breast cancer. Sadly, many of these pioneers, including Marie Curie herself, died of cancer induced by radiation – a double-edged weapon indeed. The research of Marie Curie was to have a lasting effect on the management of breast cancer.

In 1922 Geoffrey Keynes, surgeon at St. Bartholomew's Hospital London, began experimenting with the use of radium enclosed in hollow platinum needles for the treatment of advanced breast cancer. Following on from his experience with advanced disease, he then took the courageous leap of faith and started treating women with early breast cancer with local excision (lumpectomy) and radium needles inserted into the unaffected quadrants of the breast as well as and the axillary and supra-clavicular lymphatic fields. This was considered heresy at the time, yet his results at ten-year follow-up (published in the *British Medical Journal* [BMJ] in 1936) looked as good as anything that the radical mastectomy had to offer. Unfortunately, before he had a chance to popularize his technique, the Second World War broke out, and Sir Geoffrey was called to serve his country as senior surgeon to the Royal Air Force. For safety sake, his radium needles were buried deep underground; and with that, his technique was buried, only to be resurrected some twenty years after VE day.

My early surgical technique

For readers who are curious about earlier surgical conventions, I describe in full detail the technique I mastered forty years ago. (Readers who feel faint at the description of surgery may want to skip this section.)

To begin with, I had to take a skin graft from the inner thigh of the patient so as not to be tempted to compromise on the surgical incision in trying to preserve enough skin to close the wound. This meant using an instrument like an old-fashioned cutthroat razor but much longer, about 30 cm in length. The graft was then wrapped in moist saline gauze and set aside for later.

Moving to the breast, I had to cut an ellipse of skin that included the nipple with at least 3.0 cm of skin in all directions from the palpable margins of the tumor. Don't ask me why 3.0 cm. The history of radical surgery for all cancers is full of exhortations to take odd numbers of centimeters of normal tissue from the margins of the tumor. In retrospect, this seems to have had more to do with the mystique of numerology than science! Next I had to dissect skin flaps North and South so they were thin enough to transmit light like the finest porcelain – this to avoid leaving a single cancer cell behind. Then starting at the clavicle, I would cut down to the chest wall lifting a disc of tissue that incorporated the breast and the pectoralis major muscle, separating it from its origin along the edge of the sternum. This flap containing the breast and underlying muscle was then dissected off the sternum across to the armpit, taking care to control the blood vessels that perforated the muscles between the ribs and fed the breast from the internal mammary artery deep behind the sternum. Incorporated into this pound of flesh were the origins of the pectoralis minor that had to be cut by cautery from its origin over the second to the fifth ribs. All that was easy, although a little bit bloody. (On average two pints of blood loss had to be anticipated by ordering blood from the bank the day before surgery.)

Next came the tricky bit: identifying all the "clock-work" in the armpit (axilla). Starting at the first rib I learnt to identify the axillary vein, above which was the axillary artery – and above that, the cords of the brachial plexus that innervated the muscles of the arm and hand. One false move could lead to semi-paralysis. Following the lower margin along the axillary vein, I had to identify and tie off all the tiny vessels that fed the breast as they disappeared into the fat of the axilla. One false move here might tear a branch coming straight off the axillary vein, which could add another pint to the tally for transfusion. All this fatty tissue that contained the critically important lymph nodes had to be brushed downwards off the muscle walls of the axilla to be incorporated *en bloc* with the whole "specimen."

Proceeding deep in the axilla, I would identify the neurovascular bundle containing the nerve to latissimus dorsi lying on the subscapularis muscle. Damaging that would leave the patient with loss of power in the shoulder movements. Also deep in the axilla but lying on the chest wall would be the "long nerve of Bell," a dainty nerve supplying the serratus anterior, that had to be protected. Damage that and the patient's scapula would disengage from the chest wall on her back every time she tried to push open a door. I would also see the intercostal-brachial nerve adopting its curious bowstring course across the axilla to supply sensation to the under-surface of the arm. I was advised to sacrifice that nerve in the name of a radical cure, leaving the woman with quite disabling numbness and paresthesia. Finally, the skin on at the back of the armpit, was cut through and the "specimen" placed in a bucket for the pathologist to study in macroscopic and microscopic detail.

After all the bleeding was stopped, I would insert two drains and close the wound. If the wound was capable of being sutured together, it meant that I had been insufficiently radical. So, in most cases I closed what I could and covered the saucer-shaped defect with the split skin graft taken at the start. The resulting appearance was grotesque, and lymphedema (swelling of the arm) would inevitably follow as time progressed. Tightly bandaged, the patient was kept in hospital for an average of about ten days. God knows how she felt when the bandages were removed and she viewed this mutilation for the first time.

I've described this procedure in detail to illustrate the starting point of my odyssey as a surgeon. This procedure was "the treatment of choice" (oh how I hate that expression) for breast cancer all round the world until the mid-1970s. Even though I took some pride in my skills as a surgeon, I had a visceral disgust for this Halsted radical mastectomy. The story of its fall from favor is recounted in my other chapter of this book.

A New Approach: Tamoxifen and Aromatase Inhibitors

In 1972–2, my team at the University Hospital of Wales, Cardiff, were amongst the very first to use tamoxifen (known by its commercial name Nolvadex [ICI 46,474] in those days), and we were surprised and delighted at its low toxicity and efficacy. The drug produced durable remissions in about 30 percent of cases, with few side effects. This persuaded us to launch a clinical trial comparing tamoxifen with conventional chemotherapy in cases of advanced breast cancer. The *BMJ* published two papers on the direct comparison of Nolvadex with chemotherapy. In the first paper we showed that chemotherapy produced earlier and greater objective remissions; in the second paper we showed that in the longer term the survival was the same, but that Nolvadex was associated with a better quality of life (QOL). John Forbes, a co-author of these papers, repeated these studies on a much larger scale in Australia, and our original findings were confirmed. There was an important variable missing from our trials, however: knowledge of the estrogen receptor status of the tumors (ER).

To understand the significance of this variable I will have to back up a bit and describe some simple facts about endocrinology. My laboratories were next door to those of Professor Mitch Dowsett, world leader in the field of hormones and breast cancer. He was one of the pioneers in the understanding of the mechanisms of action of tamoxifen. The endocrine system consists of all the glands that produce hormones, including the thyroid that produces thyroxine, the pituitary that produces growth hormone and the ovaries that produce estrogen in premenopausal women. In postmenopausal women estrogens can be detected in the circulation but at levels about ten times lower than in younger women. The origin of estrogens in older women was a mystery until about twenty years ago. In the end it was discovered that the adrenal glands that sit on top of the kidneys and are responsible for producing cortisone, also produce low levels of the male hormone testosterone. This male hormone is then metabolized in the fatty tissue of women via an enzyme known as *aromatase*, to produce estrogen. In turn, estrogen is essential to maintain skeletal health in postmenopausal women.

All target tissues that respond to hormones have a protein in their cells that bind the hormone and present the complex to the DNA within the nucleus. These binding proteins are called receptors, and, for the purpose of this story, we should concentrate on the estrogen receptor (ER) and the progesterone receptor (PgR) that are both involved in the proliferation and function of normal breast epithelial cells. About 80 percent of breast cancer cells retain this mechanism and are referred to as hormone responsive. Hormone responsive breast cancers stop proliferating and start to die if deprived of estrogen. Tamoxifen was developed as an anti-estrogen but had a paradoxical effect of stimulating the ovaries. Professor Mitch Dowsett's work at the Institute of Cancer Research, in London, went some way to explain this in showing that like Janus, the two-faced god of ancient Greece, tamoxifen had both agonist as well as antagonist effects. As far as the breast cancer cells were concerned, the drug acted as an anti-estrogen; but as far as the endometrial cells in the uterus and the osteoblasts in the skeleton, the drug was seen as an agonist (stimulant). This then accounted for two side effects of tamoxifen, one favorable and the other unfavorable, in postmenopausal women. The favorable side effect was the protection of the skeleton from osteoporosis, and the unfavorable was the stimulus of the endometrium that can lead to postmenopausal bleeding and, rarely, endometrial cancer.

By the late 1970s assays (methods of measurement) were becoming available for human tissue to determine whether or not they were estrogen receptive. This led to separating breast cancers into two groups ER+ and ER−. ER+ tumors responded to estrogen: Estrogen "fed" the tumor. The opposite was true for ER− tumors: They had acquired resistance to estrogen. Today, it has become a routine service to classify breast cancers in these two groups in order to offer targeted therapy.

Based on my experience in using tamoxifen in advanced breast cancer and the increasing interest in the biological mechanisms of response involved in hormone therapy for cancer, I wrote a paper advocating adjuvant tamoxifen in the management of the early disease. Inasmuch as breast cancer is systemic (i.e., widespread at the point of diagnosis), it stands to reason that some form of adjuvant (i.e., added, usually after surgery) systemic therapy targeting these putative but occult micro-metastases might favorably influence the natural history of the disease. At the same time Bernie Fisher's group in the USA and Gianni Bonadonna in Milan were embarking on the first trials of adjuvant chemotherapy. I argued that tamoxifen would be less toxic but at the same time might be relevant only in about 30 percent of cases. The design of the trial was simple: Any woman eligible for surgery for early breast cancer would, at random, be placed in a group of women who took twenty milligrams of tamoxifen a day for two years, or in a group of women who did not take tamoxifen regularly but who could do so if they relapsed.

The first patient was recruited in 1977, and 1,200 patients entered the study by 1979. Our first results were published in *The Lancet* in 1983 (Baum 257–61), and I remember thinking they were too good to be true, as they showed a 30 percent relative risk reduction for relapse amongst those taking the drug. Disappointing in retrospect was our failure to demonstrate that the ER status of the tumor could predict an individual's response to tamoxifen. A year or two before this milestone publication, Fisher's group (NSABP) and Bonadonna's group in Italy had reported very promising early results from adjuvant combination chemotherapy. The stage was then set for a battle between the hawks (United States and Italy) and the doves (United Kingdom) that raged for fifteen years and was finally settled when further trials suggested that both groups had a share in the truth. If the patient's tumor was ER+, a combination of both approaches, could improve relapse-free survival by about 50 percent. From a peak in 1985, breast cancer mortality in the UK for both pre- and postmenopausal women started falling rapidly, and about half that benefit could be attributed to tamoxifen.

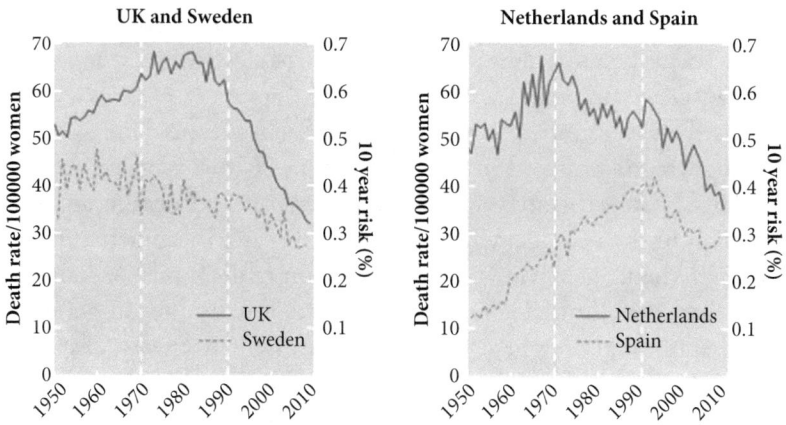

Trends in breast cancer mortality from 1970s until now

Aromatase Inhibitors

Without doubt the most important component of my work in the years 1980–2000 whilst I was working at the Royal Marsden Hospital and Institute of Cancer Research, London, was the development and launching of the ATAC trial (see below). In the meantime, the pharmaceutical industry had developed pure aromatase inhibitors (AIs) that, in theory, could shut down estrogen production completely in the older woman. These drugs were investigated in the lab by Professor Mitch Dowsett, and in the clinic by Professor Trevor Powles. As our labs were close to each other, we shared a coffee room and our conversations strayed to consider the possibility of an AI being superior to tamoxifen as adjuvant therapy for early breast cancer. Early experience with the AIs showed that they were extremely well tolerated and active in the advanced disease. On a train coming back from (I think) Edinburgh after a meeting of the British Breast Group, a number of us that included Joan Houghton, Jeff Tobias, Tony Howell, Mitch and myself, designed the ideal trial on the back of a coffee-stained envelope.

We hawked this idea around the pharmaceutical companies that produced the AIs, and Astra Zeneca (AZ) accepted our ideas with the obvious proviso that we use their drug anastrozole (Arimidex). This involved a great leap of faith, as we had yet no idea if Arimidex was more effective in advanced disease than tamoxifen. The trial involved randomizing postmenopausal women with operable breast cancer to Arimidex (A), Tamoxifen (T) or Arimidex and Tamoxifen Combined (AC) – hence the acronym ATAC. One-third of the women would get A, one-third T, and one-third AT. Astra Zeneca were to provide the drugs free and finance the infrastructure for the Cancer Research Campaign clinical trials unit, but an independent international steering committee would supervise the conduct of the trial and, independent of that, would be a data monitoring and safety committee (DMSC) who had the power to stop the study if there were any suggestion of statistically significant differences in serious adverse events or efficacy between any two of the three arms.

This trial was hugely ambitious, as we were challenging the "gold standard" of cancer treatment for this class of patient. Secondly, we were looking for evidence not only of improved effectiveness in cancer outcomes but also improvements in toxicity and tolerability so that in the end we might draw up a balance sheet of benefits versus harms. We therefore had our statisticians estimate how many patients we needed to recruit in the ATAC trial so that there was only a 10 percent chance of missing a clinically important result (i.e. 90 percent power) whilst also having the power to detect important differences in predetermined toxic side effects. Ultimately our chief of statistics, Professor Jack Cuzick, came up with the sobering news that we would need over 9,000 patients – in other words, over 3,000 patients in each arm of the study. To recruit 9,000 patients within a reasonable time period was a huge and expensive challenge.

Astra Zeneca were well aware that their competitors Novartis and Pfizer were hot on their heels, so they plunged in with a major financial gamble and gave us the green light. With adequate funding we were able to rapidly recruit the staff to support the trial at home and abroad, and I packed my bags to set off on the first of a number of global travels to recruit centers from all round the world for this massive task. It took all my powers of diplomacy to persuade new centers that they were equal stakeholders, and to an extent this was achieved by a publication policy that would recognize everyone's contributions equally. The main publications were to be in the name of the ATAC trialist group with a very long appendix naming all centers and all contributors. In the end we recruited from 381 centers in twenty-one countries, making it the largest collaborative effort in clinical cancer research on record.

We reached our target in about three years and I was able to report our preliminary results at the premier breast cancer event, the San Antonio Breast Cancer Symposium, in 2001. Standing up in front of an expectant audience of about 10,000 of my peers, I thought a little theatre might be in order as I only had ten minutes to put the message across. Five minutes were used up describing the rationale, methodology and statistics of the study. The first "result" slide showed the "life table" curves for recurrence-free survival (i.e., percent of patients in each cohort alive and free of cancer recurrence). As a tease, I showed the curve for tamoxifen – and then after a pause of a second or two, I unfolded the result for anastrozole that was significantly superior. After I sat down, the audience went mad; and I savored the moment that is experienced maybe once in a lifetime by only a minority of scientists. Funnily enough I didn't feel the least bit smug or complacent. In fact, I felt a sense of caution, whilst at the same time remembering the "wounds of battle"

I'd suffered on the road to this point. (These data were published in *The Lancet* in 2002 (ATAC trialist group).

A few more details are needed here to make sense out of a massive set of data. The toxicity profiles of the two drugs, tamoxifen and anastrozole, were strikingly different. Tamoxifen was associated with more gynecological problems that lead to a four-fold excess of hysterectomies and also an increase in the risk of thrombosis (blood clot). Anastrozole was better tolerated in the short term, but its use was associated with an increased risk of osteoporosis and fractures. In addition, the AI patients described an increase in joint pain (polyarthralgia) and vaginal dryness. To put all this into perspective, however, only 7 percent of the patients on anastrozole had to stop taking the drug because of side effects; and the group as a whole enjoyed a 92 percent chance of remaining recurrence-free at five years. Furthermore, the most important side effect of the aromatase inhibitor can be dealt with by avoiding its use in women who are osteoporotic at the time of diagnosis and by monitoring the bone density (BMD) annually in the other women. If the BMD falls, there are a number of agents that can be used (e.g., bisphosphonates) to reverse the trend of bone loss. After all, we don't withhold chemotherapy for fear of a drop in white cell count; we anticipate the event and correct it should it occur.

With further maturation of the data, the American Society of Clinical Oncology changed its guidelines, and Astra Zeneca started enjoying a return on its investment. The most recent results of the ATAC trial, published in 2010, showed a 4.3 percent improvement in recurrence-free survival for Arimidex against the tamoxifen control. [10] Trials of other AIs (Novartis' letrozole and Pfizer's exemestane) have shown similar outcomes and there now remains a turf war concerning whether any one of the three available AIs is superior to the other. Personally, I think it unlikely. Another unresolved issue is whether two years of tamoxifen followed by three years of an AI is superior to five years of an AI, but this is all fine-tuning that follows any scientific breakthrough. As of today, the National Institute of Clinical Excellence in the UK (NICE) recommends that all postmenopausal women with ER+ breast cancers receive an AI as part of their care.

Bibliography

ATAC Trialist Group. "Anastrozole Alone or in Combination with Tamoxifen Versus Tamoxifen Alone for Adjuvant Treatment of Postmenopausal Women with Early Breast Cancer: First Results of the ATAC Randomised Trial." *The Lancet* 359:9324 (2002): 2131–9.

Baum, M., D. M. Brinkley, J. A. Dossett, et al. "Controlled Trial of Tamoxifen as Adjuvant Agent of Early Breast Cancer: Interim Analysis at Four Years by the Nolvadex Adjuvant Trial Organisation (NATO)." *The Lancet* 321:8319 (February 5, 1983): 257–61.

Breasted, J. H. *The Edwin Smith Papyrus.* Chicago: Chicago UP, 1930: 403–06.

Brown, John. "Rab and His Friends." <https://archive.org/details/rabhisfriends00nort/page/26/mode/2up>. Accessed February 15, 2020.

Burney, Frances. "Letter from Frances Burney to Her Sister Esther about Her Mastectomy." <https://www.bl.uk/collection-items/letter-from-frances-burney-to-her-sister-esther-about-her-mastectomy>. Accessed February 15, 2020.

Cuzick, J, I. Sestak, M. Baum, A. Buzdar, A. Howell, M. Dowsett, J. F. Forbes, and ATAC investigators. "Effect of Anastrozole and Tamoxifen as Adjuvant Treatment for Early-Stage Breast Cancer: 10-Year Analysis of the ATAC Trial." *The Lancet Oncology* 11.12 (December 2010): 1135–41.

DeMoulin, Daniel. *A Short History of Breast Cancer.* New York: Springer-Sciences + Business Media, B.V., 1983.

Halsted, W. S. "The Results of Operations for the Cure of Cancer of the Breast Performed at The Johns Hopkins Hospital from June 1889 to January1894." *Johns Hopkins Hospital Report* 4 (1894): 297–350.

Retief, F. P., and L. Cilliers. "Breast Cancer in Antiquity." *South Africa Medical Journal* 101.8 (August 2011): 513–5.

Syme, James. *Observations in Clinical Surgery.* Edinburgh: Edmonston & Douglas, 1862.

HENRY WAGNER

Radiation Therapy: Evolutions in Treatment, Consultations in Clinic

"Each piece, or part, of the whole of nature is always merely an approximation to the complete truth, or the complete truth so far as we know it. In fact, *everything we know is only some kind of approximation*, because *we know that we do not know all the laws* as yet. Therefore, things must be learned only to be unlearned again or, more likely, to be corrected. ... The principle of science, the definition, almost, is the following: *The test of all knowledge is experiment*. Experiment is the sole judge of scientific "truth." But what is the source of knowledge? Where do the laws that are to be tested come from? Experiment, itself, helps to produce these laws, in the sense that it gives us hints. But also needed is *imagination* to create from these hints the great generalizations – to guess at the wonderful, simple, but very strange patterns beneath them all, and then to experiment again to check again whether we have made the right guess." (Feynman 1)

Since I began my training as a radiation oncologist in the late 1970s, I have seen the role of radiation therapy in the management of women with breast cancer undergo dramatic changes in philosophy, clinical application and technology. There is little sense in prescribing a set of policies for its application; rather, it is better to think of radiation therapy as an evolving set of tools to be applied to our best understanding of breast cancer in the context of the individual patient. What does the woman want, and can radiation help her to achieve this goal? I will discuss this perspective in the context of experiences with a number of women I have known over the past several decades, whose experiences with breast cancer have shaped my own beliefs and approach. And while breast cancer afflicts men as well as women, I will focus almost entirely on women who make up more than 90 percent of all breast cancer patients. The technical aspects of radiation therapy for the two are generally similar, the psycho-social aspects perhaps not so much.

The past fifty years have seen sweeping changes in our understanding and treatment of breast cancer, and this is still very much a work in progress. Earlier, treatment of breast cancer had been dominated by a mutilating surgical technique and bad biology. Improvements like breast-conserving therapy (BCT) represent progress, but are also merely a way-station, not a destination.

In the early 1970s, as gap years between my undergraduate years and medical school, I spent two years working in the laboratory of cardiac biochemistry at Massachusetts General Hospital. My advisor, a cardiologist, was the classic triple threat of the time: clinician, laboratory scientist and teacher. One morning I found him to be much more withdrawn than usual, almost depressed, and over coffee he mentioned that he had just found out the day before that his mother-in-law had been diagnosed with a recurrence of breast cancer – more than fifteen years after its initial presentation and treatment with mastectomy. I was amazed, both by his candor in discussing this with me and by the long interval between initial presentation and recurrence. Like many, I had become bewitched by the American Cancer Society's emphasis on Five-Year Survival as tantamount to cure; and the idea of a cancer lying in wait for fifteen years only to return was both puzzling and ominous. How could cancer be both a rapid killer in some cases and an indolent but relentless illness in others?

My next experience with breast cancer came several years later while I was in medical school in the early 1970s. My own mother-in-law was diagnosed with breast cancer on a routine mammogram, and I, being the family medical student, was called on to obtain information about treatment options. At that point I had pretty much decided that I had an interest in oncology but didn't particularly like doing surgery. What I was able to glean from reading textbooks and journals at the time was that the old standard of "radical mastectomy" was being called into question by some surgical oncologists, and that a lesser procedure of "total mastectomy" and radiation to the chest wall was becoming more common. My mother-in-law underwent the newer treatment and did well for ten years, before succumbing to an esophageal cancer that was most likely not related to her prior breast malignancy or to its treatment.

Move four years ahead in my training and I have now firmly decided that I want to be an oncologist and that surgery is not for me. As an intern fresh out of medical school I thought I would become a medical oncologist, caring for patients by, among other things, prescribing chemotherapy. I was intrigued, however, by what was happening to my inpatients who received radiation therapy. They disappeared mysteriously to the basement and emerged several hours later with purple skin marks delineating where they had been targeted with radiation. This was a mysterious process no doubt, but it was surely no worse than injecting them with the poisons of the day. This kind of therapy intrigued me enough that I spent my one-month internship elective in the Radiation Therapy department at the Boston Deaconess Hospital, part of the Joint Center for Radiation Oncology, then chaired by Dr. Samuel Hellman. And after much thought and a year working in a state cancer hospital as a more experienced resident, I decided to specialize in radiation oncology, a subject I had had little exposure to in medical school.

I began my radiation oncology residency in 1978 at Tufts-New England Medical Center and had the opportunity to see the field begin to develop its own scientific identity. We had clearly become separate from diagnostic radiology and were in a hybrid position between surgery, with its clear anatomic approach to the eradication of disease, and medical oncology, which at that time gave drugs systemically and hoped that the kill of abnormal cells would exceed the kill of good cells. Radiation oncology was not as good as surgery for eradication of bulk tumor (in most cases) but excellent at treating microscopic amounts of residual tumor which might be left after more limited surgery. Radiation was also better at preventing local recurrences (in the breast) than treating them.

As a resident, a large proportion of cases I saw were women with breast cancer, both localized and metastatic. Historically, treatment of even early breast cancer in the majority of cancer centers in the United States and Europe entailed the surgical removal of the entire breast as well as underlying pectoral muscles and lymph nodes of the axilla (armpit). This surgical approach, known as radical mastectomy, had been championed by American surgeon William Halsted and was predicated on the theory that the spread of cancer cells from its origin in the breast was a stepwise process: From the breast, it spread first to regional lymph nodes and, from these, to other parts of the body. By completely removing the breast and regional lymph nodes, one had a chance of getting ahead of the spread of cancer and curing the patient – or so the theory held. (See also Dr. Michael Baum's essay "Understanding How Cancer Behaves" elsewhere in this book.) The downside of this approach was that removing both the entire breast and the underlying pectoral muscles of the chest wall that extended to the axilla resulted in arm weakness and swelling in a large proportion of women. Because of such unintended consequences and a shift in the understanding of how cancer behaves, a lesser procedure, the "total mastectomy" (also known as "modified radical mastectomy" or simply "mastectomy"), became more common. Mastectomy entails removal of all breast tissue – but not pectoral muscles – and axillary nodal metastases (if present).

By the early 1980s, women with localized disease had a seemingly new option: removal of (only) the tumor in the breast, removal of axillary nodal metastases (if present) and radiation to the breast and axilla. This approach offered women the possibility of maintaining a relatively normal breast unlike the more severely compromised form and function associated with radical or modified radical mastectomy. This approach had been proposed and tried in a small number of cases in both England and Canada but was uncommon in the United States in the 1980s (Keynes 643, Peters 1151, Cowan 50). A small minority of surgical oncologists had suggested that simple removal of the tumor without mastectomy or nodal resection might yield results similar to mastectomy in selected patients (Crile 745). But colleagues at the Harvard Joint Center, including my mentor Dr. Hellman, advocated this kind of limited surgery *followed by radiation*. There were single-institution reports of efficacy of this limited, localized surgery combined with radiation, but there were no randomized trials. We decided at New England Medical Center to adopt the approach of our Harvard colleagues and offer this treatment to women with early-stage breast cancer who wished to avoid mastectomy.

Treatment involved local excision (removal) of the tumor in the breast – a procedure called "lumpectomy" or "partial mastectomy" – and sampling of axillary lymph nodes. Patients would then receive radiation therapy to the breast (and axilla if nodes were involved) five days per week for five weeks. This was followed by an additional boost of radiation to the part of the breast where the tumor arose (the "tumor bed"), which was initially given by implanting catheters into the breast and placing radioactive "seeds" into these catheters to deliver further localized radiation over a two-day inpatient stay. While in the hospital, with radioactive seeds inside her, the patient was in strict isolation. To eliminate the need for inpatient stay, this catheter-based boost gradually changed to external beam treatment of the tumor bed.

In current treatment, the tumor bed is typically marked with radio-opaque clips which allow it to be identified in subsequent imaging studies. Radiation treatment planning is typically performed using CT scans to delineate not only the breast but also relevant underlying normal tissues, such as the heart and lungs. In certain situations, patients may be treated in the prone rather than supine position, which allows the breast to fall away from the underlying heart and lungs, or patients may be treated while taking a deep breath and holding it (so-called Deep Inspiration Breath Hold treatment), which may further reduce radiation dose to the heart and lungs. All these techniques can help maintain a uniform radiation dose to the breast, thus avoiding "hot spots" which may cause late scarring and fibrosis and also reduce the risk of late lung and heart damage. (See also the essay by Stout and Fantom elsewhere in this book.)

Breast conservation plus whole breast irradiation had been shown to produce rates of local control and overall survival comparable to those achieved with mastectomy (Winchester 134), but these trials left many other questions about local treatment of early breast cancer incompletely answered:

- What is the optimal radiation dose to the breast? How should this total dose be divided into multiple daily treatments to strike a good balance between effectiveness against residual tumor cells and minimizing the potentially harmful effects of radiation on normal breast tissue and surrounding normal organs, including the lungs and heart?
- Should the tumor bed receive an additional boost dose of radiation?
- Might the tumor bed be the only portion of the breast requiring RT?

- Is there a role for surgery alone, without RT, for selected patients based on patient characteristics, tumor characteristics or some combination of these two?
- Should lymph nodes in the axilla or internal mammary chain (along the breastbone) also receive radiation in some patients?

Such trials and the questions they created altered belief about the biology of breast cancer. We came to realize that metastases usually occur because cancer cells had already spread before surgery and/or radiation. Therefore, adding hormonal or chemotherapy could delay or prevent their growth. (See also Dr. Michael Baum's essay "An Historical Overview of Breast Cancer and Its Treatments" elsewhere in this book.) We also learned that radiation was not necessarily needed in all patients, particularly in older women with biologically favorable tumors.

While these issues were being addressed in multiple single-institution and cooperative group trials (often but not always randomized), I had settled into a practice in which the majority of my patients had lung cancer or lymphoma. But breast cancer came back into my life when my wife was found on a routine mammogram to have a left breast mass, which turned out on initial biopsy to be a small breast cancer with axillary node metastases. Surgeons removed the tumor bed and positive (malignant) lymph nodes, and obtained "negative margins," which means that no know tumor cells remain at the edge of the tumor. My wife was also free of additional positive nodes.

By this time, in the early 2000s, there were clear data that the best survival results were with adjuvant (therapy applied after initial treatment, especially to suppress secondary tumor formation) chemotherapy, radiation to the breast and axilla and ten years of anti-estrogen therapy. Following lumpectomy, my wife underwent this regimen and has continued to do well for more than eighteen years. What came into question for me at the time was whether my apparent certainty in the recommended treatment was enough: Had I reviewed the literature well enough? Should I trust my colleagues or get a second opinion? And what if doing all the right things didn't work and the cancer persisted or recurred? I worried for a while, then not so much, and now think more about the specter of late recurrence of hormone-positive tumors and late effects of radiation on lung and heart function, particularly with left-sided tumors. During treatment I became keenly aware of the physical and psychological impact of all of my wife's treatments – surgical, chemotherapeutic, radiotherapeutic and hormonal – and how each of these has both short- and long-term consequences, both for the patient and her family.

What I Like to Do in My Initial Consultation with a Patient

The choices facing a patient, usually a woman, with newly diagnosed breast cancer are multiple and complex. For purposes of discussion, let's assume that a postmenopausal 55-year-old woman had been found on routine mammogram to have a breast mass about 2 cm in diameter. There were no palpable lymph nodes. She underwent core needle biopsy of the breast mass and it was found to be an infiltrating ductal carcinoma (also referred to as an "invasive ductal carcinoma" to distinguish it from a carcinoma *in situ*), moderately well-differentiated, estrogen and progesterone positive and Her-2 negative. She wants to explore treatment options, and, like many patients, has been told a variety of stories, some encouraging and some frightening, by well-meaning friends. She is in good general health, works as an IT professional in a company close to where she lives and has little background information on breast cancer or cancer in general. After the initial diagnosis at a local hospital in a rural area, she has come to the Cancer Institute for consultation and possible therapy. How do I approach meeting the medical and psychological needs of this patient?

My preference is first to meet with the patient to talk while she's wearing street clothes, before she has been "prepped" and gowned as a patient. This may be easier to accomplish when a nurse or other clinical assistant does not see the patient before I do. I first try to find out from the patient what she understands about her disease and treatment options – why she's meeting with me today and what she hopes to gain from our meeting. Some patients view cancer as an unfortunate but natural process that may occur to any organism; others view it as a malevolent enemy to be battled. Many will be quite unsure of what their options are, in terms of both initial logistics and potential longer-term consequences, but some will have exhaustively researched their care and come prepared to discuss technical aspects of radiation. Getting a clear sense of where the patient stands in these matters is key for successful further discussion and should precede physical examination. Talk first, palpate later.

With this personal background to complement the information in the patient's medical record, (which I will have reviewed prior to meeting her), I then discuss my understanding of her case in the context of what we generally know about pertinent risk factors in breast cancer and treatment options. This discussion, which really should be a mutual discussion rather than a lecture, can be one of the most enjoyable aspects of my practice. Helping people better understand their disease and make better and more informed decisions about their treatment is an enduring pleasure of medical practice (Tamir 1114). The discussion should include a general presentation of breast cancer: its biology, the patterns by which it might spread and the ability of radiation to impact this. Individual risk factors – including stage, histology (how the tissue looks under a microscope), hormone and molecular determinants such as Oncotype – need to be discussed, in terms of their relevance for local control (Boyages 576, Harris 21, Woodward), as well as their role for overall risk of recurrence.

I then obtain a focused medical history, concentrating on factors such as prior cancer history; any prior experience with surgery and radiotherapy; smoking, general physical activity, family history, occupation, and living status. After this, I examine the patient with particular attention to the breasts, the degree of asymmetry as a result of prior surgery, and regional lymph nodes in the axilla and around the collarbone and neck.

In most cases, prior surgery will have removed the tumor in the breast with "negative margins," meaning, again, that the outer edges of the excised tumor are clear of detected disease. Thus, any treatment given at this time is "adjuvant," designed to eliminate possible residual (but currently undetected) tumor. While this concept has become better understood in the context of hormonal and chemotherapy, it may be foreign to patients in the context of radiation. Patients may ask how I will know, when they have completed radiation, if it has been effective. I explain that since I can't detect any cancer cells when they begin radiation, I will need to follow them closely after completing radiation therapy. If they do not develop local recurrence, it means either that adjuvant radiation was not necessary or that it was necessary and effective. This concept – that we are using invisible beams of radiation to destroy tumor cells that may or may not be present in the breast – not infrequently baffles patients.

Explaining Radiation

After presentation of the general options of mastectomy (with or without breast reconstruction) or lumpectomy followed by radiation to the breast, I include some discussion of the effects of radiation on normal tissues. I explain why radiation, which can kill all cells, can be used wisely and selectively to kill cancer cells with modest and generally acceptable effects on normal tissues. I typically show a picture of one of the treatment linear accelerators (our machines) and describe how we focus the radiation and calculate the dose we deliver. I also explain that the way we divide that total dose into daily doses (on weekdays) can make a difference in the relative impact of radiation on the cancer cells we want to kill and the normal cells that are essential to one's ability to live a long and relatively normal life.

Radiation kills cells. Killing cancer cells is called therapy. Killing normal cells is called "collateral damage" and produces side effects. Some side effects – like skin reddening and blistering – are annoying, usually not too severe, and last a relatively short time. Others – such as skin and subcutaneous tissue fibrosis and scarring, and damage to lung and heart tissue that may be within the radiation field – may be more severe and tend to increase with time. Cosmetic results tend to be worse in women with small breasts and larger tumors – as well as in women with larger breasts, where there tends to be more fibrosis (thickening and scarring from surgery and radiation therapy) and therefore greater difference in appearance between treated and untreated breasts. Newer radiation techniques may be helpful in these circumstances: Deep inspiration breath-hold and prone positioning can reduce unintentional radiation dose to the heart and lungs as well as more closely regulate dose in women with larger breasts. It is important that I remember the common fears that many patients have of radiation and try to relate these to actual patient experiences (Brownlee 371, Shaverdian 1673).

Choosing Between Mastectomy and Lumpectomy plus Radiation

Despite the advantages of breast conservation therapy for many patients, mastectomy might be the better choice for some patients for whom convenience is a primary concern. In this setting, mastectomy will achieve low risks of recurrent disease and minimize or eliminate the need for radiotherapy. Local resection alone will yield somewhat higher rates of local recurrence, but these may still be relatively low in carefully selected patients. A number of years ago I received a phone call from a dear aunt, then in her eighties, who told me that she had been diagnosed with a small breast cancer and wanted to know whether she should undergo mastectomy or lumpectomy and radiation. After discussion of the pros and cons of both approaches, she opted to have mastectomy. She had no residual disease or involvement of axillary nodes, was started on adjuvant anti-estrogen therapy and died of unrelated causes several years later without recurrence at the age of 96. Her rationale for this choice of treatment was that she would not object to surgical loss of the breast but would be significantly inconvenienced by daily radiation therapy for four to six weeks.

In women who undergo lumpectomy and do not receive radiation therapy, the majority of local recurrences, if these do occur, are in the same general location of the breast as the original tumor, suggesting that they are not new, independent tumors but rather recurrence of microscopic disease inadvertently left behind at the time of the original surgery. This led to the suggestion that the appropriate radiation therapy target might not be the entire breast but rather the tumor bed, and several single-institution trials showed good results with this approach. Several recent randomized trials have compared this strategy with whole-breast radiation therapy and have shown similar, but not identical, survival. The advantage of partial breast irradiation for patients is that it is typically completed in one week, rather than four to six. Overall rates of local recurrence in these favorable patients have been low for both study populations (Correa 73, Vicini 4, Whelan 3).

How physicians present data can make a huge difference in how patients interpret information relevant to their diagnosis and treatment. A large enough trial may show "statistical significance" between two treatments even if one achieves tumor control on 95 percent of patients and the other in 98 percent. If the more effective treatment were also more expensive and less convenient, many patients might opt for the statistically less effective treatment and be willing to trade off a 3 percent gain. But if the same data are presented as one treatment having more than twice as many failures than the other (5 percent versus 2 percent), patients might well be inclined to choose differently. Honest disclosure of data requires that we not mislead patients or befuddle them with statistics that they may not understand. Most studies suggest that presenting actual event rates rather than ratios or probabilities is the better understood approach to allow patients to make truly informed choices.

When discussing options of more conservative therapy with patients, it is important to make sure that they do not equate lack of aggressiveness with poorer outcomes. Patients will sometimes come in wanting to have "everything done," and they may resist the scientific evidence that they are as likely to do well with local excision and adjuvant hormonal therapy as with radical mastectomy. Especially for an older patient with a biologically favorable tumor (small, well-differentiated, hormone receptor-positive), less aggressive therapy can reduce both physical and psychological side effects (Courdi 4571).

Only after presenting and discussing these relatively standard and data-supported options do I discuss the option of investigational protocol treatment with patients who might qualify. I try to make a clear distinction between "therapeutic" and "investigational": The former is for the sole benefit of the patient; the latter may or may not benefit the patient, as its primary purpose is to obtain new knowledge.

The Process of Informed Consent

In discussing treatment options, it becomes clear at times that the patient has strongly held opinions with which I do not agree. I see my role as helping the patient develop sufficient understanding of her disease and the available treatment options to allow her to make a treatment choice most consistent with her preferences. Whether this is the decision I would make is not germane; it is not my decision to make. From my perspective, the greater concern arises when I believe that the patient does not have a good understanding of the relevant issues and is making an uninformed choice. At this point I need to take a deep breath and try to resolve the situation. Just as a patient cannot receive treatment without agreeing to it, I worry about uninformed *refusal* of treatment.

What doesn't typically work well in this setting is getting more technical. Drawing more survival curves, relapse-free survival curves, or God forbid, Venn Diagrams (all things I have done in the past and don't do any more) were dismal failures. I have found the most effective way for me to understand what the patient understands is to ask her to tell me, in her own words, what she perceives are her options and why she is choosing one over the others. This may help me to identify situations in which the patient believes something which I think to be demonstrably wrong, or identify patients who are truly lost in the complexities of decision- making.

After discussing therapeutic options and coming to an agreement with the patient about a planned course of treatment, it is sometime useful to defer signing the informed consent document until the patient returns for treatment planning on a subsequent day. While this can be discouraged by administrators in busy departments like mine, it emphasizes that informed consent is a process, not a document, and allows me to ask the patient when she comes for her second visit whether she has any additional questions that might have arisen since our last meeting. This process allows the patient more time to reflect and perhaps to solicit additional questions and opinions from family and friends. It can also provide an opportunity to discuss, if the patient asks (and most do), what I would recommend if the patient were my mother, sister, wife or other close relative. In this situation, I think about the patient's values (as she has described them) and how those values might impact the advice I would give to a close family member.

Beyond Initial Radiation Therapy

The end of radiation is often the end of major active treatment for patients, but the end of radiation is not the end of care by the radiation oncologist. Despite the burden of daily radiation over several weeks, some patients view the experience as a source of support, and they build strong and sometimes enduring relationships with fellow patients, therapists, nurses and physicians. While current insurance plans often limit reimbursement to one or two visits after the completion of radiation treatment, both patients and physicians benefit from longer-term follow-up. This is especially true for patients who have recurrent disease: They can rest assured that further palliative radiation will be given by someone who has come to know them as a person rather than simply a clinical problem to be solved.

Indeed, even for patients with very favorable clinical presentations of breast cancer, 20 percent or more will develop metastatic disease. Depending on the number, location and timing of the development of metastases, there may be roles for surgery, radiation or systemic hormonal or chemotherapy in their management. Though the majority of patients with metastatic disease are not curable with present treatment modalities, it is often possible to extend survival for years, so considerations of both duration and quality of life are highly important. The development of metastases heralds a change in treatment goals, but it is not the end of the world. I find it helpful to let patients know at our first meeting that, should there be evidence that their cancer has metastasized, I will let them know this and discuss what new treatments may be most appropriate for them to consider. Some basic information about metastases of breast cancer include:

- When breast cancer spreads, the most common sites are bone, brain, liver, lung and lymph nodes.
- Some patients, particularly women with ER+ disease with metastases limited to bone, can have a long natural history with years of good-quality life.
- Pain is often relieved or well controlled by short courses of radiation.
- Brain metastases are often effectively treated with focal radiation therapy (GammaKnife or CyberKnife). While there may still be a role for whole-brain radiation in patients with large numbers of metastases, it can be avoided or at least deferred in many cases.

Conclusion

The treatment of women with early breast cancer has undergone major changes in the past forty years, and there is good reason to expect changes of similar magnitude in the coming decades. Molecular analysis of tumor cells, the normal tissues in which they arise, and perhaps the bacteria which make up our microbiome should lead to more individualized approaches to diagnosis, therapy and prevention. In women at risk for local recurrence who may continue to benefit from adjuvant radiation, continued improvements in the understanding of radiation biology as well as limitation of radiation dose to the tissues where it is most needed should maintain its effectiveness in preventing tumor recurrence while reducing acute and late damage to normal tissues.

Bibliography

Boyages, J., and L. Baker. "Evolution of Radiotherapy Techniques in Breast Conservation Treatment." *Gland Surgery* 7.6 (December 2018): 576–95.
Brownlee, Z., R. Garg, M. Listo, et al. "Later Complications of Radiation Therapy for Breast Cancer: Evolution in Techniques and Risk over Time." *Gland Surgery* 7.4 (August 2018): 371–8.

Correa, C., E. E. Harris, M. C. Leonardi, et al. "Accelerated Partial Breast Irradiation: Executive Summary for the Update of an ASTRO Evidence-Based Consensus Statement." *Practical Radiation Oncology* 7.2 (March–April 2017): 73–9.

Courdi, A., and J.-P. Gérard. "Radiotherapy for Elderly Patients with Breast Cancer." *Journal of Clinical Oncology* 31.31 (November 1, 2013): 4571.

Cowan, D. H. "Vera Peters and the Conservative Management of Early-Stage Breast Cancer." *Current Oncology* 17.2 (April 2010): 50–4.

Crile, G. "Simplified Treatment of Cancer of the Breast: Early Results of a Clinical Study." *Annals of Surgery* 153.5 (May 1961): 745–61.

Feynman, R. P. "Atoms in Motion: Introduction." *The Feynman Lectures in Physics* (1963) Volume I, Lecture 1. New York: Basic Books, 2011.

Fisher, B., C. Redmond, R. Poisson, et al. "Eight Year Results of a Randomized Clinical Total Comparing Total Mastectomy and Lumpectomy with or without Irradiation in the Treatment of Breast Cancer." *New England Journal of Medicine* 320.13 (March 30, 1989): 822–8.

Harris, J. R. "Fifty Years of Progress in Radiation Therapy of Breast Cancer." *ASCO Educational Book* 2014: 21–5.

Hughes, K. S., L. A. Schnaper, J. R. Bellon, et al. "Lumpectomy Plus Tamoxifen with or without Irradiation in Women Age 70 years or Older in Early Breast Cancer: Long-Term Follow-Up of CALGB 9343. *Journal of Clinical Oncology* 31.19 (July 1, 2013): 2382–7.

Keynes, J. "Conservative Treatment of Cancer of the Breast." *British Medical Journal* 2.4004 (October 2, 1937): 643–7.

Lin, A. "Omission of Adjuvant Radiotherapy in Early-Stage Breast Cancer: Have We Identified a Subgroup?" *Translational Cancer Research* 5 (2016): S1380–2.

Peters, M. V. "Wedge Resection with or without Radiation in Early Breast Cancer." *International Journal of Radiation Oncology, Biology and Physics* 2.11–2 (November–December 1977): 1151–6.

Shaverdian, N., X. Wang, J. V. Hegde, et al. "The Patient's Perspective on Breast Radiotherapy: Initial Fears and Expectations Versus Reality." *BMC Cancer* (February 26, 2018): 1673–81.

Tamir, D. I., J. Zaki, and J. P. Mitchell. "Informing Others Is Associated with Behavioral and Neural Signatures of Value." *Journal of Experimental Psychology: General* 144.6 (2015): 1114–23.

Veronesi, U., A. Luini, M. Del Vecchio, et al. "Radiotherapy after Breast-Preserving Surgery in Women with Localized Cancer of the Breast." *New England Journal of Medicine* 328.22 (June 3, 1993): 1587–91.

Vicini, F. A., R. S. Cecchini, J. R. White, et al. "Primary Results of NSABP B-39/RTOG 0413 (NRG Oncology): A Randomized Phase III Study of Conventional Whole Breast Irradiation (WBI) Versus Partial Breast

Irradiation (PBI) for Women with Stage 0, I, or II Breast Cancer: Proceedings of the 2018 San Antonio Breast Cancer Symposium." *Cancer Research* 79 (2019): GS4–04.

Whelan, T., J. Julian, M. Levine et al. "RAPID: A Randomized Trial of Accelerated Partial Breast Irradiation Using 3-Dimensional Conformal Radiotherapy (3D- CRT): Proceedings of the 2018 San Antonio Breast Cancer Symposium." *Cancer Research* 79 (2019): GS4–03.

Winchester, D. P., and J. D. Cox. "Standards for Breast-Conservation Treatment." *CA-A Cancer Journal for Clinicians* 42 (1992): 134–62.

Woodward, W. A. "Using Oncotype DX for Radiotherapy Decisions in Breast Cancer." Presentation at UT MD Anderson Cancer Center, November 11, 2018. <https://www.accc-cancer.org>presentations>7-woodward-hsco-2018>. Accessed on January 27, 2020.

MICHAEL BAUM

Understanding How Cancer Behaves: Implications for Paradigm Shifts in Treatment

In this essay I wish to concentrate on the natural history of breast cancer – that is, what happens if cancer is left to its own devices – and on the evolution of conceptual models to explain its behavior. I propose that all this is fundamental to improving the lot of our suffering patients for the simple reason that our treatments are the therapeutic consequence of our belief in the underlying mechanisms of disease. In other words, belief systems and treatment modalities are two sides of the same coin. In order to consider what would happen if breast is left untreated – and, more importantly, *why* it would happen – I wish to describe two anecdotal case histories, one from the seventeenth century and one from the twenty-first.

The Louvre in Paris houses a large and beguiling masterpiece by Rembrandt, *Bathsheba at Her Bath*. Completed in 1654, the painting shows a naked Bathsheba looking wistfully into the middle-distance left, whilst holding a letter in her right hand. Her attendant bathes her feet in a pool, and the background is dark and ambiguous. Perhaps she has just learnt of her husband's death in battle as a result of King's David's treachery. About thirty years ago whilst I was working as a senior lecturer in the department of surgery at the Welsh National School of Medicine in Cardiff, a young Australian research fellow, Peter Braithwaite, drew my attention to the dimple in the upper outer quadrant of Bathsheba's left breast. I had to agree with him: The model for this painting has the classical stigma of breast cancer, a detail that I have confirmed on subsequent visits to the Louvre to see the painting in the flesh, so to speak. I encouraged him to research the history of the painting and its model. His work on this subject ultimately appeared in print and, since then, Bathsheba has become an icon of the breast cancer movement (Braithwaite and Shugg). Rembrandt's presumed model, Hendrekje Stoffels, was both his mistress and housekeeper. She was in her thirties when the picture was completed, and she died nine years later. Her mode of dying was characteristic of breast cancer with secondaries (i.e., metastases, or the spread of cancer) to the liver. There is no record of her being treated, but in any case, treatment in those days was a futile hocus pocus based on the doctrines of Aristotle and Galen. Even so, she lived nine years after the clinically obvious disease (perhaps unknowingly portrayed in the painting) became apparent. (See also Professor Conaty's discussion of *Bathsheba at Her Bath* elsewhere in this book.)

More recently a woman booked into my clinic in central London as a "long-standing patient," yet my secretary had no record of her. It transpired that I had seen her on only one occasion, eight years previously at The Royal Marsden Hospital. Piecing the story together, I suddenly recalled the visit. She was 49 at the time but was now 57. I had diagnosed multi-focal carcinoma of the left breast at biopsy and recommended a mastectomy to be followed by five years of tamoxifen. She firmly but politely declined my advice and, as she put it, placed herself in the hands of Jesus and the prayers of her evangelical community. Not believing in the power of prayer to heal (almost no one dies of breast cancer without an attempt at intercessory prayer), I confessed surprise at seeing her alive and wanted to know how I could help. The only complaint to which she confessed was swelling of the left arm. Exchanging glances with her attentive husband and daughter, I asked her to disrobe in the examination room, bracing myself for the worst. While it wasn't the worst I've seen, it was pretty gruesome, nonetheless. Both breasts were now replaced by hard nodules of cancer and both axillae (armpits) were full of the disease. This caused massive lymphedema (swelling due to the accumulation of tissue fluid) of the arms, yet there was no evidence of distant metastases. Not wishing to push my luck too far by asking for another biopsy, I made the assumption that the tumor was hormone responsive and advised her to start on anastrozole – suggesting that Jesus now needed a little help from modern medicine, as prayer alone would no longer hold the cancer in check. She politely took my prescription and promised to return in one month to check on progress, but she did not return.

Despite having undergone no treatment for breast cancer, women in both these cases had survived at least eight years. Just how typical are these examples, then, and what do they suggest about whether to prescribe treatment – and what kind?

In 1970, whilst working with Dr. Bernard Fisher in Pittsburgh, Pennsylvania, I visited the library of the National Institute of Health (NIH) in Bethesda, Maryland, with the goal of completing an historical review for my doctoral thesis. Whilst searching for one reference, a more important one fell in my lap (a process that we scholars describe as library gremlins at play): a treatise on breast cancer by one Dr. Gross of Philadelphia, published in 1880 (Gross). Latterly I've recognized that this was the same Dr. Gross immortalized in Thomas Eakins' masterpiece *The Gross Clinic*, which I was fortunate to see in an exhibition at the Metropolitan Museum of Art in New York the summer of 2004.

Gross's treatise provided a clear insight into the status of breast cancer in the era immediately before developments in anesthesia and antisepsis allowed surgeons to attempt a radical cure. He describes 616 patients, most of whom had skin infiltration on presentation (that is, when they were originally seen by a physician). In 25 percent of the patients, cancer had ulcerated through the skin. About two-thirds had extensive involvement of axillary nodes. Accepting that the meagre benefits of surgery seldom outweighed the risks in those days, Gross judged it ethical to follow the natural course with ninety-seven patients who received nothing other than "constitutional support."

He describes how skin ulcers appeared, on average, twenty months after a tumor is first detected, with growth into the chest wall itself after a further two months and direct invasion of the other breast (if the patient lived) an average of three years after the lump first appeared. In a quarter of all these untreated cases, patients went on to develop obvious secondaries in vital organs within a year, and another quarter after three years. In the end, only one in twenty patients survived more than five years.

In the century and a half since Gross's findings, other data about untreated breast cancer have been reported. The study that has attracted the most attention during this time was that of the great English oncologist Dr. Julian Bloom, published in 1968 (Bloom). His data came from the records of 250 women dying of breast cancer in the Middlesex Hospital Cancer ward between 1905 and 1933. It should be noted that almost all of the women presented with neglected disease and many already had secondaries in vital organs. The survival rates from the "alleged onset" of symptoms were 5 percent at five years, with only two patients alive at fifteen years. The reasons for withholding treatment are also worthy of note: Most of them were too old or infirm to withstand treatment, and 20 percent refused treatment.

It would of course be inconceivable to suggest we study an untreated group today, and the closest approximation we can find comes from a report of the Ontario cancer clinics between 1938 and 1956, just preceding a jump in breast cancer incidence in the developed world (MacKay and Sellers). Close on 10,000 cases were analyzed in the province of Ontario during this period. Amongst this group were 150 well-documented cases who received no treatment of any kind. One-hundred of these cases were untreated because of the late stage of presentation or poor general condition; the rest were unable or unwilling to attend for treatment. A careful note was made of the date the patient first became aware of the lump, from which point survival rates were computed. About a third survived for five years from first recorded symptom, and the average survival of the whole group was four years. The most surprising figure was a near 70 percent five-year survival for the small group presenting with stage I disease. Let me emphasize that nearly three-quarters of those we see today in the Western world diagnosed with "early" breast cancer survive five years without treatment. That said, we cannot quantify the *quality* of that survival.

The influence of surgery on the natural history of breast cancer

From the popularization of the classical radical mastectomy at the very end of the nineteenth century until about 1975, almost all patients with breast cancer who had potentially curable disease were treated with modifications of the radical mastectomy. To those with an open mind, without commitment to a prior conceptual model of the disease, this allowed for new insights about the nature of the malignant process. Before considering this matter, it's worth revisiting the conceptual model that allowed the radical operation to reign supreme for seventy-five years.

In 1840, Dr. Rudolph Virchow of Berlin, the founding father of the discipline of pathology, described a revolutionary model of breast cancer building on the development of microscopy and post-mortem examinations of the cadavers of breast cancer victims (Virchow). He suggested that the disease started as a single focus within the breast, expanding with time and then migrating along lymphatic channels to the lymph glands in the axilla. These glands were said to act as a first line of defense in filtering out the cancer cells. Once these filters became saturated, the glands themselves acted as a source for tertiary spread to a second and then third line of defense, like the curtain walls around a medieval citadel. Ultimately, when all defenses were exhausted, the disease spread along tissue planes to the skeleton and vital organs.

Armed with the teachings of Virchow, a decade of progress in anesthesia and antisepsis and prodigious surgical skills, William Halsted, a brilliant and famous surgeon at the Johns Hopkins hospital, Baltimore, developed in the mid-1890s the operation that carries his name to this day (Halsted). He believed it inevitable that his patients would be cured by radical operations that cut away all of the breast, the overlying skin, the underlying muscles and as many lymph nodes as possible whilst still preserving the patient's life. So convincing were his arguments and so charismatic their chief proponent, the Halsted operation was adopted as default therapy all round the world for generations to come. At this long perspective, however, we are entitled to ask to what extent did the radical operation add to the curability of the disease, and what can we learn about the nature of the beast by its behavior following such mutilating surgery?

Halsted operated at a time when the triumph of mechanistic principles was at its peak – when the common man had begun enjoying the fruits of the Industrial Revolution. Naturally, Halsted's "complete operation" was based on mechanistic concepts about the nature of cancer. His surgical expertise was remarkable, and for the first time, breast cancer seemed curable, with recurrence rates of only 10 percent at three years, very low compared to what surgeons were generally achieving at that time. Unfortunately, though, only about a quarter of patients treated by Halsted survived ten years (Lewis and Rienhoff 336). The natural reaction to this failure was not to question the belief system, but to attempt even more radical treatment. Halsted's "complete operation" did not include removal of internal mammary lymph nodes under the sternum although these nodes receive about 25 percent of the lymphatic drainage from the breast. It seemed logical to remove those nodes as well, and by the mid-twentieth century, these "super-radical" operations became fashionable (Meier et al.). Alternatively, post-surgery radiation was applied to large areas of the chest in an attempt to kill off these hypothetical residual foci of the disease (McWhirter 599). Given mature data on survival rates, we now know that this process merely increased peri-operative deaths (i.e., around the time of surgery) and added a swollen arm (lymphedema) to the gross disfigurement of the chest wall (Early Breast Cancer Trialists "Effects"). There was no improvement in cure rate. Thus, even when the tumor seemed to have been completely "removed with its roots," the patients still developed distant metastases and succumbed; about half of all patients eventually died of the disease over ten years, and those who survived up to twenty-five years were not "cured" but lived with breast cancer as a chronic disease.

A seminal study by Diana Brinkley and John Haybittle, published in *The Lancet* in 1975, illustrates this conclusion (Brinkley and Haybittle). The study described a group of over 700 breast cancer patients treated by radical surgery in Addenbrooke's Hospital, Cambridge and followed up for twenty-five years. The patients continued to demonstrate an excess mortality rate compared to a population matched for age, and this excess mortality was principally related to breast cancer that continued to recur (in spite of it "all being taken away") for up to twenty-five years.

The biological revolution of the late twentieth century

Prompted by the failures of radical and super-radical operations to cure patients with breast cancer, Professor Bernard Fisher from Pittsburgh, Pennsylvania (my mentor) proposed a revolutionary hypothesis that rejected the mechanistic model that had prevailed since Virchow, replacing it with a biological model based on ten years of painstaking work with laboratory mice (Fisher). From these animal experiments he postulated that cancer spreads via the blood stream first of all – bypassing the lymphatic channels – and that this process can occur even before the lump is first detectable. That is, the rate of growth and the rate of spread are determined by the nature of the malignancy at its inception – whether aggressive (poorly differentiated) cancers that grow and spread rapidly, or indolent (well differentiated) cancers that grow and spread at a pace measured in years rather than months. Furthermore, Fisher speculated that the patient is not a passive host to the disease but has the capacity to mount a defense against its incursion via a natural immune response. Putting this all together, Fisher argued that the outcome of treatment by surgery alone was predetermined by the biology of the cancer and immune response interactions. Indirect evidence of success or failure of this battle could be deduced by the status of the glands at surgery. Negative lymph nodes (those showing no signs of cancer) might suggest an intact host defense, whilst positive nodes likely represent an exhausted system that has allowed the cancer cells to maraud unchecked around the body. To put it succinctly, positive glands (showing evidence of cancer) in the axilla are the expression rather than determinant of a poor prognosis.

I've coined the term "biological predeterminism" to describe this theory, from which one can make the following predictions:

(A) The extent of local treatment by surgery and radiotherapy might control the disease on the chest wall but have no effect on survival – the horse (cancer) having bolted before the stable door (radical surgery) was slammed shut.

(B) If the outcome of treatment was predetermined by the extent of microscopic (occult) secondaries present at the time of diagnosis, then the only chance of cure would be with "adjuvant systemic therapy" – that is, drugs that target these putative sites of disease – even for patients with "localized" tumors, seemingly limited to one place. Adjuvant therapy could be tailored from drugs known to produce responses in advanced disease, such as a combination of cytotoxic agents (chemotherapy) or drugs that could interfere with production or uptake of estrogens by the tumor (hormone therapy).

As regards the extent of local treatment, many trials have tested less versus more surgery. A recent world overview of these trials concluded that more radical local treatment does not have any influence on the appearance of distant disease or overall survival. Bottom line: Although radical surgery and/or postoperative radiotherapy has a substantial effect on reducing *local* recurrence rates, it does not improve overall survival. Furthermore, as predicted, breast cancer survival can be influenced favorably with adjuvant systemic therapy (Early Breast Cancer Trialists "Systemic").

All the above can be taken as powerful corroboration of Fisher's theory that metastases of any importance have already occurred *before* the clinical or radiological detection of most breast cancers. Therefore, to this day the standard of care includes surgery and radiotherapy to control the local disease and systemic therapy to control the putative occult micro-metastases. Among other things, the surgery might involve a simple lumpectomy or even a total mastectomy with or without reconstruction – all this depending on the size of the tumor relative to the size of the breast. Surgery to the breast is usually combined with some degree of exploration of the axillary contents, as much as for prognostic reasons and selection of systemic therapy as for local control.

Apart from Herceptin (trastuzumab) that was approved by the FDA in 1998, no new systemic therapies for breast cancer have been shown to improve length or quality of life (Romond et al.). [14] There is an illusion of progress, however, because of the plethora of new drugs that have been evaluated according to "surrogate outcome measures" – that is, anything other than length or quality of life. A good example might be progression-free survival (PFS), the period of time when there is no measurable progression of overt metastatic disease and also no impact on time of death or quality of life (Hudis et al.). Apart from being hugely expensive, some of these drugs have little or no benefit from the patient's point of view, although the pharmaceutical industry and some clinicians with conflicts of interest are making loads of money. This scandal is amplified by the fact that many patients who are desperate for a cure bankrupt themselves in the process (Ward). Even so-called "personalized" or "precision" medicine based on the molecular profile of the cancer has not lived up to its promise (Masys and Altman).

On the horizon: the next paradigm shift

My sister developed widespread bone metastases twenty-five years after her "successful" treatment – lumpectomy, axillary node sampling, whole-breast radiotherapy and five years of tamoxifen – for the primary disease. What does that tell us? This personal anecdote represents just one of many inconsistencies in the conventional biological model of breast cancer. When I first involved myself in conducting research into cancer about fifty years ago, it was taught that after malignant transformation, cancer cells grew exponentially with the doubling time of the tumor reflecting the speed of growth. (The doubling time is based on the assumption that the time taken for a tumor to double in size from, say, 0.5 cm to 1.0 cm is the same for a tumor of 1.0 cm to become 2.0 cm.) In due course this model was modified to fit the data by factoring in another variable, the access of oxygen to the cells in the center of the growing spheroidal tumor. It was estimated that a tumor cannot grow beyond 10^7 cells without inducing its own blood supply (angiogenesis), after which it continued growing; but as a result, the cancer cells could gain access to the circulation and disseminate metastases to vital organs (Skipper). For all that to happen, you must postulate three or four mutations in the malignant cells. The first for unlimited proliferation, the second for the induction of angiogenesis, the third to allow the cells to migrate out of the vascular channels and the fourth for the process of invading other organs. If all these events are time-related, then it is reasonable to assume that the tumor will grow from an *in-situ* phase to an invasive stage (Stage 1 "early cancer"), from this stage to local or regional spread (Stage 2) and ultimately to the invasion of distant vital organs (Stage 3/4).

This concept of the biological nature of breast cancer has generated a catchphrase, almost a mantra, that goes something like "Catch it early, save a life and save a breast!" This simplistic translation of a complex subject has done much indirect harm to many women who have been coerced into having screening mammograms. Despite the huge increase in the detection of ductal carcinoma *in situ* (DCIS) at screening, the incidence of invasive cancer has not declined in the screened population (Welch). Up to 50 percent of "cancers" detected at screening are now recognized as overdiagnosis (Jørgensen and Gøtzsche). The rare deaths from the toxicity of treating these lesions cancels out the rare cases of breast cancer deaths avoided. Screening is therefore considered by some (myself included) a zero-sum game, and more and more countries are now seriously considering de-implementation of the program (Adami et al.).

Another alarming inconsistency concerns the hazard rate for recurrent disease. Instead of a steady state of recurrence over time – as might be predicted if there is a spectrum with extremes where good tumors grew slowly and bad tumors grew fast – we see a hazard rate that peaks at about thirty months after surgery (Saphner et al.). It is now accepted that the very act of surgery itself may in some way provoke the outgrowth of occult disease, which would account for the initial peak of hazard two to three years after surgery (Baum et al.). Following any trauma, including surgery, a whole cascade of genes is switched on for the healing response. The healing response releases chemicals into the blood which can stimulate cancer cells to grow and can activate the growth of little blood vessels at the wound site. The same natural process also might kick-start metastases from a latent state to an active state of progression (Retsky et al.).

Cancer is a complex system, nesting in a complex system, with treatments adding to the complexity of interactions. Any progress in the future must address this challenge, and this demands open minds free of conflicts of interest as well as utilization of artificial intelligence that can harness chaos theory to augment our innate wisdom ("Complex System").

Bibliography

Adami, Hans-Olov, et al. "Time to Abandon Early Detection Cancer Screening." *European Journal of Clinical Investigation* 49.3 (December 19, 2018): e13062.

Baum, M., R. Demicheli, W. Hrushesky, and M. Retsky. "Does Surgery Unfavourably Perturb the "Natural History" of Early Breast Cancer by Accelerating the Appearance of Distant Metastases?" *European Journal of Cancer* 41.4 (March 2005): 508–15.

Bloom, H. J. G. "Survival of Women with Untreated Breast Cancer-Past and Present." In *Prognostic Factors in Breast Cancer*. Eds. APM Forrest and PB Kunkler. Edinburgh: E&S Livingston Ltd., 1968.

Braithwaite, P. A., and D. Shugg. "Rembrandt's Bathsheba: The Dark Shadow of the Left Breast." *Annals of the Royal College of Surgeons* 65 (1983): 337–9.

Brinkley, D., and J. L. Haybittle. "The Curability of Breast Cancer." *The Lancet* 306:7925 (July 19, 1975): 9–14.

"Complex System" <https://en.wikipedia.org/wiki/Complex_system>. Accessed February 20, 2020.

Early Breast Cancer Trialists' Collaborative Group. "Effects of Radiotherapy and Surgery in Early Breast Cancer: An Overview of Randomized Trials." *New England Journal of Medicine* 333 (November 30, 1995):1444–56.

———. "Systemic Treatment of Early Breast Cancer by Hormonal, Cytotoxic or Immune Therapy: 133 Randomized Trials Involving 31,000 Recurrences and 24,000 Deaths Among 75,000 Women." *The Lancet* 339.8785 (1992): 71–85.

Fisher, B. "Laboratory and Clinical Research in Breast Cancer: A Personal Adventure. The David A. Karnofsky Memorial Lecture." *Cancer Research* 40 (1980): 3863–74.

Gross, S. W. *A Practical Treatise of Tumours of the Mammary Gland*. New York: D. Appelton & Co, 1880.

Halsted, W. S. "The Results of Operations for the Cure of Cancer of the Breast Performed at The Johns Hopkins Hospital from June 1889 to January1894." *Johns Hopkins Hospital Report* 4 (1894): 297–350.

Hudis, C. A., W. E. Barlow, J. P. Costantino, et al. "Proposal for Standard in Definitions for Efficacy End Points in Adjuvant Breast Cancer Trials: The STEEP System." *Journal of Clinical Oncology* 26 (2007): 2127–32.

Jørgensen, Karsten Juhl and Gøtzsche Peter C. "Overdiagnosis in Publicly Organised Mammography Screening Programmes: Systematic Review of Incidence Trends." *British Medical Journal* 339 (2009): b2587.

Lewis, D., and W. F. J. Rienhoff. "Results of Operations at the Johns Hopkins Hospital for Cancer of the Breast." *Annals of Surgery* 95.3 (March 1932): 336–400.

MacKay, E. N., and A. H. Sellers. "Breast Cancer at the Ontario Cancer Clinics, 1938–56: A Statistical Review." Medical Statistics Branch, Ontario Department of Health. 1965.

Masys, Daniel R., and Russ B. Altman. "The Incidentalome: A Threat to Genomic Medicine." *Journal of the American Medical Association* 296.2 (2006): 212–5.

McWhirter, R. "The Value of Simple Mastectomy and Radiotherapy in the Treatment of Cancer of the Breast." *British Journal of Radiology* 21 (1948): 599–610.

Meier, P., D. J. Ferguson, and T. Karrison. "A Controlled Trial of Extended Radical Mastectomy." *Cancer* 55 (1985): 880–91.

Retsky, M., R. Demicheli, W. Hrushesky, M. Baum, and I. Gukas. "Surgery Triggers Outgrowth of Latent Distant Disease in Breast Cancer: An Inconvenient Truth?" *Cancers* 2 (2010): 305–37.

Romond Edward, H., Edith A. Perez, John Bryant, et al. "Trastuzumab Plus Adjuvant Chemotherapy for Operable HER2-Positive Breast Cancer." New England Journal of Medicine 353 (October 20, 2005): 1673–84.

Saphner, T., D. C. Tormey, and R. Gray. "Annual Hazard Rates of Recurrence for Breast Cancer After Primary Therapy. *Journal of Clinical Oncology* 14 (1996): 2738–46.

Skipper, H. E. "Kinetics of Mammary Tumor Cell Growth and Implications for Therapy." *Cancer* 28 (1971): 1479–99.

Virchow, R. *1862–1863 Die Krankhaften Geschwülste*. Berlin: Hirshwald Publishers, 1978.

Ward, Lisa. "The High Cost of Cancer Care May Take Physical and Emotional Toll on Patients." <https://www.wsj.com/articles/the-high-cost-of-cancer-care-may-take-physical-and-emotional-toll-on-patients-1455592260>. Accessed on February 20, 2020.

Welch, H. G. "Overdiagnosis and Mammography Screening." *British Medical Journal* 339 (2009): b1425.

MARIA J. BAKER

Genetic Counseling and Testing for Hereditary Breast Cancer: A Genetic Counselor's Perspective

Genetic Counselor: A medical professional with specialized education in genetics and counseling who helps individuals and their families make personal decisions about their genetic health. Genetic counselors guide and support patients (aka "clients") who are seeking information regarding how a condition may be inherited within their family. Genetic counselors coordinate genetic testing when appropriate, as well as interpret subsequent test results and provide supportive resources as needed to help individuals adjust to this newfound knowledge.

The Evolution of Genetic Counseling

Now that we're all on the same page about the role of a genetic counselor, I'd like to share a historical perspective about the field of genetic counseling and, in particular, cancer genetic counseling, as it has evolved over the past fifty years. The first genetic counselors graduated with their Masters degrees from Sarah Lawrence College in 1971. At the time, most genetic counselors specialized in the areas of prenatal/pediatric genetics and/or public health genetics. Today, thanks in large part to the Human Genome Project, genetic counselors also practice in various subspecialties such as cancer genetics, neurogenetics and cardiovascular genetics, and even serve a vital role in "direct-to-consumer" genetic testing by helping individuals understand test results from companies such as 23andMe and Ancestry. And although genetic counselors have historically worked mostly for academic medical centers and government-funded programs, such as those for newborn screening, today they also work for genetic testing laboratories, health insurance companies, telephone- and web-based counseling services, etc. Some even work in private practice settings as their specialized skills increasingly become recognized by major health insurers.

In 1998, I returned to an academic medical center to develop the Penn State Cancer Genetics Program, whose mission is to help individuals concerned about a personal and/or family history of cancer. Two major breast cancer susceptibility genes, BRCA1 and BRCA2, were discovered in 1994 and 1995, respectively, and clinical testing became available in 1996. In addition to breast cancer, these two genes also predispose a person to a number of other cancers: ovarian, fallopian tube, primary peritoneal cancer, male breast and prostate cancers, pancreatic cancer in both men and women, and melanoma (BRCA2 only). During the early days, much effort was spent educating people – not only the public but also healthcare providers – about the potential benefits of cancer genetic counseling and testing to help prevent cancer and/or detect it at an earlier, more curable stage. Simply by identifying those individuals with a hereditary predisposition to cancer due to a mutation in a cancer susceptibility gene, now referred to as a "pathogenic variant," we could offer various management strategies such as positive lifestyle changes (e.g., maintaining a healthy body weight and limiting alcohol consumption to lower one's risk of breast cancer), enhanced surveillance (e.g., incorporating breast MRI on an annual basis, alternating with mammography, beginning at a younger age to promote early detection), chemoprevention (e.g., prescribing medications such as tamoxifen or raloxifene to lower breast cancer risk) and the option of prophylactic surgery (e.g., bilateral mastectomy, whereby most of the breast tissue is surgically removed in order to significantly reduce one's risk of developing breast cancer).

Early on, there were significant concerns about the potential for genetic discrimination, as well as the cost of genetic testing. Fortunately, in the years since, a number of federal laws have been enacted to protect against health insurance discrimination: the Health Insurance Portability and Accountability Act, known as HIPAA; the Genetic Information Non-discrimination Act, known as GINA; and the Affordable Care Act, or ACA. In addition, the Americans with Disabilities Act (ADA) and

GINA both protect against employment discrimination. With regard to the cost of genetic testing, most insurance companies now reimburse for these services when there is sufficient concern for a genetic predisposition. Furthermore, the cost of genetic testing has decreased exponentially over time, due not only to improvements in technology, but also because in 2013 the US Supreme Court overturned the patent protection on the BRCA1 and BRCA2 genes, thus enabling other qualified laboratories to offer this testing. Just as competition helps lower our gas, electric and cable bills, so does choice in the genetic testing arena!

An additional barrier that has limited the public's access to cancer genetic services has been the lack of recognition of genetic counselors by major insurers. Without this recognition, genetic counselors historically could not bill for their services, which significantly limited the growth of the genetic counseling profession for many years and hindered patient access to these services when not covered by health insurance ... this despite board certification and now licensure in twenty-nine states! Although state licensure has enhanced the recognition of genetic counselors, the Centers for Medicare and Medicaid Services (CMS) still does not permit genetic counselors to bill for their services. Therefore, individuals with Medicare, Medicaid and other federal plans, such as those covering federal employees and the military, must pay out-of-pocket for genetic counseling services even when they have health insurance! The National Society of Genetic Counselors sought bipartisan support to eliminate this financial barrier and improve access to genetic counseling services – advocacy that has resulted in the proposal of H.R. 3235 – Access to Genetic Counselors Services Act of 2019. For those of you who are politically minded, contact your representative and ask them to support this effort!

Patient – Counselor Experiences

I'll never forget the first patient I officially met with for cancer genetic counseling and testing. Her mother and her sister, as well as more distant relatives on the maternal side of her family, had been diagnosed with breast and/or ovarian cancer. She had teenage children and was prepared to have both her breasts and ovaries removed, should she test positive for the BRCA mutation that had previously been identified in her sister. Fortunately, she tested negative for the familial mutation, and it was not necessary for her to choose between losing that which society viewed as defining her femininity and the privilege of raising her children and seeing them become adults. Years prior to the advent of cancer genetic testing, though, many women had no choice but to make that decision based solely on their family history and the anxiety that the threat of breast cancer understandably evoked – without the benefit of knowledge regarding their genetic predisposition, or lack thereof.

I also recall the first patient I met with whose life was saved because she had the courage to explore her genetic destiny and, as a result, had the good fortune to rewrite her future. This woman was of Ashkenazi Jewish ancestry and had already developed and survived bilateral breast cancer approximately twenty years prior. Unfortunately, her sister had died from ovarian cancer. Although genetic testing had not been available when she was initially diagnosed with breast cancer, she continued to be followed by her oncologist who, in time, referred her for cancer genetic counseling and testing. We know from population-based studies that approximately 1 in 400 (0.25 percent) individuals carry a mutation in either the BRCA1 or BRCA2 gene. By contrast, approximately 1 in 40 (2.5 percent) individuals of Ashkenazi Jewish ancestry carry one of three common Jewish founder mutations, which they typically inherit from either their mother or father (National Cancer Institute). However, due to the prevalence of these founder mutations in this population, Ashkenazi Jews sometimes inherit two mutations, one from each parent or both from the same parent.

Testing in my patient revealed that she did indeed carry a BRCA mutation, so I referred her for a consultation with one of our gynecologic oncologists to discuss prophylactic removal of her ovaries and fallopian tubes. Because she had pursued TRAM (Transverse Rectus Abdominis Myocutaneous) flap reconstruction of her breasts years earlier, she was hesitant to undergo additional abdominal surgery. Fortunately, despite her ambivalence, she elected to pursue the surgical intervention. Pathology on the surgical specimen revealed the presence of an occult (hidden) fallopian tube cancer. The prophylactic surgery was curative and, due to the early stage at diagnosis, she was able to safely avoid the sometimes toxic effects of chemotherapy. I was once again reminded of how fortunate I am to work with individuals and families who face very difficult decisions and somehow manage to come through on the other side.

I have also experienced some surprising reactions by patients and their family members to both positive and negative test results. The experiences have taught me never to assume one's reaction to either "good" or "bad" test results but rather to spend my time preparing them for results that none of us have control over, given that the specific variations in our genes were determined years ago when we were conceived. In the first case, my patient was thrilled to discover that her breast cancer was hereditary: She actually clapped when I disclosed her test results, which took me by surprise. Exploring her reaction, I learned that her family had blamed her diagnosis on her past lifestyle and that she now felt vindicated because genetic testing had proven that heredity was the major driving force that resulted in her diagnosis of breast cancer.

In the second case, I met with a woman who was one of five sisters. She was the only sister who did not have children and, as the laws of Mendelian genetics would have it, she was the only sibling who did not inherit the familial BRCA mutation. Her sisters were not at all supportive and, in fact, they resented her good news since each of them now faced the possibility of having passed on the predisposition to cancer to at least some of their children. We explored her feelings of survivor's guilt, as past relatives had succumbed to cancer, and we discussed how she no longer looked to the future with the same perspective that was shared by her sisters. She felt isolated. We explored FORCE (Facing Our Risk of Cancer Empowered), a national nonprofit organization devoted to helping families at risk for hereditary breast, ovarian and related cancers; and we discussed the option of meeting with a trained professional to better understand the variety of human responses to situations not under our control and how to navigate the changes in her family dynamics that had resulted from discovering each relative's genetic information. All of these experiences, with my patients as honorary teachers, have molded and shaped me as a genetic counselor – one who is, I hope, better able to help the next person as we pull back the various branches of their family tree.

The Current Landscape of Genetic Testing for Hereditary Breast Cancer

Historically, the cancer genetic counseling process consisted of a series of three visits over the course of several months. During the first visit, I elicited the family history and created a family tree, either drawn by hand or generated by a computer software program. Also during that first visit, I discussed our current understanding about the genetics of breast cancer. Together, we – the patient, family (when present), and I – reviewed the risks, benefits and limitations of genetic testing and discussed how test results might impact medical management. For those patients who expressed interest in pursuing genetic testing, we then looked into insurance coverage, and I sometimes wrote letters of medical necessity to justify coverage for the $3,400 to $4,000 test. (Remember, these genes were patented, and testing was performed at only one laboratory until mid-2013. Many laboratories today bill much less for the testing ... as low as $1,500 for up to eighty-four genes; some provide a self-pay option of as little as $250, while also offering very generous patient assistance programs to help ensure affordable access to genetic testing.) If insurance approved coverage, a follow-up appointment was scheduled during which a consent form was reviewed and signed, and a test requisition form was completed. Once test results became available – usually within four weeks – a third appointment was scheduled to disclose the results and discuss next steps based on the patient's identified risk(s) for cancer.

Now, in part due to our fast-paced society, this process has been distilled into a one- or two-visit model. In many centers, only one in-person visit is required, as all results are disclosed over the telephone. Should a cancer-predisposing mutation be identified, a follow-up appointment may be offered to discuss the results in further detail, including an overview of the current management recommendations, implications for family members and available support resources.

Not only has the cancer genetic counseling process undergone changes, but so has the technology and the number of genes for which testing is available. When testing of the BRCA1 and BRCA2 genes was initially introduced in 1996, laboratories utilized a method called Sanger sequencing in which the DNA sequence was proofread in both the forward and reverse direction. (DNA is a double-stranded helix of basepairs comprised of adenine [A], guanine [G], thymine [T] and cytosine [C].) The testing underwent enhancements in 2003 and then again in 2006 with the addition of laboratory methods to detect large deletions and/or duplications of genetic material – where whole chunks of DNA were either missing or extra within the gene, thus disrupting its normal function in protecting against the development of cancer.

Fast forward to 2012 and the whole approach to genetic testing changed overnight! No longer were BRCA1 and BRCA2 the only genes to be interrogated; rather, a whole panel of breast cancer susceptibility genes, and possibly other genes as well, could be analyzed simultaneously to explore one's personal and/or family history of cancer. Some of the genes included on these "next generation sequencing" (NGS) panels are high-susceptibility genes, which pose a significant increased risk for cancer, like BRCA1 and BRCA2. Others genes included on the panels pose only a moderate increased risk for cancer and may or may not influence medical management recommendations at this time. Still others have lesser-known significance for one's risk of developing cancer, which prompts patients and healthcare providers to work together, developing and participating in research studies, such as PROMPT (Prospective Registry of MultiPlex Testing) and ICARE (Inherited Cancer Registry), to better understand their impact.

Quandaries Caused by Genetic Testing

Multi-gene panel tests, as the NGS panels are called, certainly increase the possibility that uncertain results may be found. In addition to the steep learning curve associated with offering newer genes on these panels for which we're still trying to appreciate the full spectrum of cancers and their respective lifetime risks, testing a greater number of genes increases the likelihood of identifying one or more variants of uncertain significance, referred to as a VUS. Simply put, a variant of uncertain significance is a genetic difference or spelling in a gene that may or may not increase one's risk of developing cancer. In fact, one laboratory reported such an experience with the first 10,000 NGS panels they completed: As the size of the panel grew with respect to the number of genes included, more variants of uncertain significance were identified, ranging anywhere from 7.4 percent to 34.7 percent. However, the likelihood of identifying a pathogenic variant or mutation in the patient, which is the goal of the test should a predisposition exist within the family, also increased, ranging from 3.8 percent to 13.7 percent (Susswein 828–9). In other words, the more genes included on the panel, the better chance of identifying a genetic predisposition to cancer within the patient, but at the expense of possibly identifying one or more uncertain variants or findings.

A word of caution: Not all genetic testing laboratories interpret a particular genetic variant the same way. Whereas one laboratory may classify a variant as a VUS with uncertain significance, another laboratory may interpret the variant as pathogenic or likely pathogenic. Variant interpretation is not an exact science, and discrepancies may sometimes be due to internal data that a laboratory may possess which sways their interpretation from one end of the spectrum to the other. So what's a patient and the genetic counselor to do?!? When in this situation, I disclose the discrepant results – not just the results of the laboratory where the sample was sent but also the sometimes conflicting interpretations from other laboratories about the same genetic variant. Fortunately, most labs submit their data regarding the interpretation of each of these variants into a database called ClinVar. If a patient has a VUS identified by one laboratory but a search of ClinVar reveals that another laboratory classifies the same variant as a mutation, I disclose this to the patient and offer repeat testing for the variant at the other laboratory so the patient has an actionable test result (i.e., mutation positive) that can now be used to influence medical management recommendations, provide medical necessity for insurance coverage, and justify offering testing to relatives at risk. Yes, the variant still has discrepant interpretations by different laboratories, but the patient now has the option to pursue heightened surveillance – such as breast MRI or prophylactic removal of the ovaries if she chooses – rather than wait for the first lab to update their interpretation based on additional data ... especially if multiple other laboratories already classify the variant as pathogenic.

Multi-gene panel tests are here to stay until if and when whole exome sequencing (WES), which involves analyzing all the genes that form the blueprint to create a human being, becomes standard of care. Despite the inherent uncertainty that comes with analyzing an increasing number of genes, a greater number of families are gaining clarity regarding the clustering of cancer within their family. Some families who previously tested negative for a BRCA1 or BRCA2 mutation are now testing positive for a mutation in one of the other breast cancer susceptibility genes such as ATM, CHEK2 or PALB2. Other families who previously had a BRCA mutation identified, but for whom that single variant did not explain all the cancers within the family, are now being identified with one or more additional predispositions to cancer. Armed with this knowledge regarding the pathogenic variant(s) that segregate within a specific family, we then have a predictive test to determine which relatives carry one or more of the genetic predispositions and need to be managed appropriately and which, despite the strong family history, are not at increased risk for cancer and can safely go back to screening guidelines for the general population.

Challenges Facing Genetic Counselors

As technology improves and new genes are discovered, genetic counselors are faced with how best to notify prior patients about new developments in the field. One survey conducted about patients' experiences with the Penn State Cancer Genetics Program asked whose responsibility it would be to notify them regarding the discovery of a new gene. Although 39 percent of respondents stated that it was either the patient's personal responsibility or the responsibility of her referring provider, 61 percent stated it was the responsibility of the genetic counselor to notify them regarding a new gene discovery (Baker 413). But because genetic counselors typically meet with patients only one or two times, after which a summary letter is written, follow-up notification presents a significant challenge for genetic counselors whose programs are typically short-staffed and who don't have the benefit of meeting with patients on a regular basis to provide such updates. Additionally, most of the variants of uncertain significance that are identified by genetic testing will eventually be reclassified (greater than 90 percent are downgraded to a likely benign or benign variant) and the laboratory will issue an amended report, after which the genetic counselor will notify patients regarding the updated interpretation. Lastly, the National Comprehensive Cancer Network (NCCN) updates its patient management recommendations two, three or even four times per year. For example, females with a BRCA mutation were told years ago to start mammograms at a younger age to address their increased risk for breast cancer; not a mention was made of breast MRI. Now, women with a BRCA mutation are advised to pursue breast MRIs on an annual basis beginning at twenty-five years of age and to add mammography at thirty years of age, alternating the two imaging modalities every six months. Again, who takes responsibility for alerting patients to these new recommendations?

Some solutions have been developed to address these challenges. For example, some programs have developed a longitudinal high-risk program in which patients with a hereditary predisposition to cancer are followed on at least an annual basis by a physician or nurse practitioner with expertise in the management of hereditary cancer syndromes. Patients are updated on new screening recommendations, as well as any new cancer risks that may be identified. In addition, these patients may be notified about new research studies that become available to further our knowledge about specific hereditary cancer syndromes. One web-based service, My Gene Counsel, markets itself as a digital health company that serves to update patients on current, evidence-based information regarding their genetic test results. Another web-based service, Check Your Genes, provides a secure, free notification service to help notify family members about one's positive BRCA test results. Notification of relatives at risk is of vital importance. Fortunately, a number of laboratories now offer free testing for the familial mutation identified to any biologic relative (referred to as "cascade testing") for up to ninety days. (I don't know about you, but if I have a coupon with an expiration date, I'm more likely to use it.) And notification of relatives at risk, leading to cascade testing, has the potential to save lives! Genetic counselors discuss with patients one's moral and ethical obligation to attempt to share this information with relatives at risk, despite a number of barriers which have become quite commonplace – for example, relatives separated by miles; rifts in the family, where one branch of the family does not talk to the other; and simple lack of knowledge about one side of the family due to an absent parent. If patients do not attempt to communicate their positive test results to relatives at risk, we lose the opportunity to prevent cancer and/or detect it at a more curable stage. Imagine a worst-case scenario in which a relative develops an incurable ovarian cancer that could have been prevented if information regarding one's positive test results had been shared in a timely fashion.

Looking Toward the Future

Although I practiced for many years as a prenatal and pediatric genetic counselor, being a cancer genetic counselor has become an integral part of my identity – much more than a means to provide for my family. Genetic counseling is a rewarding helping profession that is dynamic and constantly changing. For example, the recent addition of RNA analysis to DNA analysis in 2019 marks the next advancement in genetic testing, and testing guidelines are becoming more comprehensive. Sometimes these new testing guidelines create their own controversies as, for instance, when the American Society of Breast Surgeons (ASBrS) recently recommended that all patients with a diagnosis of breast cancer should be offered genetic testing, regardless of age, ethnicity or type of breast cancer. Not everyone believes this course of action is appropriate, especially considering rising healthcare costs. And, of course, there will always be new genes to discover for the foreseeable future. Although we've sequenced the human genome and know all three billion base pairs that make up our DNA, we've yet to appreciate the respective function of each of those genes. My recommendation ... fasten your seatbelts! New discoveries regarding the genetics of breast cancer, as well as other types of cancer and myriad other health conditions, will occur at a rapidly increasing pace. Although it took thirteen years to map and sequence the first human genome, we can now sequence a newborn's DNA in the neonatal intensive care unit in less than a day to shed light on his or her care. The ultimate goal is personalized medicine. Rather than treating all patients with breast cancer in a similar fashion – as was done years ago before testing of the estrogen and progesterone receptors and measurement of HER2/neu overexpression became available – the goal is to treat a patient's breast cancer based on the specific genetic signature of her (or his) tumor. That goal, as well as elucidating other hereditary causes of breast cancer, is within our reach.

Bibliography

American Society of Breast Surgeons. "Consensus Guideline on Genetic Testing for Hereditary Breast Cancer." (2019) <https://www.breastsurgeons.org/docs/statements/Consensus-Guideline-on-Genetic-Testing-for-Hereditary-Breast-Cancer.pdf>. Accessed February 7, 2020.
Check Your Genes. <https://www.checkyourgenes.org/>. Accessed February 7, 2020.
FORCE. "Facing our Risk of Cancer Empowered." <https://www.facingourrisk.org/index.php>. Accessed February 6, 2020.
GINA. "Genetic Information Nondiscrimination Act." (2010) <http://www.ginahelp.org/GINAhelp.pdf>. Accessed February 6, 2020.
ICARE. "Inherited Cancer Registry." <https://www.inheritedcancer.net/>. Accessed February 7, 2020.
Kausmeyer, Dana T., Eugene J. Lengerich, and Kluhsman, et al. "A Survey of Patients' Experiences with the Cancer Genetic Counseling Process: Recommendations for Cancer Genetics Programs." *Journal of Genetic Counseling* 15.6 (December 2006): 409–31.
My Gene Counsel. <https://www.mygenecounsel.com/>. Accessed February 7, 2020.

National Cancer Institute. "Genetics of Breast and Gynecologic Cancers (PDQ®)–Health Professional Version." (2020) <https://www.cancer.gov/types/breast/hp/breast-ovarian-genetics-pdq#_113_toc>. Accessed February 6, 2020.

NCCN, "National Comprehensive Cancer Network." <https://www.nccn.org/professionals/default.aspx>. Accessed February 7, 2020.

National Conference of State Legislatures. "The Affordable Care Act: A Brief Summary." (2011) <https://www.ncsl.org/research/health/the-affordable-care-act-brief-summary.aspx>. Accessed February 6, 2020.

PROMPT. "Prospective Registry of MultiPlex Testing." (2018) <http://promptstudy.info/>. Accessed February 7, 2020.

Susswein, Lisa R., Megan L. Marshall, Rachel Nusbaum, et al. "Pathogenic and Likely Pathogenic Variant Prevalence Among the First 10,000 Patients Referred for Next-Generation Cancer Panel Testing." *Genetics in Medicine* 18.8 (August 2016): 823–32.

"The HIPAA Guide. HIPAA for Dummies." (Copyright © 2007–2018) <https://www.hipaaguide.net/hipaa-for-dummies/>. Accessed February 6, 2020.

U.S. Department of Education. "Americans with Disabilities Act (ADA)." (1990) <https://www2.ed.gov/about/offices/list/ocr/docs/hq9805.html>. Accessed February 6, 2020.

VICTORIA O'DONNELL

The Marketing of Metastatic Breast Cancer: A Cultural Analysis of the Ibrance Commercial

Introduction

In 1978 two horror movies were released. One was *Halloween*, a slasher film about a serial killer who breaks out of a mental institution and goes on a killing rampage. The other was a docudrama on television, *First You Cry*, based on a 1976 book by television news correspondent Betty Rollins about her experience with breast cancer. There is a scene in the movie in which Betty, portrayed by Mary Tyler Moore, home from the hospital after a mastectomy, disrobes and looks in the mirror. The audience does not see her reflection; instead, the camera focuses on Betty's expression, which is one of complete and utter horror. The made-for-television movie tells the story of Betty's struggle as her husband, Arthur (Tony Perkins), leaves her because he cannot support her emotional neediness. In the end, Betty finds happiness in a new life with David (Richard Crenna). Rollins' book, and subsequently the movie, were intended to encourage public awareness about breast cancer. Four years earlier, in 1974, First Lady of the United States Betty Ford made public that she had undergone a mastectomy due to breast cancer. Two weeks later, Happy Rockefeller, who would become the Second Lady of the United States, announced that she too had breast cancer and had undergone a double mastectomy. Ironically, it was Betty Rollins who covered their announcements on television.

The words "breast" and "cancer" had rarely been spoken on television in 1974, as the media mostly avoided them. There were no breast cancer centers for information, exercises or classes. There were no walkathons for breast cancer, no pink ribbons, shirts or bracelets. There was no October Breast

Cancer Awareness Month. There were no special programs for free mammograms for low-income women. Support groups like "Bosom Buddies" did not exist. Breast cancer was feared, but people, especially women with the disease, did not talk about it. Our culture, and especially the media, was very different then.

"Culture," defined as "actual practices and customs, languages, beliefs, forms of representation, and a system of formal and informal rules that tell people how to behave most of the time," enables people to make sense of their world through a certain amount of shared meanings and recognition of differing meanings (Jowett & O'Donnell 177). Today breast cancer is talked about in our culture, and both fiction and fact about it regularly appear in newscasts, newspapers, magazines, pharmaceutical advertisements, television series, sporting events, movies and even billboards. Films such as *Terms of Endearment* and *The Family Stone* highlighted breast cancer in their narratives. Well-known television series such as *Sex and the City*, *Murphy Brown*, *Parenthood* and *Jane the Virgin* included episodes in which featured characters had breast cancer. In the opening season of *Chicago Med* in September 2019, the character Maggie (Marlyne Barrett), who is the head ER nurse on the series, is diagnosed with metastatic adenocarcinoma of the breast and undergoes a lumpectomy and chemotherapy. At first, she does not want her colleagues to know because she doesn't want pity or obligation; but a friend who once had cancer convinced her that having a support community is healing. At the end of the episode, Maggie reveals her balding head to her colleagues, who surround her with compassionate hugs.

Various television episodes have featured women's different reactions to having been diagnosed with breast cancer and realistic portrayals of breast cancer treatments, such as mastectomies and chemotherapy. In October 2018, to remind women to schedule their mammograms, Ali Meyer, a 42-year-old television reporter in Oklahoma, chose to live-stream her own mammogram on Facebook Live. When the radiologist found non-invasive ductal breast cancer, Meyer chose to have a mastectomy. A Fox News journalist interviewed Meyer, who said, "I will never stop telling women to take care of their bodies and schedule their mammograms" (Farber).

One of the most startling stories occurred in the 2003 film *Ice Bound*, a true story about Dr. Jerri Nielsen (played by Susan Sarandon) who was stranded at an outpost in the South Pole where everything was on lockdown. There were no flights available out of the Amundsen-Scott station, but daring rescue flights dropped medical supplies so that Dr. Nielsen could administer chemotherapy to herself. Finally, she was air lifted to a hospital where she could receive medical care.

Since 2009, television viewers of National League Football games have seen players, coaches, referees and cheerleaders wearing all kinds of pink paraphernalia in honor of October Breast Cancer Awareness month: from pink jerseys, gloves, decals, shoe laces, sideline towels and wristbands to tutus, whistles and kicking tees. Through these efforts, the NFL has raised more than $3 million for the American Cancer society.[1]

Public service announcements (PSAs) encourage women to get mammograms. Often these are not somber warnings that discuss dire consequences but instead are clever, light-hearted and catchy. "Day with the Girls" is a likeable PSA that features a young, attractive African American woman getting out of bed in the morning. She shakes her long, curly hair and puts on a lace bra. A female voice-over says, "Dress 'em up." Wearing a pretty, flower-print dress, she smiles at a woman walking past her on the street as the voice-over says, "Show 'em off." The last scene is in a doctor's office where she sits on an examination table, swinging her legs and smiling at the doctor when he walks in and shakes her hand. The voice-over says, "Get 'em checked." This PSA is emblematic of how commonplace it is now to hear about breast cancer in the media, especially as it relates to screening.[2]

---

1 Beginning in 2020, the NFL will change its activities to support cancer in general with each team given the option to choose which type of cancer they prefer to highlight. (NFL)
2 The multitude of breast cancer awareness television and Internet public service announcements reflect various national campaigns to encourage mammograms. A few of the commercials target men, but most aim at women.

Television Advertising

Television advertising, an essential income source for broadcast television, markets products targeted to viewers based on demographics and types of television programming. Frequently seen on television are advertisements for pharmaceutical drugs. These commercials usually feature happy people doing ordinary, fun activities with their loved ones while voice-overs can be heard discussing treatment, warning of serious side effects and encouraging viewers to "Talk to your doctor." As of 2018, prescription drug makers spent $4.5 billion a year on television advertising (Thrush and Thomas). Notably, the public responds favorably to this tactic. A study by *Prevention* magazine found that one out of every three consumers who sees pharmaceutical ads on television or in magazines has spoken with a doctor about an advertised medication (Wamsley).

In late 2019, there are three commercials on network television for drugs that treat metastatic breast cancer: Verzenio, by Lilly Pharmaceuticals; Piqray, by Novartis; and Ibrance, by Pfizer. Verzenio's tag line is "An everyday treatment for a relentless disease" and its commercial is entitled "Relentless." Three women refer to their metastatic breast cancer as "MBC." An African American woman says, "MBC is relentless, but I'm relentless too." A Hispanic woman says, "MBC doesn't take a day off, and neither will I." A Caucasian woman says, "I treat my MBC with new everyday Verzenio, the only one of its kind that can be taken every day." Buried in the commercial is a message that claims this drug gives women "significantly more time." Piqray, approved by the FDA in May 2019, began to advertise on television in October 2019. Entitled "Hope," the commercial features a senior Caucasian woman walking outdoors while a female voice-over says, "They say life is all about making choices. Well, I didn't choose metastatic breast cancer, not this type, not this mutation; but I choose Piqray and also clarity." It ends with a male voice-over saying, "Discover Piqray, the first and only treatment that targets MBC," while the visual is of an African American woman speaking in front of an audience. The caption says women with advanced MBC who test positive for the PIK3CA mutation will be eligible for the biomarker-driven therapy by Piqray. Ibrance commercials claim that their product "helps slow the progression of cancer." Ibrance commercials appear frequently on television with scenarios that tend to change with the seasons. In what follows, I offer a cultural analysis of an Ibrance commercial that appeared on television in late 2019, entitled "Your Moment."[3]

The Ibrance Commercial

Founded in 1849 and based in New York City, Pfizer is a multinational pharmaceutical company and one of the largest corporations in the United States. On September 23, 2019, Pfizer co-sponsored the television show *Bob ♡ Abishola*, a new half-hour comedy series about a patient who falls in love with his nurse. The original version of the Ibrance commercial, which appeared near the end of the pilot episode, was entitled "In the Moment." The target audience would have been the 160,000 women in America living with metastatic breast cancer. Kate Pickert, author of *Radical: The Science, Culture, and History of Breast Cancer in America* (2019) writes:

> Despite the billions of dollars collected and spent on breast cancer research over the past half-century, relatively little has been devoted to studying metastatic breast cancer patients or their particular forms of the disease. Doctors do not know why some breast cancers eventually form deadly metastases or how to quash the disease once it has spread. Patients with metastatic disease are typically treated with one drug after another. Eventually, nearly all patients with breast cancer metastases run out of options and die, although in recent years, many have been living longer. (46)

Thus, "In the Moment" should appeal to patients who understand that their disease is fatal but who want to enjoy life as long as possible.

The placement of the commercial is deliberate. The new television program was highly anticipated because its creator, Chuck Lorre, is known for

---

3   <https://www.ispot.tv/ad/ZLFN/ibrance-your-moment> Accessed December 16, 2019.

other high-quality comedies including *The Big Bang Theory*; such timing optimizes the number of people who would potentially see the commercial. Further, because the first episode of the show is set in a hospital where the character Bob is having a heart attack but is also attracted to his nurse, Abishola, the show perhaps appeals to the largely female demographic who watch medically themed romance dramas. The viewer is likely to be relaxed while enjoying the program and therefore may not pay attention to the list of possible side effects. She might instead perceive only the pleasant images and the message that Ibrance can delay progression of metastatic breast cancer.

A cultural analysis reveals that the Ibrance commercial is emblematic of the complexity in representing ideas through visual images and verbal discourse. The commercial emphasizes a range of ages, multiple family relationships and racial diversity. It was produced in a particular medium, within a certain period of time, and in certain social context. The medium is television, although it can also be found on the Internet; the time is the present (the beginning of the fall season) and the social context is a world of positives – accomplishment, togetherness, ordinary domestic family activities and new beginnings. These elements are important aspects of culture, and the commercial relies on viewer familiarity with these aspects of culture. Culture enables us to make sense of our world through some shared meanings and recognition of differing meanings. The meaning that a person derives from a cultural artifact, like a television commercial, depends on her or his individual "subjectivities," including socio-cultural background, political perspectives and a range of other similarly broad contexts. Multiple meanings are at the heart of cultural analysis. Before investigating the particulars of this Ibrance commercial, let's take a step back to consider how to go about our analysis and the theories behind the process.

Cultural Analysis

Cultural analysis is derived from cultural studies, an interdisciplinary field of inquiry that explores the production and consumption of meaning. Cultural analysis asks the question: "How does a work relate to the shared living conditions of the time?" because the intended and derived meanings of a work are dependent on the current social, political and economic contexts. Sometimes the meanings are durable; sometimes they are transitory. Consequently, multiple meanings are possible, and this phenomenon is known as polysemy.

A key concept in cultural studies is that meaning does not reside in any given visual or verbal symbol but in the relationship between sender and receiver, the encoder and the decoder. Cultural critics work in a manner similar to literary critics, but their texts are the messages in the media. They "read" the "text" to determine meanings as might be differently constructed by various individuals, and polysemy exists because various individuals incorporate their own experiences, lifestyles, values and other cultural practices into their interpretations of a symbol. In his classic book *Ways of Seeing* (1972), John Berger wrote, "The way we see things is affected by what we know or what we believe" (8). Meaning lies in the power of a symbol to signify something and in the individual's potential to derive meaning from the symbol. People bring to their understanding of cultural artifacts (a television commercial, for instance) other aspects of their culture (images in the media, for example) that link the artifact to a recognizable context. This largely unconscious process enables a person to make sense of an expression or a representation. A visual image and a verbal discourse may coalesce into meaning for one person but seem contradictory to another person.

Raymond Williams, a pioneer in cultural studies, said that culture is the symbolic life of peoples. He was especially concerned about the symbols of the customs of the working class. In one of his lectures on BBC Television, Williams discussed an eighteenth-century painting of sheep peacefully grazing while a little girl dressed in a pretty shepherd's costume sat against a tree nearby. He asked, "Where are the real shepherds?" His point was that the workers upon whom the running of the estate depended were invisible. Williams insisted that cultural texts be inclusive, that everyone in a particular culture be involved in "a shared practice of making meaning" (Couldry 24). Williams' work encourages the analyst to ask, "Who is present and who is absent?"

Stuart Hall, perhaps the most prominent cultural studies scholar, broadened the scope of Williams' inquiries to include matters of race and immigration in the United Kingdom. Hall theorized that symbols are associated with power relations – whether driven by economics, politics or social discrimination – because they determine who is and who is not represented and what issues are or are not important. A key power-related term is "hegemony," the power or dominance that one group or groups hold over others. Significantly, subjugated peoples also have power – power to resist the way they are represented. Hall recognized that audiences are therefore not necessarily passive, but rather active consumers who decode symbols and make their own meanings.

Hall believed we decode symbols by interpreting through various lenses – "from the family in which you were brought up, the places of work, the institutions you belong to, the other practices you do" (Cruz and Lewis 270). In this way, a person could place him- or herself inside a representative image, identifying with it – or not – to varying degrees. When we belong to the same communities, we may derive similar meanings. And when people have some control over the production of meaning, they are likely to experience pleasure because they have maintained their own social identity – even when they resist the dominant (intended) meaning.

Hall developed an encoding/decoding model that enables us to see how an individual may prefer the intended or dominant meaning and thus become the subject within the (dominant) cultural hegemony. He said that a symbolic representation "hails" an individual as if it were hailing a taxi. In other words, it calls to the person. To answer the "hail," a person recognizes the social position that has been constructed in encoding the symbol, and, if the response is cooperative, the meaning is adopted. On the other hand, if an individual resists the dominant meaning, that person has the power to oppose it and find a meaning that is contradictory to the intended one. The opposite meaning may be a refutation or argument against the dominant meaning, a refusal to accept what one sees and/or hears as any kind of truth, logic or reality.

When an individual fits into the dominant ideology but resists certain elements of the intended meaning, a negotiated meaning results. Negotiated positions are popular with various social groups that question their relation to the dominant social, political and economic ideology of the time. Negotiated meanings tend to be what most people take out of messages most of the time.

The Codes of Television

A television commercial depends upon visual representation of people, places and action. A representation tries to be recognizable as "real"; it is an imitation that attempts to evoke a response as if to the real thing. In order to develop representations, certain codes are utilized.

John Fiske, an Australian academic, amplified Hall's model by describing the coding process in a television production in his book *Television Culture*, thus providing the cultural studies analyst with a set of categories to examine. He defined "code" as "a rule-governed system of signs, whose rules and conventions are shared amongst members of a culture, and which is used to generate and circulate meanings in and for that culture" (Fiske 3). Fiske said that television casting directors use these codes most conventionally and, subsequently, stereotypically.

Take social and ideological codes, for example. Social codes include appearance, sound, setting and behavior. Appearance includes skin color, hair, make-up, speech, facial expressions and gestures. Sound includes natural sounds such as wind, and artificial sounds, such as sirens or music. Settings may be indoors with objects intended to denote taste and social class and to promote certain feelings such as comfort or tensions. Outdoor settings may suggest tranquility or danger. Physical behaviors may be easily recognized, such as kissing or hugging; others may require contextual information. Social codes are conveyed through technical means including camera placement, lighting, music and editing to convey a narrative and the preferred meaning while also appearing natural. This is called "representation." Ideological codes such as materialism, success, class, capitalism, equality etc. are also at play in the media. Including characters of diverse races and ethnicities, for example, can be coded as equality.

A cultural studies analysis enables us to understand the range of cultural implications in a work. It recognizes that many meanings can be made by different recipients of that work. It also allows us to reflect upon the ideals and contradictions of our culture and to realize how very complex that finding meaning can be. A television commercial is not just a plea to buy certain goods and services; it also aims to create a recognition of a need, problem, lack or desire. If a person identifies with the images and narrative of a commercial, then she or he may recognize that the advertised product can fulfill the need, solve the problem, supply what's lacking or satisfy the desire. A television commercial "hails" or summons us, and if we recognize that it is speaking to us, we respond to it, thus acknowledging the social position that is encoded within it and within us. In this way we become its subjects.

The Ibrance Commercial[4]

Soft melodic music plays and birds chirp as the commercial opens with the words "I CAN DO THIS MOMENT" (in capital green and white letters) superimposed over a long shot[5] of women carrying bright yellow t-shirts. The scene immediately transitions to a medium long shot of the women adjusting their t-shirts that have "MBC" and a logo of a woman walking on the front. The women appear to be in their early 30s. One has short brown hair; the other is wearing a wide headband that covers most of her dark hair. Behind them is a banner that says "Metastatic Breast Cancer 3K Walk."

The next scene begins with the word "PROUD MAMA MOMENT" in front of a medium long shot of a young man opening a car trunk. There is a "WELCOME" banner hanging to the left above the car, and a "FRESHMEN" banner on a building in the distant back. Young people

4 <https://www.ispot.tv/ad/ZLFN/ibrance-your-moment> The version of the Ibrance commercial I use here for analysis was shown on November 4, 2019, a little over a month after the original version aired on September 23. See Footnote 6 for a comment on slight modifications in the commercial over a short period of time.

5 A long shot creates a full picture of a person, groups or a landscape. A medium shot lets a person's torso and head fill the picture, while the legs and feet are out of the picture. There is a strong tendency in television toward medium shots because they lend themselves to what is considered most natural, as they let the viewer concentrate on the interaction between characters. A close-up focuses on a single, magnified dimension of an object. (See O'Donnell 58–9)

are walking by on screen-right with laundry baskets and other bags, and we hear a bell toll twice to signal the half-hour. Next there is a medium shot of a late middle-age smiling woman, who is obviously the young man's mother, holding a tennis racket. Mother and son are dressed casually – he in a gray hoodie jacket, she in a peach-pink top and light tan sweater. She is wearing a gold necklace, earrings, bracelet and watch. They have medium brown skin and may be African American or perhaps of mixed ethnicity. A female voice-over says, "Thousands of women with metastatic breast cancer, which is breast cancer that has spread to other parts of the body, are living in the moment and taking Ibrance."

Next is a close-up of a Caucasian woman propping her face on her left hand and looking at another person who is blurred. Another close-up of her right hand with a pen reveals that she is working a crossword puzzle. Then in a medium shot we see her and a Caucasian male, both of whom have grey-white hair, sitting in a kitchen as the words "UNWIND MOMENT" flash on the screen. Plants line the window sills, and green plants are visible outside the windows. Fruit, a teapot, a newspaper and a book are on the kitchen counter where the couple sit. A female voice-over is heard while the same words appear at the bottom of the screen: "IBRANCE with an aromatase inhibitor is for postmenopausal women or for men with hormonal receptor-positive (HR+), human epidermal growth factor receptor 2-negative (HER2-) breast cancer that has spread to other parts of the body (metastatic) as the first hormonal based therapy." IBRANCE appears in bold blue letters beside the word "(palbociclib)."

During this voice-over, we shift to a close-up of a hose and then medium close-up of the same older couple washing a Border Collie dog on an outside patio. She is wearing a red tweed sweater while holding the dog's head and laughing. He is in a dark shirt, holding the hose on the dog. The couple towel-dries their dog, and the scene shifts again.

The voice-over proceeds as the words at the bottom of the screen reinforce it: "Ibrance plus letrozole SIGNIFICANTLY DELAYED DISEASE PROGRESSION versus letrozole … ." Numerical data appear in small white print at the bottom of the screen: "Median of 24.8 months for IBRANCE and letrozole vs. 14.5 months for letrozole, in a clinical trial." While hearing and seeing this, we observe the mother and son walking into a dormitory room, both with duffle bags over their shoulders. They turn and look around smiling. As we see them put sheets on one of the two single beds in the dorm room, the voice-over continues: "... and SHRANK TUMORS in over half of patients" as the overlying text mirrors what we hear and small white text at the bottom reads, "55% of patients who took IBRANCE plus letrozole vs. 44% who took letrozole."

In a medium shot, the young man, his back to the viewer, arranges books on his desk while his mother sits beside his bed smiling and folding a green shirt. In a close-up, the mother is seen hanging clothes in a closet, and then the son sits down on the bed beside his mother. They look at each other and smile, and look around the room with satisfaction that they've done good work. The female voice-over continues: "Patients taking Ibrance can develop low white blood cell counts, which may cause serious infections that can lead to death. Ibrance may cause severe inflammation of the lungs that can lead to death." Small white text at the bottom of the screen presents briefer information that complements the words we hear: "IBRANCE may cause serious side effects. Your doctor should take blood tests before you start and while taking IBRANCE. [....] IBRANCE may cause serious side effects."

The commercial comes back to a medium long shot of four Caucasian women in the foreground walking. Still wearing yellow t-shirts, they smile and appear well pleased with themselves. More women are walking behind them. The voice-over continues with the advice to "Tell your doctor right away if you have new or worsening symptoms, including trouble breathing, shortness of breath, cough or chest pain." The next shot, a close-up, shows a Caucasian woman and an African American man standing behind a table, handing out water to the walkers, presumably as the women finish the walk. The people serving drinks are wearing yellow MBC t-shirts as well. Then the walkers, who have flushed cheeks, are seen in a close-up shot drinking water.

Transitioning to the next scene, the female voice-over says, "Before taking Ibrance, tell your doctor if you have fever, chills, or other signs of infection, liver or kidney problems, are pregnant, breast feeding or plan to become pregnant." The screen returns to a medium shot of the senior couple who are sitting on the sofa, watching television and snacking on popcorn. Warm light emanates from two lamps in the room, and photographs – including one of their dog – sit on a table behind them. Their dog jumps over the man and settles down between the couple, who then pat the dog.[6] Small white print on the bottom of the screen reads, "Tell your doctor about medical conditions you have and all medicine you take." The scene ends in a close-up of their three profiles.

The walkers return in a medium close-up. A banner behind them says, "FINISH." They are talking, smiling, clasping hands, and hugging one another and family members. One of the women poses for a photograph with two young adults who are presumably her daughter and son. The voice-over says, "Common side effects include low red blood cells and low platelet counts, infections, tiredness, nausea, sore mouth, abnormalities in liver blood tests, diarrhea, hair thinning or loss, vomiting, rash and loss of appetite." The small white print reads, "These are not all the possible side effects of IBRANCE. For more information, ask your doctor."

Two brief medium close-up shots finish the commercial. First, in front of a college building the mother and son are hugging; we see her say "okay" then we hear her say "good" as her son says, "Bye, Mom." The voice-over says, "Be in your moment," and the small white print reads, "IBRANCE will not work for everyone. Results may vary. By prescription only." In front of a background sign that says "Walk for MBC," the second shot shows the female walker with her daughter and son looking at a cell phone picture. As the voice-over says, "Ask your doctor about Ibrance," the caption on the screen reads, "IBRANCE (in bold blue-purple font) #1 prescribed FDA-approved oral combination treatment for HR+/HER2- metastatic breast cancer. Ibrance.com 844–9Ibrance. Visit IBRANCEpricing.com for cost info."

The commercial lasts only seventy-five seconds, but it has a wealth of visual and aural information.

6   The segment of the dog jumping on the sofa and settling down between the couple was inserted into the earlier (September) version of the commercial in which the dog was already seated between the man and woman. This is but one of the slight modifications in the commercial over a short period of time. While one would expect substantive changes in a commercial as a product or as media conventions evolve, such slight changes pique curiosity: Why did the producers choose to add these elements? How did they imagine the additions might change consumer response?

Cultural Analysis of the Ibrance Commercial

Reflecting on the Ibrance commercial demonstrates how a cultural analysis enables us to understand cultural implications – implications that may also impact us on a personal level. Produced for television transmission, the images in the commercial are carefully designed and controlled by cameras, camera angles, camera movement, direction, lighting, digital manipulation and editing. Television images are production attempts to construct images that resemble the real; therefore, they are representations. Just as people can interpret "reality" to mean different things, so too can they interpret representations of reality in different ways. The practice of looking and seeing images on television rests on complex conditions of existence. Viewers may imagine themselves or someone they know in the televised representations, and their perceptions may change within a short period of time. The recognition of the self in an image, whether the viewer accepts or resists the representation, is an indicator that viewers make active choices as they decode.

Visual Codes and Representation

Social Codes

The Ibrance commercial aired in late September 2019, and the outdoor scenes are coded as pleasant fall weather when women engage in a walk-athon, a couple washes their dog outside, and a mother and son arrive on a college campus for the fall semester. The participants in each of the scenes are dressed casually in shirts, sweaters and, in the case of the walkers, t-shirts with appropriate logos. Their hair is loose and casual as well. Facial expressions include a lot of smiling and eye contact. There is hugging and touching as well. Smiles indicate that the people are happy and satisfied, while hugging and touching signify caring and loving. The majority of the actors are Caucasian with the exception of the mother-son duo who appear in the college scenes and one African American man distributing water at the walkathon. The mother is probably African American, but the son may be racially mixed. Various ages are represented – from the thirties to late sixties. The senior couple and their dog are depicted in a pleasant kitchen with plants and fruit, suggesting a comfortable, middle-class home. It is not unusual to see a dog in a commercial because visuals of dogs tend to evoke positive emotions. The mother appears able to afford to send her son to college; they arrive in a late-model car and she is wearing nice jewelry. The women at the walkathon are probably economically comfortable enough to have the time to participate in it. One of the walkers is shown at the end with (we assume) her proud son and daughter looking at the photos that were taken earlier on a cell phone. Their behavior is leisurely, fun and ordinary.

Representation

Camera use is of particular interest in this commercial. Camera placements are mostly medium shots with several close-ups and medium close-ups. There are only a couple of long shots. This combination suggests intimacy and identification, allowing the viewer to identify with the representations of the people and become subjects of the message. The lighting is soothing, both indoors and out. It is daylight in each outdoor scene; and, with the exception of the scene where the senior couple is watching television, the indoor lighting is bright and natural. Soft music plays in the background, which suggests peacefulness and comfort. Attractive, unblemished actors have been cast in the various roles. There is no overt dialogue, only a woman's voice-over talking about Ibrance. She says nothing about the activities on the screen. The message is predominantly visual, as variations of the word "MOMENT" pass over the sequences.

What is represented here is normalcy – happy people engaging in ordinary, pleasant activities and enjoying life together. In every scene, the characters are interacting with one another. No one is alone.

Ideological Codes

An ideology includes a set of beliefs, values, attitudes and behaviors that are agreed on to the point that they constitute a set of desirable norms for society. Ideology is a form of consent to a particular kind of social or economic order. The following are the ideological codes in the Ibrance commercial: equality, middle class, community, togetherness, family, devotion, love, education, success and time. The presence of racial diversity can be coded as equality. Middle class is coded in the settings, clothing, jewelry, car and activities. A strong sense of community is depicted in the walk-athon scenes. Togetherness, family, devotion, love and comfort are coded in all three scenarios. The importance of education is coded in the mother-son scenes at a university. Success is established when the walkers reach the finish line. The words "significantly delayed disease progression" is a verbal code that tells the viewer that she can have more time if she takes this drug.

The characters in the commercial represent women who presumably have metastatic breast cancer engaging in activities that are ordinary and normal. The viewers who are "hailed" are women who might be a thirty-something married mother of young children, a happily married senior, or a proud mother of a college-bound son. The viewer might be a woman with metastatic breast cancer; she could be a caregiver; she could know someone with MBC. If the viewer identifies with one or more of these representations, she becomes the subject of the commercial.

The Dominant Ideology and the Preferred Meaning

The dominant ideology of this commercial is "Live for the Moment." It is coded in words that prominently appear in bold letters on the screen: "MOMENT," "I CAN DO THIS MOMENT," "PROUD MAMA MOMENT" and "UNWIND MOMENT." The preferred meaning, therefore, is that women with MBC who take Ibrance can live normal lives in the present while engaging in ordinary activities. Rather than focus on one's mortality because the disease is incurable, the subject of the commercial is encouraged to fix her attention to the here and now, appreciate her family and friends and enjoy life while she can. She is reassured that she can do all this – with the help of Ibrance. It is an optimistic message that can buoy positive emotions.

The hailed viewer may respond by saying, "I want to take Ibrance." If she is already taking it, she may respond by saying, "I'm glad I'm taking Ibrance," or she may be reminded to take her dose. Her response to the side effects may be to ignore them or to rationalize that the risks are worth the benefits. A caregiver or friend who accepts the preferred meaning may encourage a woman with MBC to try the drug.

Negotiated Meanings

Viewers who generally accept the ideologies of equality, middle class, community, togetherness, family, love, devotion, education, success and time may nevertheless tweak their positions to fit their own individual identities. A negotiated position might include acceptance of equality but question the commercial's depiction of it, thinking that there should be more representation of race and ethnicity. Another negotiated position might accept family but prefer the inclusion of nontraditional families, such as gay or lesbian couples and their children. A further negotiated position might prefer representation of a different social class, such as working-class women or single mothers struggling to balance work and family. While there could be many other negotiated meanings, if the "Live in the Moment" message is not accepted, then the viewer will oppose the preferred meaning.

Oppositional Meanings

Focusing on the many side effects, for instance, a viewer could reject the preferred meaning, believing that the risks of infection, fatigue, diarrhea and vomiting, trouble breathing and death outweigh the extra time that the drug might provide. A viewer may believe that it is important to think about the future, not just dwell on the present, asking questions such as "Will the mother live to see her son graduate from college?" and "To what extent would a family milestone like that influence her decision to take Ibrance?" Because the disease is incurable, a viewer might ask, "How can life be normal and ordinary when I have metastatic breast cancer? There are many days when I am too sick to do anything that is normal. How can I be happy when I know I'm going to die?" A viewer may recognize the discrepancy between the happy, smiling people in the commercial and the voice-over's rapid listing of negative and serious side effects. A person with a low income may oppose the meaning because Ibrance is very expensive[7] and there is currently no generic form. Although most insurance programs cover some of the costs, co-pays might be prohibitive. What about patients who have no insurance? How can they afford to pay for the drug? The viewer may also oppose the preferred meaning because the commercial could be misleading or even deceptive. This viewer may ask whether the drug is effective. Knowing that production costs for advertising are very high and believing that pharmaceutical companies put more money into advertising than into research, the viewer may reject the commercial altogether by making a meaning that is opposite of the preferred meaning.

Positioning Viewers as Subjects and Pleasure Derived from Viewing

In order for a viewer to derive meaning from a television commercial, a connection must be made that unifies the different elements within the cultural context of the viewer and the viewed – between the

[7] In 2019, one month's supply of Ibrance cost $13,000, up from $9,850/month in 2015. A 20 percent co-pay would be $2,600 a month. (Patients for Affordable Drugs)

signification of the images and the viewer's ability to interpret meaning. Put another way, cultural contexts can enable viewers to make the connection between the elements of the commercial and the message they derive from it. In the Ibrance commercial, the images "hail" viewers with culturally identifiable scenes: a walkathon for breast cancer, ordinary life at home, and beginning college in the fall. It enables viewers of different ages to identify with one or more of the actors and scenarios. It gets viewer attention with the play on the word "Moment" and immediately sets up the idea of living in the moment and enjoying life right now. Viewer recognition of and identification with the images in the commercial empowers them, giving them pleasure from understanding the preferred meaning, negotiating an individual meaning, or opposing the dominant meaning. Furthermore, some viewers may gain pleasure from looking at the characters (including the dog) and observing their contentment.

Making Sense of Social Experience

The Ibrance commercial is easy to understand, and it emphasizes happy family life, community and success, all of which are common American values. Viewers of television commercials are used to seeing physically attractive actors in programs and commercials; therefore, the absence of less attractive or sick women is not unusual and perhaps not even noticeable. Nonetheless, viewers may question what symptoms of metastatic breast cancer are not being shown. A viewer who has MBC may or may not see herself in the commercial, but she may be encouraged to want to be like the characters she is observing. If she believes that she is or can be represented by the characters in the commercial, then she is likely to "ask her doctor." If not, she may challenge the representation and protest the ways in which she believes her condition is being misrepresented.

Conclusion

Critically examining how breast cancer is represented in the media and in other cultural artifacts[8] as we have done here yields important insights about how we conceive of the illness, and it raises important questions about how we as individuals relate to the messages that are being presented to us. These questions can, in turn, lead us to make certain choices or behave in certain ways. In short, representations like the Ibrance commercial provide an affective framework in which we can reflect on our own beliefs and experiences in order to better determine how we want to respond to breast cancer in the present and future. In the essay that follows, health communication researcher Ariane Anderson utilizes precisely this approach of cultural analysis as she examines an online MBC social media support group.

Bibliography

Barker, Chris. *Cultural Studies: Theory and Practice*. 3rd ed. Thousand Oaks, CA: Sage, 2008.
Berger, John. *Ways of Seeing*. London: Penguin, 1972.
Couldry, Nick. *Inside Culture: Reimagining the Method of Cultural Studies*. 2nd ed. London: Sage, 2008.
Cruz, Jon and Justin Lewis. *Viewing, Reading, Listening: Audiences and Cultural Reception*. Philadelphia: Westview Press, 1993.
Farber, M. Oklahoma news anchor diagnosed with breast cancer after streaming first-ever mammogram on Facebook Live <www.foxnews.com/health/oklahoma-news-anchor-diagnosed-breast-cancer-facebook-live>. Accessed November 1, 2019.
Fiske, John. *Television Culture*. London: Methuen, 1987.

8   See the selections by Johanna Shapiro (poetry), Kimberly Myers (comics), Rachel O'Connor, Wendy Palmer and Kimberly Myers (multimedia exhibit), Siobhan Conaty (visual art) and Ariane Anderson (social media) elsewhere in this book.

Hall, Stuart. *Essential Essays: Foundations of Cultural Studies & Identity and Diaspora (Stuart Hall: Selected Writings)*. Durham: Duke UP, 2018.
Jowett, Garth and Victoria O'Donnell. *Propaganda and Persuasion.* 5th ed. Thousand Oaks, CA: Sage, 2011.
NFL supports Breast Cancer Awareness Month <www.nfl.com/news/story/0ap000000068474/article/nfl-supports-breast-cancer-awareness-month>. Accessed November 1, 2019.
O'Donnell, Victoria. *Television Criticism.* 3rd ed. Thousand Oaks, CA: Sage, 2017. Patients for affordable drugs.org <www.patientsforaffordabledrugs.org/2019/01/16/pfizer-statement/>. Accessed November 1, 2019.
Pickert, Kate. "Radical: The Science, Culture, and History of Breast Cancer in America." *Time* (October 14, 2019): 44–50.
Thrush, Glenn and Katie Thomas. "Drug Prices Will Soon Appear in Many TV Ads." *New York Times* (May 8, 2019).
Wamsley, M. (2006, May 3). "A Soft Sell for Hard Drugs." *Media Education Foundation* <www.mediaed.org.>. Accessed November 1, 2019.
Williams, Raymond. *The Country and the City.* London: Hogarth Press, 1958.

ARIANE B. ANDERSON

The New Normal: Metastatic Breast Cancer Patient Experiences of Survivor Identity

Note: Ariane Anderson succumbed to metastatic breast cancer shortly after beginning this essay. We are honored to include her ideas here, though incomplete (and unedited), for two reasons: to acknowledge that breast cancer renders some things unfinished and, more importantly, to celebrate the life and work of a remarkable woman. Dr. Anderson was awarded her Ph.D. posthumously.

Many of us are familiar with current pharmaceutical commercials featuring metastatic breast cancer (MBC) patients coping with the disease (thanks to Ibrance®, letrozole and Verzenio®), beginning with the words "It's a normal day for Carla." Merck's branding slogan is unmistakable for MBC patients: This is your "new normal."

These messages suggest to the metastatic breast cancer patient that while in treatment with these drugs, he or she too can have a fulfilling life as a late-stage breast cancer patient. But do these messages actually resonate with the majority of those of us who are living with MBC? Based on their personal experiences, many patients might say that living with chronic disease is inexact at best.

Moreover, do we, with MBC, adopt the term *survivor* in the way that it has been commonly marketed to the public through the American Cancer Society, Susan G Komen and advertisers? Are *we* "sheroes" (Sulik, 2012), constantly doing battle with our foe? Or, as is apparent in this and other recent marketing, are we now being given a new cancer identity to adopt? Do we ascribe to either of these identities – the hero-survivor or new normal? As a patient, a health communication researcher and a patient-provider communication teacher for the past ten years, I have been trying to make sense of this disease and how to live with it as I move through each day in all of my interactions. In this essay, I set about to discuss ways we MBC patients are making sense (Weick, 1995) of our disease experiences in one online MBC social media support group. Thirteen interviews with fellow patients (myself included) reveal that members' understandings of their disease vary, not just among one another but also with regard to popular discourses about breast cancer, including the "new normal."

"Now don't get me started."

Nadine, a four-year member of the MBC support group that I attended every Tuesday, got my immediate attention when she said this. She said it in response to what another member had commented on about the latest series of TV commercials about Ibrance and the "new normal" that the women portrayed in each commercial were (theoretically) experiencing. The room became loud with numerous responses affirming Nadine's comment. I was relatively new to the group and feeling like I had missed out on a previous discussion, so I asked Nadine what she meant by that comment.

She said, "Those ads are not realistic. They make me *really* want to vomit! They don't show the stuff we really go through. My plans constantly change because I don't know how I am going to feel from one hour to the next. Tomorrow morning, I could wake up and not feel like I can even get up. Other days, I make plans, feel okay, then three hours later I have to lay down."

Another member chimed in: "How about the fact that most of the time I can't even eat and hold my food down, let alone share an ice cream cone with my granddaughter, like in the one where she goes to the ball game?!"

Lisa, who had been NED (no new evidence of disease) for about three years, said, "Those commercials remind me that my own family forgets that I am still dealing with the side effects of my treatments and they assume

I can keep up with them with my neuropathy. I can't! I am constantly having to remind them that I can't do theme parks all day and night long."

As we were discussing this, I could feel everyone's frustration with the disconnect between what was being portrayed to the masses and our own lived experiences as women with metastatic breast cancer who indeed looked like patients with bald heads, scars all over our bodies, puffy faces from steroids and/or invisible marks of pain such as our perpetual existence as economically disadvantaged women who can neither work nor survive on social security disability. Instead of showing these truths, the commercials feature well-dressed, able-bodied women, hair intact, cheeks a bit rosy, faintly smiling, surrounded by family and friends, easily ambulating around a baseball stadium, lecturing in a college classroom and enjoying family out by the lake. True, some of us looked healthy on the surface, but all of us in this group were there because we needed each other's stories to help us cope individually with the treatments and impairments that we all had in common.

Naturally, our group was full of different experiences, challenges and backgrounds, but we all shared a similar diagnosis. Some of us had had very recent diagnoses; others had been dealing with MBC for five years or more (as I had). Some were triple negative, thus having fewer treatment options; some were on promising immunotherapies; some had significant breathing issues; some were on their fifth or six course of treatment and were running out of options. And yet, whatever our differences, we all felt similar disdain for the commercials, even angry because they are misleading.

I left the meeting that day contemplating exactly how all of us (and many others I had met during the past five years) from our various walks of life were actually coping with our individual diagnoses of stage IV breast cancer. Many of us used the supportive care and behavioral medicine services provided by our cancer hospital as well as our own forms of alternative therapies such as CBD (cannabidiol), specific diet regimens and spiritual approaches. But it seemed that we kept returning to the same theme week after week: How difficult it was to cope with a chronic and uncertain disease trajectory.

Us and Them

MBC patients have unique, evolving physiological and psychosocial needs (Cardoso, Harbeck, Mertz & Fenech, 2016). They experience ongoing isolating effects of diagnosis and treatments as well as shorter prognoses. MBC patients are often encouraged by their psycho-oncologists to seek and join supportive networks. Those who do often find that they can engage in freer expression, sharing less socially desirable stories. For instance, in Vilhauer's study of mixed-stage groups, MBC members described feeling alienated because earlier-stage members did not want to hear their fears about dying. Yet later-stage members felt support from each other because of seeing each other "living well despite MBC," which in turn made them feel more hopeful (Vilhauer 2012).

Surely the group I am attending functions as a place where we can say just about anything and not feel rejected, because we know we are surrounded by people who are going through what we are going through on some level. Contrast this with having MBC and being in a group of earlier-stage breast cancer patients who might talk about their "firsts" such as losing their hair, or early rounds of chemo, or getting reconstructive surgery. It would be harder to feel support from the earlier-stage patients because not only are they not going through things MBC patients have already been through numerous times, but they also have an end in sight; most MBC patients don't have that perspective. Although studies indicate that MBC patients report that they are most satisfied with support from spouses, family and friends, the need for support from fellow patients remains (Cardoso, Harbeck, Mertz & Fenech, 2016). MBC patients need each other for support in ways that clinicians, family members and friends cannot provide.

LISA KATZ

Support Group

Five women are counting women
one by one, they want to count to five,
five cups, five eggs,
five oranges, five pearls,
five days a week to work.

Five women are counting women
one by one, they want to count to five.
And their children count the fingers on each hand:
father, mother, father, mother, father,
father, mother, father, mother, father.

There are so many new things to count.
The doctor who frowns *for your own good*
and the one who cuts
and the one who builds with plastic.
Time spent waiting.
For the first infusion
the second the third the fourth the fifth the last.
For hair to fall,
to grow back again;
cells and nodes and empty hands,
counts from bone and counts from blood.

How time dies in the waiting room:
months weeks
days minutes
seconds.

You'd counted on
longer, hadn't you?

Four women are counting women
One by one, they want to count to four.

Notes on Contributors

In the spirit of considering each of the following people a companion who illuminates breast cancer from the inside out, we use first names below instead of formal titles.

ARIANE B. ANDERSON earned her PhD in Communication from the University of South Florida. She was a health and interpersonal communication scholar and instructor of interpersonal communication and public speaking at USF and several other institutions. Ariane used feminist perspectives on health within the research of actual and cyber-mediated platforms of chronic illness and acute disease. More specifically, she participated in, and examined, a stage-four breast cancer online support group in terms of individual/organizational sense-making regarding survivorship. Ariane's research included the study of dominant discourses of survivor identity, citizenship philanthropy and end-of-life communication.

MARIA J. BAKER, PhD, MS, is a diplomate of the American Board of Medical Genetics and Genomics and the American Board of Genetic Counseling with dual certification as a genetic counselor and medical geneticist. In her roles as Professor of Medicine at Penn State College of Medicine and Director of the Penn State Cancer Genetics Program, Maria has launched leading cancer initiatives: the Penn State Cancer Genetics Program, which provides genetic counseling and testing to individuals concerned about a personal and/or family history of cancer; a universal screening policy for Lynch syndrome, the most common hereditary cause of both colorectal and endometrial cancer; and the Pediatric Cancer Genetics Program. Maria's scholarship focuses on improving the identification of hereditary cancer syndromes, as well as ethical, legal and social implications of cancer predisposition testing.

MICHAEL BAUM, MD, qualified in medicine at Birmingham University Medical School in 1960. He has held Chairs of Surgery at Kings College London (1980–90), the Institute of Cancer Research (1990–5) and University College London (1995–2001) and has served as Chairman of the British Oncology Association, the European Breast Cancer Conference and the psychosocial committee of the National Cancer Research Institute. Having now retired from surgery, Mike is currently Professor Emeritus of Surgery and Visiting Professor of Medical Humanities at University College London, where he teaches and promotes the medical humanities, including fine art, literature and philosophy.

DEBORAH BOWMAN, MA, PhD, is Professor of Bioethics and Clinical Ethics at St George's, University of London. Her academic interests concern the application of ethics to policy, clinical practice, public involvement in ethical debate, and healthcare regulation. She comments widely about medical ethics in both academic and popular publications and is currently serving as Chair of the General Medical Council's working group, whose revised consent guidance for doctors will be published in 2020. Deborah also works as a radio broadcaster, including as a presenter of *Test Case, Patient Undone* and as a regular panelist and program consultant to *Inside the Ethics Committee*, all for BBC Radio 4. Deborah's honors include Most Excellent Order of the British Empire and Fellowship of the Royal Society of Arts.

DAVID CARNISH, MA, MDiv, is an ordained, board-certified chaplain with thirty years of experience in chaplaincy ranging from nursing home care, community hospitals, hospice, mental health and academic medical centers. He is Manager of Clinical Pastoral Education with Penn State Hershey Medical Center and serves on the Board of Directors of the national Association of Clinical Pastoral Education. David has focused his career on aspects of religious humanism, including art, literature and particularly poetry as ways in which persons convey the depths of their lives.

SIOBHAN CONATY, PhD, is Associate Professor of Art History at La Salle University, where she teaches courses on art and medicine, politics and gender. Her scholarship in health and medical humanities has appeared in the *Journal of Humanities in Rehabilitation*, *Woman's Art Journal*, *The International Journal of the Humanities*, and as book chapters in *American Women Artists: Gender, Culture, and Politics* and *Research Methods in Health Humanities*. Siobhan's research has been supported by the Doctors Kienle Center for Humanistic Medicine at Penn State College of Medicine, the National Endowment for the Humanities, the J. Paul Getty Research Institute and the American Academy in Rome. Siobhan serves on steering committees for the Section on Medicine and the Arts at the College of Physicians of Philadelphia, the Health Humanities Consortium and ARTZ Philadelphia.

LYNN FANTOM, RN, BSN, CBCN, is a clinical nurse coordinator at the Penn State Milton S. Hershey Medical Center, where she educates and assists breast cancer patients throughout their journey. Lynn has worked as a nurse navigator/coordinator since 2003.

DANIEL R. GEORGE is Associate Professor of Humanities at Penn State College of Medicine. He earned a BA in English and philosophy from the College of Wooster and an MSc and PhD in medical anthropology from Oxford University. Danny's main research focus concerns issues related to aging and dementia, and he is co-author of *The Myth of Alzheimer's* (St. Martins Press, 2008), and *American Dementia* (Johns Hopkins University Press, 2021).

DEBRA REX GEORGE, MA, MEd, is semi-retired and currently serving as an executive advisor to not-for-profit leaders in the social services and behavioral health fields. During her forty-two-year career, Debra has worked as CEO of an award-winning child welfare and children's behavioral health nonprofit organization in Northeast Ohio and has been recognized for her leadership both locally and nationally, including Leader of the Year by the National Alliance for Children, Families, and Communities and by Behavioral Health Today. Debra remains active with several state and local groups that strive to help vulnerable children and families and serves as a mentor and coach to leaders who seek to carry out their work strategically and with heart.

JENNIFER HAYDEN is a graphic novelist based in New Jersey. Her breast cancer memoir, *The Story of My Tits*, was nominated for an Eisner Award and has been translated into Italian and Spanish. Her first collection, *Underwire*, was excerpted in *The Best American Comics 2013*. She is currently working on a graphic travel novella about France called *Le Chat Noir*, as well as an anticookbook – her first work in color – called *Where There's Smoke There's Dinner*. She has lectured at Columbia, Princeton and Harvard Universities and regularly speaks to breast cancer organizations, women's groups, art students, and comix and literary audiences from California to New York City, Miami to Toronto, and London.

MICHAEL HAYES, PhD, is Assistant Professor in the Departments of Psychiatry & Behavioral Health and Medicine at Penn State College of Medicine, Psychosocial Services Coordinator for the Penn State Cancer Institute's Cancer Committee and founding Program Director of Penn State Cancer Institute CARE (Cancer Assistance and Resource Education) Center. Michael is a licensed psychologist whose clinical practice is dedicated to caring for patients diagnosed with cancer and those undergoing bone marrow or solid organ transplantation. Additionally, he is a teacher and facilitator of Mindfulness-Based Stress Reduction, certified by the University of Massachusetts School of Medicine Center for Mindfulness. Michael's scholarship focuses on social determinants of health, the impact of creative writing on mood in cancer patients, and the use of tablet-based supportive care interventions for women with metastatic breast cancer.

ELIANA V. HEMPEL, MD, is Assistant Professor of Medicine at Penn State College of Medicine, where she serves as Associate Program Director for Ambulatory Medicine and Director of the Primary Care Track. In her various roles, she explores the value of relationships in the development of learners, the care of patients, and the fulfillment of physicians. Eliana's scholarship focuses on primary care and health systems science-related medical education and narratives on grief. Her work appears in professional journals including 2020 publications in the *New England Journal of Medicine* and *Obstetrics & Gynecology*.

AMY HOLIDAY is a stage-two breast cancer survivor living and working in New York City, where she serves as Deputy Chief of Staff at the College Board. Amy is a graduate of Tulane University. This is her first publication.

MARK L. HUNNICUTT has served local churches the Southeast U.S. since 1991. A two-time cancer veteran, Mark now lives and works in Dalton, Georgia. He loves people and connecting them to life in Christ.

KATE JOLLIE retired seven years post-treatment after thirty-five years in insurance and information technology. Her journey has taken her from being the office manager for a surgical practice (where she was treated) to exploring voice-over work, working part-time in the pro-shop of a large golf course, singing for the pure joy of sharing music and, most recently, relocating to southern Maine to become the Executive Director of a community senior center whose primary goal is to bring people together to enjoy, learn and grow.

LISA KATZ earned her PhD from Hebrew University and teaches translation, most recently at Ben Gurion University. In 2018, her translation of *Late Beauty*, poems by Tuvia Ruebner, was a National Jewish Book Award finalist. Lisa serves as Israeli editor of *Poetry International Archives* and, since April 2017, as (interim) Central English editor of the *PIA* site in Rotterdam, the Netherlands. In the fall of 2017 she was translator-in-residence at the Iowa MFA program. Her poetry collections *Are You With Me* and *Reconstruction* (*Shikzur*) have been published in English and in Hebrew translation.

GORDON L. KAUFFMAN, Jr., MD, is Emeritus Professor at the Pennsylvania State University. His primary appointment was in the Department of Surgery, but he also held joint appointments in the

Departments of Physiology, Humanities, and Medicine. The majority of his publications are in the scientific literature. He was a member of the inaugural Penn State Hershey Physician Writers Group organized by Kimberly Myers. Gordon continues to explore narrative writing that broadens the scope and deepens the understanding of patient-physician/physician-patient interactions.

KEVIN B. KNOPF, MD, is Division Chief of Hematology/Oncology at Highland Hospital, a "safety net" hospital in Oakland, California. He has been a practicing oncologist for twenty years and a health economist/health services researcher and Assistant Clinical Professor of Medicine at University of California San Francisco School of Medicine, where he is a member of the Institute for Health Policy Studies. Kevin has written many articles on the economics and public health aspects of delivering oncology care. He attended college at the Massachusetts Institute of Technology, where he was an English minor.

JEFFREY M. KOWALESKI, MD, is a Staff Physician for the Veterans Affairs Boston Healthcare System and Clinical Instructor in Medicine at Harvard Medical School. Jeff wears several clinical hats, attending on the Hospice and Palliative Care Unit, the subacute rehab service and the inpatient Palliative Care consult service. His scholarly interests range from reflective writing to quality improvement, and he has published in professional journals including *Journal of the American Medical Association* and *Journal of Palliative Medicine*.

JULIE A. MACK, MD, is Division Chief of Breast Imaging in the Department of Radiology at Penn State Hershey Medical Center and co-director of the Penn State Hershey Breast Center. She lives in Lancaster, Pennsylvania with her husband and enjoys spending time with her four adult children and her grandson.

KIMBERLY R. MYERS, MA, PhD, is Professor of Humanities and Medicine and Distinguished Educator at Penn State College of Medicine, where she co-created and co-directs the "Medical Humanities" course required of all first-year medical students. Kimberly founded and hosts the Penn State Hershey Physician Writers Group and serves as Program Director of Schwartz Center Rounds for the Penn State Cancer Institute. Kimberly's scholarship, which focuses on medical education, illness narratives and graphic medicine, appears in professional journals including *Journal of the American Medical Association, British Medical Journal, American Medical Association Journal of Ethics, Annals of Internal Medicine, Literature and Medicine*, and *Academic Medicine*, as well as lay periodicals including *The Chronicle of Higher Education* and *The Atlantic*. She is author or editor of six books.

RACHEL O'CONNOR, MA, is a curator, educator and art historian. She is Curator for the Art Association of Harrisburg, where she works to bring professional, cutting-edge exhibitions to the state capital and surrounding area. Rachel is particularly interested in creating socially relevant exhibits that challenge audiences' world views and perceptions about topics such as feminism, race and illness. Rachel is an adjunct Art History professor at Messiah University, where she teaches Art History Survey I & II, as well as an interdisciplinary non-Western Topics course that focuses on Women Artists from Eastern and Indigenous cultures.

VICTORIA O'DONNELL, PhD, was Professor of Communication and Director of the University Honors Program for twelve years at Montana State University, as well as Professor and Chair of Communication Departments at the University of North Texas and Oregon State University. She authored four books and numerous articles and book chapters on a wide range of subjects concerning persuasion, the social effects of media, women in film and television, British politics, Nazi propaganda, collective memory and cultural studies theory. She was also a Danforth Foundation Associate and a Summer Scholar of the National Endowment for the Humanities and received numerous research grants, honors and teaching awards. Victoria passed away while on Safari in Africa on March 8, 2020, due to events unrelated to cancer.

WENDY PALMER earned dual degrees in Physiotherapy and Sports Science from the University of Cape Town, South Africa. She is a professional photographer whose work has been displayed nationally, and a review of her photographs chronicling a journey with breast cancer was published in the *Journal of the American Medical Association* in 2018. Wendy regularly leads portrait and lighting workshops at community colleges and currently lives in Naples, Florida.

JOHN D. POTOCHNY, MD, is Associate Professor of Surgery at Penn State Health Milton S. Hershey Medical Center, where he specializes in plastic and reconstructive surgery, including breast reconstruction. In addition to clinical practice, John participates in medical student and resident education and began a multidisciplinary microsurgery training program for resident physicians and graduate students to introduce trainees to the basic skill sets required to master complex microsurgery. In recognition of his outstanding contribution to medical and graduate education, John received a 2019 Dean's Award for Excellence in Teaching.

ELIZABETH REID, MS, RDN, LDN, is an advanced practice dietitian at the Children's Hospital of Philadelphia, where she works with children with cystic fibrosis. She has published and presented nationally on pancreatic enzyme replacement therapy, the feeding relationship, disordered eating and sports nutrition in people living with cystic fibrosis.

IAN R. ROSS, MD, is a staff physician at the John Cochran VA Medical Center in St. Louis, Missouri. His scholarship focuses on education for medical students, residents and practicing internists, specifically regarding diagnostic and procedural point-of-care ultrasound. His research and medical creative writing have been published in professional journals, including *Annals of Internal Medicine*, *Journal of General Internal Medicine*, and *PLOS One*, and he co-authored a chapter of *The Washington Manual of Critical Care*.

KATHRYN H. SCHMITZ, PhD, MPH, FACSM, is Professor of Public Health Sciences at the Pennsylvania State University's College of

Medicine. She is a clinical trialist who has led many exercise trials and has translated her work into clinical practice. Kathryn has served as president of the American College of Sports Medicine, currently chairs the Global Exercise In Medicine Governing Committee and is founder of the Moving Through Cancer Initiative of the American College of Sports Medicine. She has published over 260 peer reviewed scientific papers and was the lead author of the first ACSM Roundtable on Exercise for Cancer Survivors. In March, 2018 Kathryn co-chaired an International Multidisciplinary ACSM Roundtable on Exercise and Cancer Prevention and Control. The physicians, outpatient rehabilitation specialists, researchers, and exercise professionals in the room broadly agreed it is time for exercise oncology to go prime time. The question is how. Kathryn's professional mission is to answer that question.

JOHANNA SHAPIRO, MA, PhD, is Professor of Family Medicine and Founder/Director of the Program in Medical Humanities & Arts, University of California Irvine School of Medicine. She has received many teaching honors, including the Society of Teachers of Family Medicine's Humanism in Medicine Award in 2020. Johanna's research focuses on the process of professional identity formation in medical education, including the impact of training on student empathy, on medical student-patient relationships, and on the management of difficult clinical encounters. She is widely published in the field of medical humanities and serves as editor for several professional medical journals. Her book, *The Inner World of Medical Students: Listening to Their Voices in Poetry*, is a critical analysis of important themes in the socialization process of medical students as expressed through their creative writing.

GEORGE R. SIMMS, MD, PhD, MTS, trained at the University of Zurich Faculty of Medicine in Switzerland and subsequently practiced primary care and palliative care medicine for fifty years in Hong Kong, California, Oklahoma, Pennsylvania and Massachusetts. George served as Professor and Chair of the Department of Family & Community Medicine at Penn State University College of Medicine where, though now retired, he continues to mentor students and faculty. His training in medicine, human behavior and theology stems from a lifelong commitment to practice whole-person medicine.

MARK STOUT, PA-C, is a Physician Assistant who has worked for over thirty-five years in the fields of family practice, substance abuse, bone marrow transplant and, currently, radiation oncology at Penn State Cancer Institute. Mark serves as a committee member for the Penn State Cancer Institute Schwartz Center Rounds. This is his first attempt at scholarly writing.

HENRY WAGNER, MD, is Professor of Radiation Oncology, Radiology, and Medicine at Penn State College of Medicine. He served as Director of the Division of Radiation Oncology for twelve years and was the founding Physician Director of Schwartz Center Rounds for Penn State Cancer Institute. Henry's clinical and research activities have been devoted to the multimodality management of cancer, with studies published in *Cancer*; *International Journal of Radiation Oncology, Biology, and Physics*; *Journal of Clinical Oncology,* and *British Journal of Hematology* and chapters in *Clinical Radiation Oncology* and *Cancer Screening*, among others.

ELVA J. WINTER, PhD, is a certified sex therapist and retired Professor of Psychiatric/Mental Health Nursing at York College of Pennsylvania. A member of the American Association of Sexuality Educators, Counselors and Therapists, Elva has practiced psychotherapy and sex therapy for over thirty years. Her research and publication interests have been in women's health, human sexuality and the educational and therapeutic use of poetry.

Index

adjuvant therapy 391, 402, 404, 419–20
 see also chemotherapy, adjuvant therapy; aromatase inhibitors
advance care planning 100
aesthetic concerns 9, 51, 205, 288–9, 312–3, 327, 360, 405
 see also reconstruction
African-American 217, 222, 226–7
agency see autonomy
alcohol 165
Amazon warrior 232, 241, 327, 334–6, 361–2
anastrozole (brand Arimidex) see aromatase inhibitors
anger 81, 103–4, 250, 267, 462
anti-estrogen therapy see hormonal therapy
anxiety 18–9, 21, 22–3, 25–6, 44–5, 48–9, 100, 147, 152, 255–65, 318–9, 359–60
applied humanities 4
Arimidex see aromatase inhibitors
aromatase inhibitors (AIs) 34, 69, 144, 374, 389–96, 414, 449, 461
artistic representations of breasts and breast cancer 331–67, 413–4
 Baroque 345–50
 Best, Clare 359–64
 classical period 333–6
 Eakins, Thomas 351–4, 363–4, 415
 medieval period 336–41
 Michelangelo 342–5, 363
 Postmodern 354–63
 prehistoric period 331–3
 Raphael 342, 369
 Realism 350–4, 363
 Rembrandt 345–50, 363, 413–4
 Renaissance 341–5
 Spence, Jo 357–9, 364
 Stevens, Laura 360–1
 Stieglitz, Alfred 288–9
 Venus of Willendorf 332–3
 Wilke, Hanna 354–6, 359, 364
Astra Zeneca 393
ATAC trial see research / clinical trials
autonomy 10, 65–6, 101, 142–8, 172–3, 197, 199, 203–7, 210–1, 327, 363, 408
axilla see lymph nodes

baldness see hair loss
Bathsheba at Her Bath see artistic representations of breasts and breast cancer, Rembrandt
behavior see lifestyle changes
being present see listening
biopsy 8, 24, 31, 136, 142, 263–4
blastema theory 384
body image see self-image / self-identity
BRCA1 and BRCA2 33, 47, 54, 56, 180, 373, 426–8, 430–1, 433–4
 see also genetics
breast cancer marketplace 11, 224–5, 375, 439–41
breast conservation therapy 374, 398, 400–2, 406–8
 ongoing clinical questions 401–2
 technique 401
 see also lumpectomy
breast exam see physical exam

breast-feeding 55, 82, 336
Burney, Frances ("Fanny") 381–2

cancer research 139, 144
Cancer Research Campaign 393
cancer risk management 152, 155–70, 426, 429
    Reid; Schmitz
CAT scan *see* CT scan
chaos story *see* Frank, Arthur
chaplain 77–83
chemotherapy 33–5, 45, 270, 372, 465
    adjuvant therapy 69, 419
    fever 87
    hydration 165–6
    neoadjuvant therapy 53, 69, 199
clinical trials *see* research / clinical trials
cognitive-behavioral therapy (CBT) 126–7, 183
comics *see* graphic medicine
coming out *see* diagnosis, sharing with others
communication *see* doctor-patient relationship, communication
confidentiality 74
core needle biopsy *see* biopsy
covering *see* diagnosis, sharing with others
critical humanities 4, 7
CT scan 37–9, 401
cultural studies 444–59

death and dying 97–102, 103–5, 113–4, 133–4, 135, 198, 235, 238–40, 273, 356, 392
delivering bad news *see* diagnosis, emotional impact
denial 29, 61
dense breasts 22–4
depression 126–7, 152, 304, 378
diagnosis 1–2, 8–9

data presentation 54, 407–8
diagnostic mammogram 21
emotional impact 8, 25, 30, 61, 81, 108–9, 112, 136, 138, 147, 148, 198, 255–8, 265–6, 277, 429
    informing others 63–5, 121, 136–8, 265, 267, 371
    initial consultation 37, 44, 53, 403–5
Diagnostic and Statistical Manual of Mental Disorders (DSM) 19
diet *see* nutrition
disclosure *see* diagnosis, informing others
doctor-patient relationship 17, 43–50, 92–4, 100, 220, 222, 255, 403
    body language 43–5, 48, 89–90, 176, 198–9, 200, 264
    communication 12, 17, 24, 26, 30, 45, 55–6, 146, 198–200, 204, 249, 264, 265, 270, 407–9
        barriers 99–100, 222–3, 227, 286, 403–5
    delivering bad news 92–4, 95, 112, 198, 257
    trust 17, 20, 92, 223–4
doctors, perceptions of 222–4
ductal carcinoma
    in situ (DCIS) 75, 136, 146, 403, 422
    invasive 115, 172, 277, 403

Edwin Smith surgical papyrus 376
Egypt, ancient 11, 331, 376
emergency room 390, 391
empathy 8, 46, 72, 255
    see also doctor-patient relationship
endocrine system 390
endocrine therapy *see* hormonal therapy
end-of-life care *see* hospice; palliative care
environmental factors 227–8

Index

ER/PR + (estrogen-receptor and progesterone-receptor positive) 68–9, 178, 390–1, 395, 410
ethics *see* medical ethics
exercise 126–7, 130–1, 144, 147, 151–4, 155, 167–8, 270, 318–9
    exercise oncology 10, 151–2
existential concerns 46, 75, 100, 101, 103–5, 121, 235–6, 274, 294–5, 320–1, 463, 465
    see also purpose and meaning
expanders *see* implants
expressive humanities 4

family and friends 98, 118–20, 135–8, 173, 253, 255, 268, 270, 277, 371–3, 429, 439, 452–4, 462
    motherhood 8, 32, 53, 82, 137, 148–9, 348–9
fatigue 100, 117–8, 151, 155, 165, 174
fear 78, 82, 132, 135, 198, 206, 258, 261, 267, 269, 294, 359
    see also anxiety
feminism 334, 354–64
fertility 10, 32, 47, 82, 171–8, 179, 332–3, 336
Fisher, Bernard 391, 415, 418
Frank, Arthur
    chaos story 217
    quest story 216, 237, 241
    restitution story 216, 230–1, 240

Galen 379, 414
genetics 33, 47, 359–60, 374, 425–37
    Ashkenazi Jewish ancestry 373, 428
    discrimination 426–7
    next generation sequencing 431
    relatives at risk 119, 434–5
    RNA analysis 435
    see also BRCA1 and BRCA2
Google *see* internet

graphic medicine 11, 249–54, 255–71
gratitude 25, 207, 322–3
Greece, ancient 333–6, 377–9
grief 180
    see also depression
guilt 183, 196, 429

hair loss 34, 234–5, 270, 275, 300–1, 303, 305, 306–7
Halsted, William *see* mastectomy, radical
healing 72–3
    see also resilience
health humanities 4–7
health insurance *see* insurance
HER2/neu 34, 68–9, 74, 420
Herceptin *see* HER2/neu
Hippocrates 377
hope 9, 44–5, 202, 277, 312–3, 392
    see also survivorship
hormonal therapy 12, 30, 31, 33–4, 68–9, 178, 180, 390–6, 402
    see also aromatase inhibitors
hospice 87–8, 98–9, 103–5, 374
    see also palliative care
hospital
    admission 85–6
    hospitalist 85–8
    hospital medicine 86–8
    perceptions of 220–2
humor 34–5, 108–10, 275, 306–7
humoral medicine 11, 377–8, 379–81
hypochondria 19–20

implants 32–3, 51, 310–1, 325, 327, 361
    exchange surgery 60
    expanders 55, 58–60
    sensation 54, 184
    see also reconstruction
informed consent 56–7, 201–2, 408–9
    see also medical ethics

initial consultation *see* diagnosis
insurance 3, 33, 65, 409, 427, 430
    lack of / inadequate 9, 67, 69, 456
    see also recurrent disease,
        financial impact
interdisciplinary team 98, 100–1, 104,
    142–5, 200, 352
internet 9, 44, 62, 139, 142, 146, 147, 195,
    208, 364, 441, 444
intuition 8, 17–20, 25–7, 81

Jewish 372
    Ashkenazi 217, 226, 228, 373, 428

letrozole (brand Femara) *see* aromatase
    inhibitors
Life Review 9
    see also advance care planning;
        hospice
lifestyle changes 147, 155–6, 426
    behavior patterns 127–9
listening 78–80, 83, 125, 271
Lister, Lord 382, 384, 385
Lorde, Audre 215, 219, 225, 227, 231,
    232, 240
lumpectomy 12, 31, 69, 140–1, 357, 381,
    387, 400, 406
    see also mastectomy, versus breast
        conservation / lumpectomy
lymph nodes 44, 46, 48, 58, 92,
    116, 344–5, 379–88, 400–2,
    414, 417–9

male breast cancer 107–22, 180–1
mammogram 18, 26, 91, 136, 258–61, 422
mastectomy 11, 12, 31, 47–8, 228–32, 250,
    275, 288, 327, 338, 344, 352–4,
    359, 379, 381–3
    process described 48, 58, 387–9, 400
    prophylactic 47–8, 56, 81, 139, 204,
        360, 426

    radical 12, 345, 385–9,
        398–400, 416–8
    super radical 418
    versus breast conservation/lumpec-
        tomy 31, 406–8, 420
    see also self-image
mastitis 371, 376–7
media 12, 355, 375, 439–59
    movies 440, 441
    social media 12, 62, 253, 462
    television 12, 439, 440, 443, 461–3
    see also internet
medical anthropology 10, 139,
    140, 146–7
medical ethics 10, 71, 204–5
medical humanities 4–7
medical model 214, 217–8, 226, 231,
    233, 240
medical records 89–90, 202
medicalization of female body 230, 359
memento mori 273, 350
metastasis 72–3, 85–8, 95, 133–4, 374,
    402, 409, 421, 442–58, 461–4
    see also recurring disease
motherhood *see* family and friends
MRI 25, 45–6, 426

narratives *see* stories
National Endowment for the
    Humanities (NEH) 5
National Health Service (NHS) 3
    Carer's Allowance 4
    exemption certificate 3
National Institute of Health (NIH) 415
natural history 12
neoadjuvant therapy *see* chemotherapy,
    neoadjuvant
nipple-sparing *see* reconstruction
Novaldex *see* tamoxifen
nurse navigator 30–6, 71
nutrition 10, 144, 152, 155–70

Index

oestrogen receptor *see* estrogen receptor
Oncotype DX 34, 41
optimism *see* resilience
organic food 158–9

pain 18–9, 26, 39, 99–102, 103, 104, 117, 152–4, 314–5, 371–2, 374, 410
palbociclib (brand Ibrance) 449
palliative care 97–102, 374, 409
partial mastectomy *see* lumpectomy
partner / spouse 44, 46, 63–5, 72, 103–5, 127–8, 131–2, 171–8, 179–91, 300–1, 316–7, 324–5
  see also family and friends
paternalism 20, 93–4, 214, 222, 465
pathographies *see* stories
pathology report *see* biopsy
personalized medicine 30, 436
perspective 126–7, 128–9, 133–4
pertuzumab (brand Perjeta) *see* triple-negative breast cancer
PgR *see* ER/PR +
photographs 81–2, 273–6, 277–325, 355–64
physical exam 44, 91
  breast exam 91–2, 265–6
  screening 91
plastic surgery *see* reconstruction
poetry 51–2, 213–47, 273–6, 277–325, 327, 369, 465
post-menopausal 390
post-traumatic growth 233–5
  see also resilience
poverty 67–76
  see also insurance, lack of / inadequate; recurrent disease, financial impact
prayer 48, 275, 292, 414
  see also spirituality
pregnancy *see* fertility

primary care physician 89–96
prosthesis 33, 327
  see also implants, reconstruction
purpose and meaning 12–3, 113, 121–2, 277, 294–5
  see also existential concerns

quality of life 71, 87–8, 98–9, 129–31, 374, 390, 409
quest story *see* Frank, Arthur

radiation therapy 29, 36–41, 117–8, 144, 386–7, 397–412, 419
  explanation of 405–6
  palliative radiation 12, 409
  process 401
  side effects 39–40, 405
radiotherapy *see* radiation therapy
reconstruction 8, 11, 32–3, 51–2, 53–60, 205, 214, 228–32, 275, 310–1, 316–7, 324–5, 327
  nipple creation 312–3
  nipple sparing 58, 179
  see also implants
recurrent disease 12, 38, 398, 409–10
  fear of 35, 82–3
    see also anxiety
  financial impact of 70, 427, 463
  risk of 31, 34, 144–5, 152, 156–65, 373, 381, 392–5, 404
  see also survivorship
religion *see* spirituality
Rembrandt 413–4
Renaissance 341–5, 379–80
research / clinical trials 207–11, 393–5, 415–6, 418–20, 449–50
research ethics 208–11
resilience 34–5, 127, 133–4, 153–4, 224–5, 273, 276, 282–3, 294–5, 296–7, 298–9, 303–5, 308–9, 314–5, 322–3

resources 200
   American Institute for Cancer Research (AICR) 168
   Breast Cancer.org 168
   Check Your Genes 434
   Diet, Nutrition and Breast Cancer 168
   Environmental Working Group (EWG) 169
   Facing Our Risk of Cancer Empowered (FORCE) 429
   HIPPA Guide 437
   How to find a nutrition expert 168
   My Gene Counsel 434
   National Comprehensive Cancer Network (NCCN) 434
restitution story *see* Frank, Arthur
risk of developing cancer *see* recurrent disease, risk of
Royal Marsden Hospital 372, 414

scars 52, 54, 57, 135, 240, 310–1
screening *see* physical exam
secondaries *see* metastasis
second opinion 269
   differing opinions of doctor and patient 81, 408
   differing opinions of healthcare providers 136–7, 148, 269, 432
self-advocacy *see* autonomy
self-disclosure *see* diagnosis, informing others
self-exam 18, 195
self-image / self-identity 31, 45, 180, 196–211, 205, 228–35, 284–5, 290–1, 327, 360, 461
sexuality 10, 179–91, 275, 300–1, 316–7, 324–5, 333, 369
   resources 190–1
shame *see* stigma
siblings 89–90, 94–6
   see also family and friends

skin 39–40, 180, 183, 188, 405, 415
social construction of cancer 146, 225–6, 444–59
social media *see* media, social media
solidarity *see* support
sonogram *see* ultrasound
spirituality 104, 107–22, 339–40, 345–8
   see also existential concerns; prayer
stages of cancer 68, 75, 116, 378, 464
stigma 20, 196, 364, 373
stories 1, 78, 146, 209, 255, 265–71, 273, 278, 280–1, 327, 359, 364, 403, 463, 464
   see also Frank, Arthur
suffering 217
   see also anxiety; depression; diagnosis, emotional impact; grief; guilt
support 77, 88, 98, 101–2, 103–5, 114–5, 268
support groups 62, 270, 462, 465
supportive oncology 97, 102, 153, 409–10
surgery *see* lumpectomy; mastectomy; reconstruction
survivorship 12, 35–6, 178, 214, 237–8, 241, 392, 394–5, 409, 461–4
systemic therapy 31, 33
   see also chemotherapy; hormonal therapy

tamoxifen (brand Novaldex) 34, 143–5, 373, 374, 375, 389–92
   see also hormonal therapy
tattoos 35, 37, 52, 179, 314–5
television commercials *see* media
trastuzumab *see* HER2/neu
treatment decision *see* autonomy
triple-negative breast cancer 34, 68
trust 265
   see also doctor-patient relationship

truth-telling 45–6, 286–7, 371–2, 374, 407, 433
tumor bed 38, 401
types of breast cancer 68–9

ultrasound 22–4, 203, 261–3

voice *see* autonomy; poetry; stories

whole-person care 17, 91, 98, 103–5

youth 53–60, 172

Medical Humanities: Criticism and Creativity

Series Editors: Maria Vaccarella, MA, PhD, Lecturer in Medical Humanities, University of Bristol and
Kimberly R. Myers, MA, PhD, Professor of Humanities and Medicine, Penn State College of Medicine

This series showcases innovative research, creativity and pedagogy in the interdisciplinary field of medical humanities. Books in the series explore the complexities of human bodies, minds, illness and wellbeing through analytical frameworks derived from humanistic disciplines and clinical practice. The series publishes a range of materials, including monographs and edited collections on scholarly approaches to medical issues in culture; creative works (accompanied by analytical and educational materials) that engage with medical humanities themes; and critical, engaged or radical pedagogies on focused topics for learners in the medical and health humanities.

Medical Humanities: Criticism and Creativity is intended to provide an informative exchange across disciplines, encouraging theoretical and personal reflections on the condition of the human mind/body and contributing to debates on health-related issues from a broad range of perspectives. The series also invites research that opens up critical conversations on being human at the intersection of other forms of humanistic knowledge, such as environmental and digital humanities. We are especially interested in collaborations between academics in the humanities and healthcare professionals.

All book proposals and manuscripts undergo rigorous peer review prior to acceptance and publication.

Editorial Board: Havi Carel (University of Bristol), Gretchen Case (University of Utah School of Medicine), Siobhan Conaty (La Salle University), Cheryl Dellasega (Penn State College of Medicine), Daniel George (Penn State College of Medicine), Michael Green (Penn State College of Medicine), Jennifer Henneman (Denver Art Museum), Brian Hurwitz (King's College London), Brian Johnsrud (Adobe Education), Tess Jones (University of Colorado Anschutz Medical Campus), Lois Leveen (novelist and independent scholar), Ulrika Maude (University of Bristol), Gavin Miller (University of Glasgow), Jules Odendahl-James

(Duke University), Molly Osborne (Oregon Health and Science University), Barry Saunders (University of North Carolina School of Medicine), Johanna Shapiro (University of California, Irvine, School of Medicine), Marina Tsaplina (The Betes Organization), Craigan Usher (Oregon Health and Science University), Neil Vickers (King's College London), Martin Willis (Cardiff University), Charlotte Wu (Boston University School of Medicine)

Kimberly R. Myers (ed.), *Breast Cancer Inside Out: Bodies, Biographies & Beliefs*.
2021. ISBN 978-1-78874-733-2.